Bathsheba's Breast

WOMEN, CANCER & HISTORY

James S. Olson

THE JOHNS HOPKINS UNIVERSITY PRESS
Baltimore & London

© 2002 The Johns Hopkins University Press
All rights reserved. Published 2002
Printed in the United States of America on acid-free paper
9 8 7 6 5 4 3 2

The Johns Hopkins University Press
2715 North Charles Street
Baltimore, Maryland 21218-4363
www.press.jhu.edu

Library of Congress Cataloging-in-Publication Data
Olson, James Stuart, 1946–
  Bathsheba's breast: women, cancer, and history / by James S. Olson
    p. cm.
Includes bibliographical references and index.
  ISBN 0-8018-6936-6
  1. Breast—Cancer—History.   I. Title
  RC280.B8 O465 2002
  616.99′449′009—DC21

2001006265

A catalog record for this book is available from the British Library.

To Judy,

my wife of thirty-seven years

and my best friend

Contents

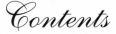

Bathsheba's Breast was born, conceptually at least, in 1981 under an electron beam, megavoltage radiotherapy contraption at the University of Texas M. D. Anderson Cancer Center in Houston. Dedicated oncologists wanted to save my left arm, and the rest of me, from the ravages of an epitheloid sarcoma. The choices seemed so bewildering, so vague and imprecise. Scientists, I naively thought, ought to be different from historians, less likely to debate an issue and traffic in contrasting personal opinions. Local physicians, after all, had urged an amputation upon me, telling me to waste no time in getting the job done, while M. D. Anderson's cadre of surgeons, radiotherapists, and physicists recommended a simple excision of the tumor—a lumpectomy—which had burrowed itself into my left hand, and then a round of radiotherapy. My long-term survival chances, they assured me, were only marginally worse with radiation than with amputation. I took their advice and went about my life—two-armed and relieved.

As a historian trying to make lemonade out of such a lemon, I decided to write a book about cancer. *Bathsheba's Breast* morphed into a sort of self-administered psychotherapy. For obvious reasons, I picked breast cancer, not soft-tissue sarcomas, as my topic. Throughout much of human history, breast cancer *was* cancer, and prominent women who endured the disease left behind a rich paper trail. The gender dynamics of the disease—female patients and male physicians—have also been a constant over time, shaping perceptions of the disease and its treatment. I was also intrigued with breast cancer's ability to reveal the subtle interactions between culture and science and how they feed off each other. Finally, in recent years, breast cancer patients have faced a series of difficult, often confusing treatment choices. All this seemed to have the makings of a good book.

In 1984, just barely into the research, I began the painful exercise of second-guessing myself. The tumor had recurred outside the radiated field. Had I made the wrong choice? Was I going to die now? I wasn't sure. Liver scans, bone scans, and lung x-rays revealed no metastases, but I was unhappy about hitching another ride on cancer's emotional roller coaster. Still, I had my arm. M. D. Anderson offered me the same choice with the same odds—radiotherapy or amputation. I agonized for several days and then underwent another lumpectomy and 6,500 rads of electron beam therapy. To no avail. By 1987 the sarcoma cells that survived inside the radiation field had multiplied into a new tumor, manifesting themselves as a painless, pea-sized lump on the top of my hand. M. D. Anderson surgeons and radiotherapists were prepared to give radiotherapy one more chance, but I was not. I wanted the lump gone, even if my arm had to go with it.

It did—a hand and fourteen inches of arm to rid me of an ornery, one-centimeter clump of aberrant DNA. So now it's 2001. I'm here but my left arm is not. I lost the battle, but it appears as if I won the war. Although I know nothing of what it is like to lose a breast, I do understand the confusion of Hobson's choices, the anxiety of confronting one's own mortality, and the trauma of saying goodbye to a body part. *Bathsheba's Breast*, I hope, will help others understand too.

Acknowledgments

There are so many people to thank, but I am especially grateful to Dr. Richard Martin, my personal surgeon at The University of Texas M. D. Anderson Cancer Center in Houston, Texas, who treated me so skillfully and so tenderly and who encouraged me in this project. Professors Randy Roberts, David Burner, Susannah Bruce, Rosanne Barker, Chris Baldwin, Terry Bilhartz, Mary Jo Richardson, and Joan Coffey read portions or all of the manuscript and offered many helpful suggestions. I also appreciate the assistance of Drs. Robert Williams, Al Gebert, David Prier, Karin Olson, and Kent Richards, who also read the manuscript with the keen eyes of physicians and helped me sort out some of my own misconceptions. Other women who critiqued portions of the manuscript include Anita Pilling, Susan Olson, Heather Beal, Carla Potter, Jayn Dickson, and Linda Pease. Professor Robert Shadle, my colleague at Sam Houston State University, has been enormously helpful in keeping me supplied with a steady stream of information from the Internet. During a recent medical crisis in my life, David and Sandra Burner generously volunteered to help finalize the manuscript. Finally, my wife Judy has been the project's most enthusiastic supporter, encouraging me when my own interest and energy flagged and supporting me during my own battle with cancer.

Bathsheba's Breast

Across Time

Flip a coin. Fifty-fifty. The twenty-year odds weren't much better than that. After more than a century of science and technology, the chances of surviving breast cancer had not improved all that much since the 1890s, when William Stewart Halsted, the brilliant surgeon at Johns Hopkins, developed the radical mastectomy. Before Halsted, the odds were only one in ten. Even if the patient had her breast removed, invisible, residual cells often remained behind, lurking in underarm lymph nodes, chest muscles, or somewhere in the bloodstream, biding their time until multiplying frantically into new tumors in new places. By removing the breast, the underarm lymph nodes, and both chest muscles, all in what he called an "en bloc resection," Halsted lifted out many tumors-to-be, reduced local recurrences of the disease, boosted survival rates, and earned himself a distinguished place in the annals of American science. He also left women feeling wounded and handicapped, though alive. The twentieth century did not produce any new Halsteds. Radiotherapy, chemotherapy, immunotherapy, and hormonal therapy came along, as did simple mastectomies, superradical mastectomies, and lumpectomies, giving cancer patients more time but not yet certifiably improving those long-term, twenty-year survival rates.

Nor had fear of the disease eased much over the years, or over centuries and millennia for that matter. Breast cancer may very well be history's oldest malaise, known as well to the ancients as it is to us. The women who have endured it share a unique sisterhood. Queen Atossa and

Dr. Jerri Nielsen—separated by era and geography, by culture, religion, politics, economics, and worldview—could hardly have been more different. Born 2,500 years apart, they stand as opposite bookends on the shelf of human history. One was the most powerful woman in the ancient world, the daughter of an emperor, the mother of a god; the other is a twenty-first-century physician with a streak of adventure coursing through her veins. From the imperial throne in ancient Babylon, Atossa could not have imagined the modern world, and only in the driest pages of classical literature could Antarctica-based Jerri Nielsen even have begun to fathom the Near East five centuries before the birth of Christ. For all of their differences, however, they shared a common fear that transcends time and space.

Atossa's father, Cyrus the Great, was the architect of Greater Persia, and in 538 BCE, after conquering much of Asia Minor and Mesopotamia, he crowned himself "King of Babylon and King of the Countries," declaring sovereignty over the entire world. Atossa married Darius of Hystaspes, and their dynastic union produced a son, Xerxes I, who inherited the mantle of emperor, expanded Persia's reach, and evolved into a living god. From her palaces in Babylon, Susa, and Ecbatana, Atossa basked in imperial glory and attracted the reverence and adoration of an empire. Aeschylus, the early Greek dramatist, hailed her as the "imperial consort of Darius . . . . The wife, the mother of the Persians' god." For all the splendor and power at her disposal, however, Queen Atossa harbored a demon, a personal terror, a gut-twisting fear of breast cancer. All the power and prestige of Persia, she worried, could not protect her. The disease respected no one, sparing neither rich nor poor.[1]

Jerri Nielsen, nicknamed "Duff" or "Duffy," had more obscure, bucolic origins, growing up in Salem, Ohio, graduating from Ohio University with a degree in zoology, and completing an M.D. in 1977 at the Medical College of Ohio. Eschewing the "female" specialties—pediatrics and family practice—Nielsen specialized in emergency room medicine. "Jerri seemed more interested in . . . excitement," recalled a medical school classmate, "wanting to see the person who gets shot in the abdomen, not the person who comes to be treated for their diabetes and hypertension." During her residency and first few years in a Cleveland, Ohio, emergency room, Nielsen married and had three children.[2]

After a nasty divorce in 1998 and an unsuccessful custody battle,

Bathsheba's Breast

Nielsen needed a reprieve, an adventure of some sort to distract her emotionally from the recent traumas. A tour of duty as a physician at the National Science Foundation's Amundsen-Scott South Pole Station in Antarctica seemed a perfect antidote. In October, she passed an exhaustive physical that included thorough mammograms. As a physician and as a woman, Nielsen understood breast cancer's dangers. Fibrocystic disease ran in the family, and when Nielsen was growing up, her mother had undergone several biopsies for what proved to be benign lesions. Jerri Nielsen suffered the same malady, lumps appearing and disappearing with the rhythms of her menstrual cycle. "I had fibrocystic breasts," she explained, "and had found small breast lumps . . . . They were always related to my menstrual cycle and went away after a few days." Over time, her alarm gave way to concern and caution, since women with fibrocystic disease are more likely candidates for breast cancer than those without it.[3]

Nielsen's concerns, however, did not match Atossa's obsession. Sometime around 490 BCE, the queen thought that the demon had come for her. She noticed a lump in her breast. Atossa kept the news to herself, hoping the growth was nothing, that it would go away. It did not. The lump increased in size and finally ruptured, releasing a filthy, alarming discharge. The lesion continued to grow, and Atossa went into hiding, staying away from Darius and bathing only in private, so her servants would have nothing to gossip about. Even 2,500 years ago, breast disease terrified women. Herodotus, the Greek historian, wrote that "so long as the sore was of no great size, she [Atossa] hid it through shame and made no mention of it to anyone." Finally, she had no choice. Worried about death and disfigurement, about sexual castration and the loss of her allure, with the growth engulfing much of her breast, Atossa called on Democêdes, a Greek slave, for medical assistance.

Democêdes examined the breast and seized an opportunity. He confidently offered the queen a cure, just what she wanted to hear. But there was a catch. He insisted that if he cured the breast, she must "grant him whatever request he might prefer." A skeptical Atossa, worried that the slave wanted into her bedroom, inquired about the nature of the request, and he assured her that "it should be nothing which she could blush to hear." As it turned out, he wanted to accompany a Persian scouting expedition to Greece, where he hoped to escape. Certain that the growth was an abscess, not cancer, Democêdes lanced it and bathed the wound in herbal potions. As expected, the infection subsided, the incision healed, and Atossa, Queen of Persia, enjoyed a new lease on life. Like most women who discover lumps in their breasts, she did not have cancer but suffered instead from a painful but temporary infection, one of dozens of benign breast diseases that, when treated, are not life-threatening. She kept her part of the bargain. Democêdes escaped Persia, and Atossa eluded the demon.[4]

Jerri Nielsen did not. She had arrived at the South Pole late in November 1998 and fell quickly into the routine, making friends in the close quarters of the South Pole. Her spirits, however, soon turned as cold as the looming Antarctic winter. Early in March, barely three months after arriving at the South Pole and six months after a clear mammogram, Nielsen detected a small, hard lump in her right breast. There was no getting off the South Pole for a trip to a major cancer center or teaching hospital, no facilities at Amundsen-Scott for biopsy, surgery, radiation, or chemotherapy. Aircraft cannot land at the South Pole in mid-winter because of gale force winds, blizzards, and 100 degree below zero temperatures. She was not one to panic. "My mammogram had been negative only six months ago," she recalled, "so I wasn't particularly worried. I decided to keep an eye on the lump and wait a month to see if anything changed."[5]

The lump changed, but for the worse. Breast lumps can be furtive and sneaky, waxing and waning with menstrual cycles or hiding out in dense tissues, appearing suddenly in spite of regular self-examinations and mammograms. Over the course of the next six weeks, the lump did not go away. In fact, it grew larger and more irregular, and Nielsen could detect a second mass taking shape beneath the first. She relayed the news to the National Science Foundation, and somebody leaked the story to the press. The wire services picked it up, and Nielsen was soon fodder for newspaper headlines, prime time network television broadcasts, weekly news magazines, and radio talk shows. At first she was only a "mystery" woman, since her name had not been released, but sleuths in the news business soon ferreted out her identity. Jerri Nielsen got her "fifteen minutes of fame" the hard way, and it soon stretched into months.[6]

The National Science Foundation arranged for an Air Force C-141 Starfighter to fly over Amundsen-Scott and by parachute drop diagnostic equipment and chemotherapy drugs. On July 11, 1998, the equipment

Bathsheba's Breast

arrived. Nielsen did not waste a minute. Because the tumor was palpable just under the skin, she performed a biopsy on herself, using ice cubes as a local anesthetic, driving a needle into the tumor, and recovering the suspicious cells. "To do one on yourself is probably not as technically difficult as it is emotionally difficult," said a friend. "Some doctors can't even inject themselves." Nielsen then prepared the tissue slides, digitalized the images, and dispatched them by satellite to radiologists in Denver, Colorado. They confirmed the malignancy and warned her, after pathologists graded the cells, that her cancer was particularly virulent and fast-growing, and that she needed to self-administer the chemotherapy drugs. Nielsen endured the anticipated nausea, and two weeks later, her hair began falling out in clumps, clogging the shower drain and tangling up in brushes and combs. Chemotherapy targets rapidly growing cancer cells, killing them during mitosis, when they are in the process of dividing. But it also kills other rapidly dividing cells, such as hair and the linings of the gastrointestinal tract, which explains the nausea and temporary hair loss many cancer patients experience. Nielsen e-mailed a photo of her Yul Brynner–Michael Jordan dome to her mother, who told a London newspaper, "I have found lumps in my breasts before, and . . . I know the fear that I went through. She is amazingly brave."[7]

She needed to be. During the rest of July, Nielsen absorbed a steady stream of bad news. Because her tumor was larger than five centimeters in size, and because it most likely did not feed on estrogen, the long-term survival odds were not good. Estrogen-dependent breast cancers are more treatable with hormonal therapy. Nor did the fact that lymph nodes under her right arm seemed swollen bode well. Perhaps the tumors had already metastasized. An e-mail from a consulting oncologist gently but clearly described her long-term survival odds: "[A]bout half the women in your situation at some point will have a recurrence of their breast cancer somewhere else in their body. That recurrence is almost always obvious in the first 5 years after diagnosis and will eventually take their lives (on average about 2 years after the recurrence is diagnosed)."[8]

Nielsen did not leave Antarctica until October 16, 1999, when an Air National Guard crew in an LC-130 Hercules aircraft flew through snow-filled polar winds and landed at Amundsen-Scott. "That was one of the most dangerous landings I've ever made, what with the wind, cold, and awful visibility," remembered pilot George McAlister. "But we were pumped." Little time could be wasted on the ground. The temperature, at 65 degrees below zero, would soon freeze hydraulic fluids. Clad in a heavy parka, Nielsen scurried aboard, and the Hercules took off again, having spent only twenty minutes on the ground. One week later, her picture was plastered on the cover of *People Weekly*. Soon after getting back to the United States, Nielsen confirmed the rumors of breast cancer, and, desperate to get more hard data on her predicament, underwent a battery of tests and made some hard decisions.[9]

At the beginning of the twentieth century, during William Stewart Halsted's day, breast cancer patients really had only one decision to make—whether or not to undergo a radical mastectomy. The operation offered many women hope for a cure, though at a terrible price, but proceeding without it meant certain death. At the end of the twentieth century, however, women enjoyed new treatment options, none more important than having a lumpectomy—removal of the tumor and the lymph nodes under the arm—while leaving the rest of the breast intact. When combined with post-surgical radiotherapy, lumpectomy did not improve survival odds, but it did not reduce them either, and women who chose it lived out their lives feeling less damaged and less wounded.

Nielsen opted for the lumpectomy, but her survival odds soon improved dramatically. The preoperative battery of liver scans, bone scans, MRIs, and CAT scans all proved negative, detecting no other tumors— no deadly metastases—and raising hopes for a long life. Equally reassuring, pathologists could find no cancer cells in the lymphatic tissues removed from under her right arm. "It was almost unbelievable," she later wrote. "I felt like a death row prisoner, clutching my pardon." For now at least, Jerri Nielsen has become a breast cancer survivor.[10]

So far. Breast cancer often seems to possess a mind of its own, confounding the architects of mortality and morbidity tables. There are no guarantees, and breast cancer is no respecter of persons, as Linda McCartney could certainly have testified. Paul McCartney, the forever boyish heartthrob of the Beatles and global pop culture icon, and his wife, Linda, had played cat and mouse games with the paparazzi throughout nearly three decades of marriage, trying to protect their privacy and insulate their four children from the public spotlight. Every family trip demanded careful tactical planning, and when they had to be alone, when they could not stand one more interview or one more flashing camera, they headed to "Santa Barbara," a code name for their secluded desert ranch outside Tucson, Arizona, where locals kept the McCartney secret.

When Linda was diagnosed with breast cancer, the McCartneys not only had to address a host of medical issues but also negotiate a public relations strategy. In December 1995, during a routine physical and a mammogram, her physicians discovered a small, malignant lump. She decided on a lumpectomy with follow-up chemotherapy and radiotherapy. She lost weight and her hair but bounced back quickly from the ordeal. Since the disease seemed to be at such an early stage, the McCartneys went public with the diagnosis and began what they thought would be a routine recovery and imminent return to Linda's successful publishing and photographic career.

Unbeknownst to anybody, the disease had already metastasized. Early in March 1998, just when Jerri Nielsen first discovered her lump, McCartney learned during a routine checkup that tumors studded her liver. The McCartneys guarded that news carefully, sharing it only with trusted friends and family. Actually, Linda was doomed. She was about to undergo what Jerri Nielsen's oncologist had described—a metastatic recurrence within five years followed by rapid decline. Nothing in the black bag of American technology could save her. McCartney spent her last days at "Santa Barbara," smelling desert flowers, riding horses, and enjoying her family. On April 17, 1998, she died there. A confirmed vegetarian, she had eaten carefully over the years, exercised regularly, and taken good care of herself. She had money, a loving family, and all the trappings of success and celebrity. "The McCartneys had all the money in the world," remarked a visitor to Arizona when learning of her death. "Enough to afford their privacy. Enough to give them a beautiful view. But all the money in the world wasn't enough to keep her alive."[11]

In 2001, more than 1.8 million women in the United States went to their doctors worried about lumps in their breasts. Like Queen Atossa, most learned, after careful physical examinations, mammograms, or biopsies, that they were just fine, that the lumps were not malignant, that they could proceed with their lives unscathed. But approximately 175,000, like Jerri Nielsen, received different news and began pondering their fates, wondering whether they would ever see a son or daughter graduate from college, or cradle a tiny grandchild, or cash a Social Security check, whether, like Linda McCartney, they were destined for premature graves. Around the world in 2001, more than two million new cases of breast cancer appeared. In the entire history of the human race, if contemporary Third World mortality rates can be extrapolated back over time, perhaps 25 million women have succumbed to the disease. Today, in doctors' offices scattered throughout the United States, five thousand or so women will have lumps in their breasts examined. Like Atossa, most will have nothing to worry about. They will sigh in relief and go about their business. But five hundred will not. When the doctor delivers the news, each woman will suck in a sharp breath and unwillingly hitch a ride on breast cancer's roller coaster.

CHAPTER ONE

Dark Ages

In 1967, T. C. Greco, an Italian surgeon and art *aficionado,* took a spring vacation in Amsterdam. At the Rijksmuseum, he strolled through a section of Rembrandts, pausing in front of *Bathsheba at Her Bath* (1654). Hendrickje Stoffels, Rembrandt's mistress, had posed for the painting. It was not Greco's first look at the work, but it was the first time he had used his surgeon's eye. He detected an asymmetry to the left breast; it seemed distended compared to her right breast. He also detected swelling, or fullness, near her left armpit. The left breast appeared discolored, and Greco saw what he thought might be "peau d'orange," a pitted section of skin with the texture of an orange peel. All signs pointed to breast cancer. With a little research, he learned that Stoffels later died after a "long illness." He was confident, and conjectured so in an Italian medical journal, that she died of breast cancer.[1]

Greco's success as a medical sleuth was not that surprising. Stoffels' tumor, and its symptoms, differed little from the breast cancer that killed Linda McCartney. Breast cancer is an old disease. It transcends race, class, time, and space, a horror known to every culture in every age. Among ancients, breast cancer *was* cancer. People died of other malignancies—ovarian tumors, multiple myelomas, bone and soft tissue sarcomas, leukemias and lymphomas, melanomas, prostate lesions, gastrointestinal carcinomas, and brain cancers—but those tumors were invisible. Friends, family members, and physicians could not see them, or could not logically correlate an external manifestation of the disease with the death that followed.

Since autopsies were not socially accepted until the seventeenth century, few physicians ever examined internal organs or understood much about the biology of death. Breast cancer, on the other hand, was clearly visible, progressing from a small lump to large tumors, wreaking havoc with the breast and the body. Establishing a causal connection between breast tumors and death was relatively simple.

Medical practitioners and patients the world over, today and eons ago, have struggled with the disease. Egyptians of the New Kingdom—more than 3,500 years ago—were the first. An anonymous surgeon, describing "bulging tumors" in the breast, gave up easily, stating simply, "There is no treatment." Other surgeons advocated cutting out the tumor or cutting off the breast. One of them was Aetios of Amida, the sixth-century court physician to Justinian I and Theodora, emperor and empress of Byzantium.

Justinian assumed the throne at Constantinople in 527 upon the death of his uncle, Justin I. Determined to recapture the ancient glory of Rome, and praying that "God will grant us the remainder of the empire the Romans lost," he sent his armies west, and they conquered North Africa, Spain, and Italy. To the east, they brought much of Persia under Byzantine control. Justinian codified Roman law, engineered a renaissance of religious arts, architecture, and literature, and presided over the greatest civilization of the West.

He also fell in love with Theodora, and their relationship scandalized the empire. She was the most common of commoners, born poor and raised by a widowed mother who encouraged her to work as a sexual acrobat at the Hippodrome circus, where chariot races and live sexual acts entertained thousands. By her early teens, Theodora was a prostitute known throughout Constantinople, if the *Secret History* of Procopius is accurate. Procopius, legal secretary to a Byzantine general, kept a journal most of his life, recording his observations and court gossip. He described some of Theodora's behavior:

> She had no sense of shame, and no one ever saw her embarrassed; rather, without any hesitation she would perform the most shameful acts . . . . She would expose naked those things, front and back, which it is customary to keep unseen and hidden from men . . . . Never was anyone more addicted to all forms of hedonistic gratification . . . . Often when she went to a bring-

your-own dinner party with ten or more vigorous young men for whom intercourse was a constant occupation, she lay with all of them for the entire night. When all of them were too exhausted to continue, she would sleep with each of their servants.

Procopius no doubt exaggerated, but Justinian did become infatuated with Theodora and set her up as his mistress in the House of Hormisdas, a miniature palace near the Hippodrome. She was twenty-five and the emperor-to-be forty-two. Justinian spent more and more time with Theodora, ignoring his wife Euphemia. When Euphemia fell ill in 525, the gossip became more vicious; Justinian's enemies preached that "there have been empresses who became harlots, but who ever heard of a harlot becoming an empress?" When Euphemia died, Justinian married Theodora the next day, preempting attempts to outlaw the union. Two years later, upon his uncle's death, Justinian and Theodora ascended to the Byzantine throne. During the next twenty years, Theodora was completely involved in the affairs of state. He was devoted to her, and she to him. After all, Justinian had moved her overnight from Hippodrome whorehouses to the splendor of the court. She had a gift for exposing court conspiracies, unraveling political intrigues, and discriminating between sycophants and supporters. Other than her frustration about not being able to produce an heir to the throne, the two enjoyed a fulfilling life together.

It ended in 548. Theodora had discovered a lump in her breast. She turned to Aetios of Amida, physician to the Byzantine court, a man Justinian and Theodora frequently consulted. He eschewed all pharmacological treatments for breast cancer. None was any good, he believed. His ideas were well-known in Constantinople. Surgery was the only answer. "I make the patient lie down," he wrote, "and then I incise the healthy part of the breast beyond the cancerous areas and I cauterize the incised parts. Then I again incise and excise the breadth from its depths and I again cauterize the incised area. And I repeat the procedure often." Aetios knew that he had to remove *all* of the diseased tissue; otherwise, the cancer would recur. The tumor had to come out; the breast had to come off.

Always her own person, Theodora chose to die. The Hippodrome's most notorious actress had one final role to perform. She continued to dress in her regal best and, with painkillers, attended to a full slate of imperial duties. Servants watched her face thin and her movements slow.

Procopius wondered why "she treats her body with great care, more than is needed. She enters the bath early, and after bathing goes direct to breakfast. Then sleep lays hold of her for long stretches." Her decline accelerated. Pope Vigilius attended her near the end. Between chest-heaving coughs and a severe burning in her throat, she hacked out a last confession, crying out at the end, as she pondered some of her past deeds, "I'm frightened." The pope lifted a sliver of cedarwood and put it to her nose. "The tree is dead, but the fragrance will never leave the wood . . . . And if this be true of the wood of a tree, is it not true of the life in our bodies? Smell of it, my daughter." Theodora did the pope's bidding, sniffing the cedarwood and accepting his blessing. She died in June 548.[2]

Aetios of Amida did not know, nor do modern oncologists, the origins of breast cancer. Ancients were certain, however, that amputation of the breast was usually not enough. They viewed cancer as a systemic, not local, disease. Tumors were manifestations of more serious problems. Cutting a tumor out might help temporarily, but most likely its first appearance would soon be followed by an encore. Amputation did not address the fundamental problem.

Hippocrates, the father of Western medicine, supplied the earliest, and by far most enduring, description of breast cancer. Born on the island of Cos around 460 BCE, he taught medicine in temples dedicated to Asclepios, the Greek god of getting well. He postulated a "humoral" theory for disease. Greek philosophers made few distinctions between the spiritual and temporal worlds; the two were just different reflections of a single reality. Confident of intricate and tangible connections between the cosmos and the body, Hippocrates searched for biological counterparts to the building blocks of nature: Air, Fire, Earth, and Water. He found them in the body's four humors, or fluids: blood, phlegm, yellow bile, and black bile. The essence of life was "inner heat," an energy produced by the heart from food people consumed. The "inner heat" not only generated energy, it also fine-tuned the body's engine and balanced its fluid levels. When the humors synchronized, not too much of one or too little of another, good health resulted. Imbalances made people sick, and the body's production of vomit, diarrhea, blood, mucous, jaundice, fevers, and pus proved the link between excess fluids and poor health.[3]

Cancer, he believed, erupted from an excess of black bile—"melanchole." Given the appearance of advanced, untreated breast cancer, humoral

Bathsheba's Breast

theory has a superficial logic. As the tumor progresses, it becomes larger, harder to the touch, and darker in appearance, pushing aside other tissues and eventually ulcerating through the skin, its necrotic tissues generating a fetid odor and dark, brackish fluids. Clarissimus Galen, the second-century Greek physician who wrote more than four hundred works on anatomy, surgery, and medicine, described the dangers of black bile: "Of black color . . . cometh cancer . . . it maketh ulceration, and for this cause, these tumors are more blacker in color, than those that cometh of inflammation, and these be not hot . . . . For less matter goeth out of the veines, into the fleshy partes . . . through the grossness of the humor, which breadeth the Cancers."[4]

Cancer's appearance provoked Hippocrates to name it "karkinos," a Greek word for crab. On close examination, tumors seemed to have tentacles, like the legs of a crab, reaching out and grasping normal tissues. From *karkinos* evolved "carcinoma," a medical term for malignant tumors developing in epithelial tissues. In the seventh century, Paul of Aegina, an Alexandrian physician, described cancer as "an uneven swelling, rough, unseemly, darkish, painful . . . it derives its origin from black bile and spreads . . . forming in most parts of the body, but more especially in the female uterus and breasts. It has the veins stretched on all sides as the animal the crab has its feet." Black bile was not confined to the tumor; it was systemic, flowing throughout the body. Surgical removal of a small tumor or of the entire breast if the tumor were larger would usually not effect a cure, since the cancer would recur near the surgical wound or elsewhere in the body.[5]

Galen, who succeeded Hippocrates as the dean of Greek medicine, accepted humoral theory but distinguished among different types of "unnatural" growths. Although he knew little about the difference between malignant and benign tumors, he realized that some lesions were more dangerous than others. He used the term "phlegmone" to describe the heat, redness, and swelling associated with curable inflammatory lesions. "Polysarkias" were painless cysts filled with clear fluid, and skin lesions issuing pus were "kolpos." Galen came up with other terms for aneurisms, warts, pimples, insect bites, bruises, leprosy, boils, glandular swellings, and varicose veins. The most dangerous lumps of all, of course, were "karkinos"—hard, painless knots which eventually ulcerated through the skin, issued black bile, and caused death.[6]

Whether or not an abnormal swelling warranted surgery, Greeks advised subsequent treatments to address the systemic problem of too much black bile. Galen harvested a cornucopia of pharmaceutical agents, including opium, rhubarb, castor oil, olive oil, barley water, licorice, turpentine, ammonium chloride, sulphur, zinc oxide, copper sulphate, valerian, cinnamon, and a variety of salves and gums. Some were bizarre folk remedies, such as burning three or five or seven (it had to be an odd number) river crabs, mixing the remains with Cyprian oil, applying the potion to the tumor with a bird's feather, and shouting incantations to the gods. Galen's favorite remedy, and an absolute prerequisite to restoring humoral stability, was the lancet: tapping into a patient's vein and draining blood and excess fluids so the "inner heat" could stimulate humoral stability. He prescribed expectorants to induce vomiting, laxatives to clear the bowel, and bloodletting, all of which, he believed, relieved vascular pressures and restored health.[7]

Within a century of his death, Galen was the godfather of medicine. By the fourth century, his scientific treatises, widely disseminated and widely read, formed the medical canon. But when the Roman Empire disintegrated and Europe broke up into hundreds of warring principalities, so did medical knowledge. Galen disappeared into the dust of history, preserved only among learned scribes and physicians of the Arab and Byzantine world. European medicine became the domain of witches, sorcerers, shamans, monks, apothecaries, and barbers.[8]

The resurrection of Clarissimus Galen took more than a thousand years. When monastic scribes translated Arab texts back into Latin in the late middle ages, Galen's star reappeared in the intellectual firmament. Humoral theories returned, undiminished by a millennium of human experience. Physicians treating breast cancer searched for telltale black bile and subjected women to pressure-relieving bleedings. Sometimes the cures worked. Tumors might disappear within days or weeks, allowing physicians and quacks alike to take credit for the recovery. What the ancients did not understand was that benign breast lesions, such as fibrocystic disease, can come and go, appearing and disappearing with the tides of a woman's menstrual cycle. Humoral practitioners succeeded in preventing the deaths of healthy women with benign breast disease.[9]

When Anne of Austria, the queen mother of France, noticed a lump in her left breast in 1663, she found herself at the mercy of physicians at the University of Paris, a conservative institution steeped in Galenic tradition. Anne, the Infanta Doña Ana Maria Mauricia, had been born on September 22, 1601, to King Philip III of Spain and his queen, Margaret of Austria. She enjoyed an unusual childhood, at least for royal children, because she saw a great deal of her parents. Anne was a bright and witty girl, popular with adults and children. She was also strikingly beautiful, considered by many to be the loveliest woman in Europe. Philip lavished her with attention, wrote regularly when he was away, closely followed her activities, and took great pride in her successes.[10]

She was also genuinely religious, a trait learned from her mother. Margaret of Austria, who supervised Anne's education, was a pious woman. They filled their days with chapel prayers, mass, school, and charitable visits to convents, hospitals, and charnel houses. Margaret revered the Roman Catholic saints, especially those of Spanish, Italian, and Austrian origin. She owned elaborate martyrologies and regularly read to Anne stories of the saints' lives. Margaret also preferred the company of nuns; she enjoyed visiting convents, inviting nuns to the royal homes, and counting nuns as her closest friends.

On November 25, 1615, when she was fourteen, Anne married Louis XIII, the fourteen-year-old king of France. It was a dynastic coupling, the result of years of diplomatic maneuvering, a union of the Spanish Hapsburgs and the French Bourbons designed to ensure stability in Europe and peace in Christendom. Mere children, they found married life difficult. The royal couple maintained separate residences at the Louvre in Paris; Louis XIII spent most of the time with Albert de Luynes, a close friend and advisor, while Anne had to deal with the machinations of Marie de Medici, the queen mother, who exercised a dominating influence over her son and, indirectly, over Anne.

Anne created a new life for herself in the Louvre, developing a close circle of friends and finding comfort in the religious ceremonies required by royal protocol and her own private devotions. Like her mother, she enjoyed being around nuns. In 1618, during a visit to Valprofond, a Benedictine convent outside Paris, Anne met Mother Marguerite de Sainte-General, the abbess. The two women became lifelong friends. Anne visited the convent often and enjoyed her time there so much that in 1621 she relocated it to Paris for convenience. She purchased property, paid for half of the construction, and had a private apartment built there. The convent became known as Val-de-Grace—a haven of privacy, friendship, and security.

The nuns at Val-de-Grace, with their royal patroness, enjoyed each other's company, debating court politics and engaging in political intrigue. They attended chapel services twice a day and participated regularly in confession and communion, but they also spent several hours each day in the convent parlor, playing cards and billiards and gossiping about each other or the latest tidbits from the royal palace. The nuns managed regular daily walks outside the convent, frequent visits to the homes of lay women, and long journeys to other religious communities. In the convents of Catholic France, and especially the Benedictine house at Val-de-Grace, Anne of Austria found a community of women who brought meaning into her life.[11]

But she was still a queen, not a nun, and reveled in her beauty and power. Although Anne was probably faithful to Louis XIII, she readily flirted with court admirers and flaunted her sensuality—tiptoeing to the edge of infidelity but never falling over the precipice. Rumors of Anne's alleged dalliances with Giulio Mazarin, the powerful French cardinal and statesman, and George Villiers, the Duke of Buckingham, titillated court society in Paris, and Anne, while self-righteously denying wrongdoing, used the rumors to political advantage.

As the years passed, Anne's relationship with Louis XIII became more tenuous. Her apparent inability to produce an heir to the throne complicated an already byzantine marriage, leaving Louis frustrated and worried about the dynasty and the young queen obsessing about whether he would send her packing to Spain. The infrequency of their sexual encounters, Anne's irregular periods, and several miscarriages left the royal couple childless. The fourteen-year-old bride had become a thirty-seven-year-old matron, the barren wife of a resentful king.

But in 1637, Anne surprised the entire realm with news that she was pregnant. The only explanation, she believed, was divine intervention; actually, Louis XIII had visited the Convent of the Visitation in Paris in December. Anne was coincidentally there. Because of stormy weather, he decided not to continue his journey to Saint-Maur. He shared Anne's bed that night. Nine months later, on September 5, 1638, Anne gave birth to the dauphin—the future King Louis XIV of France. A second son, Philippe of Anjou, soon followed.

Bathsheba's Breast

Another momentous development occurred four years later. In 1643, Louis XIII's health failed him. His decline, probably due to intestinal tuberculosis, took several weeks, giving him enough time to plan the regency. To the surprise of many, he named Anne regent until Louis XIV was old enough to succeed to the throne. Louis XIII died on May 14, 1643. When Anne learned of her husband's death, she said prayers at the chapel and walked across the garden to meet her children. There, in front of a number of dignitaries, she approached and knelt in homage to her five-year-old son, now her liege lord, King Louis XIV of France. Anne presided over a nine-year regency, a time in which she managed to preserve the monarchy and grow close to Louis and Philippe. The regency ended in 1653 with Louis's coronation.[12]

Paris was not just the capital city of France in the seventeenth century; it was the cultural and political center of the Western world, presided over by Europe's greatest prince—Louis XIV. He sat on the throne for seventy-two years, assuming during his reign the aura of a demigod. Before moving to his personal palace at Versailles in 1682, the king shuttled back and forth between a number of opulent country homes—he loved to hunt—and the royal chateau outside of Paris. Few human beings in history have enjoyed such privilege. From the moment he arose in the morning until he fell asleep at night, Louis XIV was never alone. Retinues of courtiers, sycophants, and servants shadowed his every move. In the morning, they helped him out of bed, rubbing his body with rose water and spirits of wine, shaving his face and brushing his teeth for him. They pushed and shoved for the opportunity of watching their lord squat on the chamber pot, then jockeyed about for the chance to remove the royal effluence. All the while, Louis gazed out on the starstruck audience, nodding imperiously. They watched reverently while he prayed and just as reverently while he ate. Ambitious women jostled for a night in his bed, and Louis XIV, enjoying gargantuan sexual appetites, accommodated them all, always confident that he was doing them a favor.[13]

Flush with confidence and power, Anne presided over the grandeur. The nodule she discovered in her left breast in 1663 came then as a surprise. Anne knew only too well what she might be facing. She harbored an acute dread of breast cancer, a fear born and bred in a lifetime of convent visits. On many occasions, she had seen nuns in the end stages of the disease. One visit at Val-de-Grace had been especially difficult. At a Good

Friday service in 1647, Anne and her friend and confidante Madame de Motteville visited the convent infirmary. Both witnessed a nurse change the dressings of a dying nun. The smell of death was in the air. Cancer cells not only divide rapidly, they also die rapidly, and when a patient is laced with tumors, the body is riddled with dead, necrotic tissue. Those tissues are rancid and rotten and emit a foul odor. To their horror, Anne and de Motteville saw that a tumor had destroyed one side of the nun's torso, allowing a peek into her chest cavity. It was an unforgettable scene, prompting de Motteville to record in her diary: "Having seen cancer in nuns who died all rotted with them, she [Anne] had always had a horror of this disease which she found so frightful even to imagine."[14]

When Anne noticed the lump, she tried to ignore it. The prospects of losing her breasts, undergoing bleedings and purgings, and dying after grotesque suffering terrified her. Madame de Motteville later wrote that the decision "was the cause of her doom; for if in this beginning she had looked for its cure, perhaps the unfortunate consequences would have been easier to avoid." Given the state of cancer treatment in 1663, postponement probably did not kill Anne of Austria. She was already doomed.

Procrastination where breast cancer is concerned is at best a temporary measure; tumors assert themselves eventually, demanding attention from their hosts. In May 1664, while partying at one of Louis's glamorous celebrations at Versailles, Anne felt a dull, nagging pain in her left breast. She mentioned it to de Motteville, who urged her to inform Dr. Seguín, a Spanish physician who had treated Anne for years. But the queen mother delayed again, busying herself with family matters, charitable activities, and religious devotions, visiting convents, schools, and hospitals, all the while enduring the pain and trying to ignore it.

In October 1664, pain forced a decision. The ache in her breast sharpened, leaving Anne weak and nauseous. Her complexion took on a yellowish hue, perhaps because the tumor had spread to her liver. Anne put up with the discomfort for another month, but in November she finally let Seguín examine her. He immediately consulted Dr. Vallot, the king's personal physician. Both were alarmed at the condition of the breast. Seguín had been trained by a devotee of Ambroise Paré, the legendary barber-turned-surgeon who became court physician to Francis II, Charles IX, Henry III, and Henry IV, kings of France. Attached to the French army during the Italian campaigns of 1536, Paré one evening found him-

Bathsheba's Breast

self on a battlefield littered with wounded men. Conventional wisdom insisted that the wounds be detoxified with boiling oil. Paré went ahead with the brutal treatments. Camp cooks melted lard over open fires and then poured it into open wounds. But then they ran out of lard. The rest of the wounded received a potion of turpentine, egg yolks, and rose oil. Paré could hardly sleep that night, "fearing that I would find those to whom I had not used boiling oil dead." He rose "early to visit them, where beyond my expectation I found those to whom I had applied my digestive medicine, to feel little pain, and their wounds without inflammation or tumour, had rested reasonably well in the night; the others to whom was used the said boiling oil [were] feverish, with great pain and swelling, about the edges of the wound." Paré never used boiling oil again, and medical historians consider him a leading figure in the history of surgery.[15]

But Paré had far more conventional opinions about cancer, and his ghost still stalked the Paris medical school. He recalled his experience with Mademoiselle de Montigny, a maid of honor at the royal court. It was clear to Paré that her tumor was beyond surgery, so he took her to Dr. Houllier, a distinguished faculty member, who treated her first with bleedings and laxatives, then with a lead and quicksilver poultice. The tumor kept growing, but Houllier continued the regimen, escalating it to include applications of hot towels, astringents, and salves. When the tumor ulcerated through the skin, sending forth a flow of "black bile," Houllier resorted to "caustic powders." Nothing did any good. Several months later, Paré recalled, "the Lady grew restless . . . . The heart failed and death followed."[16]

The medical faculty during Anne's day remained convinced that Galen had written the last page in medical science, that nothing remained to be discovered, that medical students need only memorize the teachings of the master at the feet of tenured, erudite, red-gowned teachers. They worshiped humoral theory, readily accepting black bile as the culprit and bleedings and purgatives as the antidotes, even if surgical removal of the tumor was possible.[17]

When Seguín showed up to treat Anne, his black bag contained only the remedies of Galen and Paré. Upon examining her, he hoped surgery would be a possibility, even though it entailed enormous risks. Physicians had no idea about bacteria and antiseptic procedures. Dirty hands and bloody tools were the rule. Most surgery patients in the seventeenth century experienced infection in the wound, and many succumbed to blood poisoning and streptococcus. The other risk was metastasis. Careless excision of a malignant tumor usually left behind, or even scattered about, malignant cells destined to evolve into new tumors. Surgeons, ignorant about cellular biology, had no idea they might increase the odds of local recurrence and metastasis. When new tumors appeared near the site of the original surgery, they blamed black bile. It was a moot issue for Anne. Thirty seconds into his examination, Seguín knew she was not a candidate for surgery. The tumor, buried deep in the breast and stretching up under her arm, was way too advanced.

In December 1664, Seguín and Vallot solicited a second opinion from the dean of the medical school, who quickly pronounced her incurable. A petty, self-possessed man who still employed astrological readings as diagnostic tools, the dean told Seguín and Vallot that Anne had nobody to blame but herself. By eating whatever she wanted over the years, and not following a regimen of periodic bleedings and purgings, she had inadvertently pushed her humoral fluids out of balance. Excessive black bile caused the cancer, and excessive yellow bile explained her complexion.

Anne had studiously avoided prophylactic humoral treatments. No doubt her reticence was at least partly rooted in her marriage. Louis XIII readily submitted to colonic purging. Between July 1640 and June 1641, he underwent 215 days of strong laxatives, 212 enemas, and 47 bleedings. He repeatedly urged Anne to cooperate and attributed her infertility to her refusal to comply. She was not about to give in. Anne felt healthy and hated the fatigue accompanying bloodletting, vomiting, and diarrhea, and in the power play of royal marriage, she took whatever victories she could. Refusing his medical advice was a tiny, but sweet, revenge.[18]

But now Anne was at the mercy of doctors. Deeply disturbed about his mother's prognosis, Louis XIV told Vallot to do whatever he could to prolong her life. The king sent messengers throughout France and Austria searching for antidotes. Vallot, certain a cure was not possible, hoped to buy Anne some more time. In his own notes, he wrote: "The extent of the queen mother's disease, combined with her advanced age, gives great reason to fear an unhappy outcome. Nevertheless, if the patient is still able to take treatment, we do not despair of being able to give her relief and keeping her alive for a number of years." It was an objective any contemporary oncologist would understand: if a cure is not possible, keep the patient alive.

Bathsheba's Breast

Seguín and Vallot focused on her fluids. They administered bleedings, daily enemas, and frequent purges. Vallot applied a hemlock ointment to Anne's breast to relieve pain. The king's appeal enticed a legion of quacks to Paris, all anxious to cure the queen mother. Seguín and Vallot evaluated each proposal and tried out a few. Father Gendron, a priest from the Orléanais, had a "secret remedy": a paste of belladonna and burnt lime to petrify the breast into a marble-like composition. Gendron applied the paste all summer, but by August 1665 it was clear to everyone that his promises were a pipedream. The tumor ulcerated, and Anne dismissed him. At the end of the month, she almost died when Vallot lanced open a new tumor that had appeared under her arm. Anne rallied, surprising even herself: "Death is so close that when I see the end of another day it seems to me a miracle which I had not expected."

Dr. Allot, a physician from Lorraine, arrived in Paris promising an arsenic poultice cure. Applied to the tumor, the poultice mortified diseased tissue, which Allot surgically removed. Every day, from August 1665 to early January 1666, he took a knife to Anne's breast, carving away dead, necrotic flesh, stopping only when he reached living tissue—normal or malignant. Anne's hopes soared, in spite of a nagging cough that appeared in October, probably the result of lung metastases. Allot's removal of dying tumor tissue seemed tangible evidence of progress against the disease. But in spite of Allot's attentions, Anne's condition deteriorated. The cough deepened and her complexion yellowed even more. Weak and nauseous, she had difficulty keeping food down and lost weight. Anne soon gave up on the caustic paste. It was time to stop thinking about how to stay alive and start thinking about how to die.

Artes moriendi, or the art of dying well, was a carefully cultivated seventeenth-century skill. People died at home, surrounded by family and friends. They sensed the coming of death and prepared for it. Unlike modern industrial society, where medical technology has reduced infant mortality, deadly infections, and epidemic disease, and in the process made death less visible, seventeenth-century people did not enjoy the luxury of denying death. They met death face to face in a way that brought them dignity and comfort.[19]

In her search for *artes moriendi,* Anne turned to the convent culture that had given her so much comfort. Among nuns, she had enjoyed friendship and refuge. Now, suffering from "nun's disease," she learned how to die. The susceptibility of nuns to breast cancer was common knowledge. Bernardino Ramazzini, professor of medicine at the University of Padua, ruminated on the puzzling epidemiology, wondering in 1713 why "tumors of this sort are found in nuns more often than in any other women . . . . Every city in Italy has several religious communities of nuns, and you seldom can find a convent that does not harbor this accursed pest, cancer, within its walls." Convents all over Europe, at any given moment, had at least one nun suffering from the disease. Like all epidemiologists, Ramazzini searched for the unique, the exception, the lifestyle difference explaining the phenomenon, and he settled on the obvious, blaming celibacy for the nun's predicament. Ramazzini had discovered the correlation; he did not have any idea, however, of the cause. Lack of intercourse, he speculated, introduced a series of "disturbances in the uterus. Cancerous tumors are [then] very often generated in the woman's breast."[20]

The conundrum intrigues modern epidemiologists. Like Ramazzini three centuries ago, they searched for elusive connections. Recent studies on the incidence of breast cancer among different groups of women shed some light on the relationship. Nuns were and are more vulnerable to breast cancer, not because they are nuns or because they are sexually inactive but because they are childless. It appears that a nun, and any other woman who never gives birth, has a greater chance of developing breast cancer than women who have children. Women who have children at an early age stand a smaller chance of getting the disease than women who postpone childbearing until later in their reproductive lives. Recent epidemiological studies hint that women who nurse their children are less likely to fall victim to premenopausal breast cancer than women who do not. Celibate Roman Catholic nuns of the seventeenth century, like childless women today, faced a tangibly greater danger of getting the disease.[21]

Breast cancer occupied a unique place in seventeenth-century convent culture. The disease was so common among nuns that convent infirmaries often had portraits of St. Peregrine on the wall. Peregrine Laziosi was born in 1265 in Forli, northern Italy. As a teenager, he joined the Order of the Servants of St. Mary. He died in 1345 at the age of eighty, and the church canonized him in 1726. Long before canonization, however, Peregrine was known among the devout as the man who had been miraculously cured of cancer. Medical historians reading descriptions of his illness suspect a serious case of varicose veins, not cancer, but the miracle

Bathsheba's Breast

story was well known in the convents of Austria and Italy, giving hope to nuns afflicted with the disease. Peregrine was destined to become the patron saint of cancer patients.[22]

Portraits of St. Agatha also adorned the walls of convent infirmaries. Nuns revered her life and sacrifice. In the third century, Decius had ascended the throne of Rome after assassinating his predecessor, Emperor Philip. Decius abhorred Christianity and unleashed a crusade against the new religion. In Sicily, where Quintinian was Roman consul, the anti-Christian mania was particularly acute. According to Roman Catholic martyrologies, Quintinian fell in love with Agatha, a wealthy young woman who had promised her virginity to Jesus. Spurned in his advances, Quintinian went into a jealous rage, consigning Agatha to a brothel. When Agatha remained true to her vow, he resorted to diabolical tortures, strapping her to the rack and burning her at the stake. Finally, in what he felt would be the ultimate indignity, he cut off her breasts. Miraculously, according to the legend, Agatha survived the torture, and in the middle of the night St. Peter appeared in a vision and restored her breasts. She died in prison the next day, apparently on February 5, 251.[23]

Agatha became the patron saint of nurses, and nursing in early modern Europe was largely the domain of Catholic nuns in such orders as Sisters of the Common Life, Poor Clares, and Sisters of Charity of St. Vincent de Paul. Such lay sisterhoods as the Beguines labored as nurses. Monks and priests abandoned such tasks, which they increasingly considered women's work, in favor of New World missionary endeavors, diocesan administration, and scholarship. By the seventeenth century, in the medical world of Anne of Austria, nuns staffed the hospitals, hospices, asylums, orphanages, and convent nursing homes of Europe.[24]

The cult of St. Agatha blossomed in the sixth century. Pope Gregory I consecrated a church in her name late in the 590s, and by the thirteenth century Roman Catholics in Sicily, Italy, Austria, southern Germany, and eastern France regularly blessed bread, candles, and fruit in her name. Beginning in the early fourteenth century, artists depicted St. Agatha carrying her severed breasts on a plate, offering them up to persecutors of the Lord, where they might satisfy a lecher's hunger but never his lust. Other portraits depicted Agatha looking plaintively to heaven during the mutilation. Permutations on the St. Agatha martyrdom became common in the Middle Ages, especially in Italy, where each village needed its own patron saint. St. Lucy, a fourth century Sicilian martyr who refused to surrender her dedicated virginity, also spent time in a brothel before having her eyes cut out. Sometimes, in the Italian villages revering her as their patroness, St. Lucy was depicted as cutting off her own breasts rather than submit to the sexual depredations of her tormentors.[25]

A thousand years later, in the seventeenth century, court fashions enthroned the breast on an erotic pedestal. During the transition from the sixteenth century, dress design evolved; sleeves blossomed and skirts expanded over multiple petticoats. Bodices tightened and necklines plunged, exposing neck, collarbones, and shoulders. At gala court parties, women tightened corsets, pushing their breasts higher and forcing them close together, creating a long, visible cleavage and revealing every square inch of flesh above the areola. Throughout her life, Anne had taken more than a little pleasure in her body. She was the most fashionable of the fashionable, and her gowns allowed for an ample display. For a finishing touch, she often wore a necklace with a crucifix as a pendant, the cross resting just above her cleavage.[26]

Now, however, like St. Agatha and St. Lucy, Anne of Austria no longer basked in physical beauty. Anne even felt she was, in some ways, dying their deaths. Just as St. Agatha and St. Lucy had lost their breasts, and their beauty, to the knife, Anne lost hers too, many times over, day after day for more than five months, as Allot carved away at the mortifying tumor. Anne believed there was a purpose to her suffering. Just as St. Agatha's martyrdom had encouraged generations of Catholic women to protect their virtue, she knew there was a lesson for others in her suffering. In the grand ceremony of seventeenth-century death, Anne symbolized how all worldly vanities come to an end, and how to endure a penance cheerfully.

The irony of Anne's demise was not lost on anybody in the court of Louis XIV. In a world of pomp and grandeur, she sat at center stage. With the snap of her fingers, the blink of an eye, she commanded wealth, respect, deference, and obedience from priests and popes and peasants and princes. But death was the great leveler. Madame de Motteville spoke with Anne about the end of life. "It was difficult," she later wrote, "to see so great a princess in such a condition without having the nothingness of created beings brought strongly to mind, and how all human aid is useless when it pleases God to destroy the highest ranking persons in the world."

Bathsheba's Breast

Anne found it particularly humiliating to be dying of breast cancer; it made her feel dirty. She was a fastidious woman, bathing regularly, changing her underwear daily, luxuriating in the most exquisite perfumes, and wearing only the finest fabrics. The ulcerating tumors discharged so much "black bile" and repulsive odors that when her bandages needed changing, servants covered her nose with heavily perfumed handkerchiefs and sprinkled perfumes in the air in a vain attempt to subdue the smell. A gentleman friend, trying to console Anne, sympathized with her plight, telling her that the disease was "a great inconvenience, especially for You who loves perfumes, because at the end these illnesses stink terribly."

There was more than humiliation to Anne's *artes moriendi;* she believed she also had to pay for her vanity. God was punishing her, and the price was accepting her fate with grace and submission. She occasionally wondered about it all. De Motteville remembered Anne's speculations: "Often she said she never would have believed her destiny would be so different from that of other creatures; that people only rotted after death, but as for her, God had condemned her to rot alive." But she subdued the anger and submitted. "God wishes to punish me," she said to de Motteville, "for having loved myself too well and having cared too much about the beauty of my body." When her son Philippe of Anjou expressed the wish that he could assume his mother's pain, Anne rebuked him: "My son, that would not be just. God wants me to do penance: I now must comply with what he ordains; I am the one who must suffer, not you."

Toward the end, priests and nuns consoled Anne, referring to the suffering of the saints, likening her demise to the deaths of St. Agatha and St. Lucy, and finding a martyrdom for her in the pain and indignity of breast cancer. Wealth, power, and physical beauty meant nothing to her now. Anne had a simple hope: "What I suffer will no doubt help my salvation; I hope that God will give me the strength to endure it with patience."

God apparently did. Anne chose to die at Val-de-Grace, under the portraits of St. Agatha and at the hands of her beloved nuns. She was carried into Val-de-Grace on a portable bed. After a few days, Louis XIV decided the convent was too inconvenient for a death vigil, and they persuaded her to take an apartment in the Louvre. Louis filled the bedroom with new furniture—a bed hung with her favorite patterned blue velvet and matching chairs and stools—and re-carpeted the hallways to muffle annoying sounds. Physicians, courtiers, nuns, servants, priests, and sons attended Anne day and night, trying to comfort her. Louis decreed that novenas and forty-hour prayer vigils take place throughout France. On January 19, 1666, Anne's priest suggested the end was near; the time had arrived for the last rites of the church. She lingered for a few more hours, long enough to say goodbye to her sons and give them a blessing. Early in the morning of January 20, 1666, Anne of Austria died, hoping that her penance had been sufficient to warrant a reward from God. If torment and suffering form the straight and narrow path to God, then Anne of Austria felt she had qualified. Perhaps St. Agatha, not St. Peter, opened to her the doors of heaven.

CHAPTER TWO

"Unkindest Cut of All"

THE ORIGINS OF THE MASTECTOMY

On September 1, 1789, President George Washington was in New York, entertaining Baron Friedrich Wilhelm von Steuben, the Prussian general who had played a key role in the American victory over Britain during the Revolution. Alcohol flowed liberally, as did toasts, nostalgic stories, and laughter. Several hours into the evening, a special courier arrived with a message for the president. His mother, Mary, was dead. Washington took the news unusually well. He remarked to his guests and later wrote in his journal, "Awful and affecting as the death of a parent is, there is consolation in knowing that Heaven has spared ours to an age beyond which few attain, and favored her with the full enjoyment of her faculties." In memory of his mother, he ordered black cockades, sword knots, and arm-ribbons for his staff, but he was not about "to go into deep mourning for her." The president's grief was restrained.[1]

Tension had long marred Washington's relationship with his mother, even though he had been the favorite of eight children. She loved him deeply but harbored a compulsion to run his life. He escaped home when he was sixteen, signing on with a survey crew working the south branch of the Potomac River. For the next forty years, Mary pelted her son with requests for money, food, servants, and slaves, complaining constantly about inconsiderate neighbors and George's dereliction in responding to her demands. The tirades embarrassed and annoyed him. The house he purchased for her in Fredericksburg became badly run-down, an eyesore compared to the other neat homes on Charles Street and a source of gossip. Mary consistently spent more money than George budgeted for her, and when he did not supplement her accounts, she spread rumors that he was unwilling to help his own mother. On one occasion, he sent her money and complained: "It is really hard on me when I am viewed as a delinquent, and considered perhaps by the world as an unjust and undutiful son."

His decision to lead the fight against the British also irritated her. In 1782 Louis de Clermont-Crevecoeur, a French soldier, visited Mary Washington just to get a look at the mother of America's hero. After the visit, he wrote in his journal, "Fredericksburg is where General Washington's mother lives. We went to call on her but were amazed to be told that this lady, who must be over seventy, is one of the most rabid Tories. Relations must be very strained between her and her son, who will always be the right arm of American freedom."

Indeed, they were strained. Mary griped constantly, condemning the rebellion, praising the British, and insisting that George reconsider his loyalties. It mattered little that her son was revered as the father of the new country, a man of distinguished bearing and extraordinary courage. All Mary wanted was more money and George's willingness to do her bidding. In thirty years, she never visited his home at Mount Vernon, even though it was only forty miles away. For his part, he saw his mother only when absolutely necessary.

In 1787 it became absolutely necessary. On April 26, the day before Washington was scheduled to depart for Philadelphia to attend the Constitutional Convention, he received a letter from his sister, urging him to come home as soon as possible. His mother was suffering from breast cancer. Describing the situation, he wrote: "I am called by an express, who assures me that not a moment is to be lost, to see [my mother] in agonies of Death." He was at her side in a few days, but he despaired of her condition, convinced that she "cannot long Survive the disorder which has reduced her to a skeleton." He misjudged her toughness. Mary survived for two years—more time to harass him. He visited twice more, once in June 1788 when she needed money and again in March 1789, a month before he was inaugurated president.[2]

Bathsheba's Breast

Four months after Washington's last meeting with his mother, an urgent letter arrived at the office of Benjamin Rush in the Pennsylvania Hospital of Philadelphia. Rush was the most famous physician in the country, a confidante of Benjamin Franklin, Thomas Jefferson, John Adams, Thomas Paine, George Washington, and John Hancock, as well as a Revolutionary hero in his own right. Elisha Hall, a doctor practicing in Fredericksburg, wanted to know about the alleged healing powers of one Hugh Martin, whose "special powder" was said to cure cancer. Hall had applied the powder to Mary Washington's breast, but it was not working. She was steadily deteriorating. When Hall learned that Martin had once been Rush's student, he wanted to check out Martin's credentials and the efficacy of "Hugh Martin's Powder."[3]

Rush's response, written several days later, reflected twenty years of treating cancer. An intellectual prodigy who had entered the College of New Jersey (later Princeton) at the age of twelve, he flirted briefly with the law but then decided on medicine, apprenticing with John Redman, a surgeon at Pennsylvania Hospital. Rush worked with him for five years and finished the apprenticeship in 1766. Redman encouraged Rush to head for Europe, especially London and Paris, to learn the latest medical theories and techniques.

A European tour was the last step in the education of well-to-do Americans. Europe was an intellectual beacon, the place to balance the pragmatic training of the New World with the sophistication of the Old. And the Enlightenment was well under way. Faith in science had never been higher, and optimism about conquering nature and human frailties abounded. Rush arrived at the University of Edinburgh in the summer of 1766. He studied there for two years, attending hundreds of lectures by physiologists, anatomists, botanists, and physicians. He earned a medical degree and studied chemistry under Joseph Black, the father of quantitative analysis. Black passed on to Rush a passion for subjecting every pharmacological remedy to rigorous chemical examination.

In September 1768, Rush left for London. Galen's ghost no longer haunted Europe's leading medical schools. By the 1760s, no physician with any self-respect offered black bile diagnoses. The death of humoral theory had been a gradual one. Information moved slowly, if at all, in the seventeenth and eighteenth centuries. Scientists working in one city had only casual contact with colleagues in another. Dissemination of new ideas was haphazard: travel was difficult and printing costs high. One man's discovery might die with him or be confined for decades to a particular region. But in the decades following Anne of Austria's death in 1666, medicine slowly changed, and the Galenic consensus entered a long period of decline. By the time Rush got to London, the collapse of Galen's edifice was well under way. Rush studied there under John Hunter, Giovanni Morgagni, John Fothergill, and Percivall Pott.

Hunter was a surgeon and an anatomist, the most unorthodox, creative physician in England. Born in 1728 in Lanarkshire, Scotland, he rebelled from the very beginning, refusing to study Latin and Greek and preferring to wander the Scottish countryside examining God's creations. A niece remembered that he "would do nothing but what he liked, and neither liked to be taught reading nor writing nor any kind of learning, but rambling amongst the woods, trees, etc., looking after bird's nests, comparing their eggs—number, size, marks, and other peculiarities." Hunter later recalled, "When I was a boy . . . . I pestered people with questions about what nobody knew or cared anything about." In 1748, he moved in with his brother William, a prominent London obstetrician.[4]

Hunter studied surgery at Chelsea Hospital, St. Bartholomew's Hospital, and St. George's Hospital and then completed a surgical stint in the British army during the Seven Years' War. He returned to London in 1763 and rocketed to fame as a surgeon, winning membership in the Royal Society. Hunter specialized in postmortem examination and developed a passion for determining, through systematic dissection and observation, the links between disease and human physiology. He ridiculed all notions of Galenic humors. In fact, Hunter wanted nothing to do with theories and speculations. Truth was to be discovered with a scalpel on the dissection table, not in the dead hand of Clarissimus Galen.[5]

Hunter's primary contribution to oncology was his description of breast cancer's spread to nearby lymph nodes. After hundreds of dissections of London women who had died of breast cancer, he informed his students that the disease migrated through the lymphatic system, and that doctors treating patients needed to examine tissues near the tumor to determine if it was spreading. His argument soon became gospel in late eighteenth- and early nineteenth-century textbooks. For several months in 1768, Hunter tutored Benjamin Rush in London.[6]

Rush also worked with John Fothergill, whose botanical garden in

Bathsheba's Breast

Essex helped him test the medicinal formulas Galenic physicians had prescribed for centuries. Many of them were bizarre remedies—wolf liver, goat and stag horns, dried vipers, crab claws, lizard intestines, urine poultices, black nightshade, frog spawn, rotten apples, lead and mercury ointments, the juices of pigeons and rabbits that were crushed or cut up alive—all mixed together with herbs and plants. Fothergill passed on to Rush his skepticism about most treatments, especially the cancer cures. He knew of no pastes or poultices that had any long-term beneficial effects.

Percivall Pott, chief surgeon at St. Bartholomew's, influenced Rush as well. Pott believed that cancer had environmental, not humoral, origins. Over the years, Pott noted the number of chimney sweeps with scrotal cancer. The cause was obvious: continual exposure to soot damaged the skin and triggered what contemporary oncologists describe as a squamous cell carcinoma. Pott scoffed at what he called "black bile bilge." Chimney sweeps got cancer from coal dust, not a bodily fluid. Infrequent bathing gave soot time to irritate the skin. He did not publish his conclusions until 1775, but his views were well known years before.[7]

Rush never met Giovanni Morgagni, his other mentor. A physician at the University of Padua, Morgagni in 1761 published *The Seats and Causes of Diseases Investigated by Anatomy*. The product of a lifetime of postmortem dissections, the book was in its third English printing by 1769 and required reading for every medical student in London. In it, Morgagni provided seven hundred case studies of diseases linking symptoms to the breakdown of an organ or physical system. London physicians elected him to the Royal Society. Benjamin Rush treasured his own copy of the book.[8]

Several of the cases described breast cancer. Starting with the Greeks, physicians had written of hard, "cold," and painless breast tumors as "scirrhus," or dangerous precancerous growths that would "usurpate" into cancer. But Morgagni urged caution; such tumors were not always dangerous. He wrote of a nun in Padua: surgeons removed a walnut-sized lump from her breast, but to the surprise of everyone, "the body consisted of many little pieces of bone, not a cancer." He was probably describing a benign calcified fibroadenoma, which was not fatal. The idea of surgically examining a tumor before removing large amounts of breast tissue was born.[9]

Imbued with the ideas of Black, Hunter, Morgagni, Fothergill, and Pott, Rush left London after six months and arrived in Paris on February 19, 1769. The city throbbed with creative intellects. Pathology labs housed dozens of carved-up cadavers surrounded by inquisitive students learning gross anatomy. On any given day, professors stood at podiums around the city, reporting recent discoveries and debating each other's ideas. In theaters with excited students looking on, surgeons demonstrated the latest techniques. Chemists and botanists worked together, conjuring up new products for apothecaries and physicians.

Galen no longer prevailed in Paris, but his demise was only recent. In the decades after the death of Anne of Austria, new theories of carcinogenesis sprouted in the gardens of Parisian science, but they were little more than humoral weeds. François de la Boe Sylvius, a French physician practicing in the Netherlands, had argued in 1680 that cancer came not from an excess of black bile but from a chemical process transforming lymphatic fluids from an acidic to an acrid nature. Claude-Deshais Gendron, a renowned Paris physician and nephew of the doctor who treated Anne of Austria, also rejected humors and insisted in the 1730s that cancer developed when nerve and glandular tissue mixed with lymph vessels. Jean-Baptiste Allot, son of the physician who had applied the arsenic poultice to Anne's breast, was Physician of the Bastille in the 1720s. He was the last respectable humoralist in Paris. Allot postulated that too much black bile produced a "scirrhus," but that scirrhus became a malignant tumor only when it mixed with salt in the blood.[10]

When Rush got to Paris in 1769, no humoralists survived, at least not among leading authorities. Students buzzed about the work of Jean Astruc, who had died just two years before at the age of eighty-two. A graduate of the medical school at Montpellier, Astruc specialized in venereal and skin diseases and became personal physician to Louis XV. In 1751 he took a piece of breast cancer tissue, along with a slice of beef, burned them both in an oven, and then chewed on both specimens. Detecting no difference in taste, he decided the tumor tissue did not contain unusual amounts of bile or acid, and he subsequently repudiated the black bile theory of cancer.[11]

With black bile discredited, physicians searched for new explanations. Many looked for a sexual origin. They knew of Bernardino Ramazzini's 1713 claim attributing breast cancer in nuns to lack of sexual activity. Celibacy was unnatural, Ramazzini argued, even if sacred and holy; without regular sexual activity, the reproductive organs, including the breast, languished and became unstable. Cancer was one outcome. But what about sexually active women who developed cancer? Astruc warned against vigorous sexual activity, especially "the complaisance with which nowadays one allows one's teats to be taken and handled, exposing them to compression." Friedrich Hoffmann, a professor of medicine in Halle, Prussia, in the 1730s, was even more explicit. Breast cancer started in a lymphatic blockage, and sexual activity could produce such an obstruction. "For thus I know women who," Hoffmann wrote in 1739, "when frolicking with their husband, because of a single rather fierce manipulation, instead of pleasure had to carry with them permanent disease and sorrow."

There was no shortage of explanations. Morgagni blamed curdled milk. Johannes de Gorter, physician to the Russian tsar in the 1750s, claimed that tumors evolved from pus-filled inflammations in the breast that mixed with blood, lodged in a milk gland, and dried into a tumor. Claude-Nicolas Le Cat, a renowned Rouen surgeon, blamed depression for causing the disease by constricting blood vessels and trapping coagulated blood. Lorenz Heister placed childless women at high risk, while others blamed a sedentary lifestyle, which brought about a slackening of bodily fluids. In fact, eighteenth-century physicians knew only a little more about the causes of breast cancer than Hippocrates and Galen and only a little less than contemporary oncologists.[12]

If the cause of breast cancer baffled physicians, they gradually became more certain about the need for mastectomy—amputation of the breast. It was the key principle Rush learned in Paris. German surgeons had called for mastectomies since the early 1600s. Wilhelm Fabry, a surgeon in Dusseldorf, had developed an instrument for mastectomies. It consisted of hand-held forceps which squeezed the base of the breast, constricting it before a sharp knife lifted it from the patient's chest. He recommended removal of visibly involved lymph nodes. Another German surgeon, Johann Schultes of Ulm, had published *Armamentarium Chirurgicum* in 1645, which was translated into several languages and became a popular medical text. His procedure involved inserting large, fishhook lances into the breast, lifting it from the chest wall by pulling on attached ropes, cutting away the breast, and cauterizing the wound with hot irons.[13]

Humoral theories always considered mastectomy a tangential treatment. If the disease was systemic, destined to return in another part of the body, women did not need to endure such surgery. But as humoral theory disappeared, physicians became increasingly skeptical about other so-called cures. By the time Rush got to Paris, several surgeons there had followed the German lead in advocating mastectomy as the only reasonable treatment. One of them was Henri Le Dran, a surgeon at the Hôpital Saint Comte in Paris. His father, Henri Le Dran, had practiced medicine in Paris from 1690 through 1720, and was the first French physician to endorse the mastectomy recommendations of German surgeons.

The younger Le Dran also became a leading figure in Parisian medicine and argued that surgery could cure breast cancer, as long as the axilla lymph nodes were removed if there was any sign of involvement. In 1757, Le Dran wrote:

> The writers who have treated this subject have represented cancer as a sordid spreading ulcer and have looked upon it as incurable; but—every cancer begins by the obstruction of one or more glands . . . . But if it increases, surgery afforded no other remedy but extirpation and where that is practicable we may be assured of success. Also, if just becoming painful, provided the operation is not delayed, we may hope for a perfect cure . . . . If only a few axillary glands are found involved, be sure to remove them along with the breast or it might give rise to a fresh cancer.

Claude-Nicolas Le Cat was even more adamant. Only the scalpel could cure cancer. In addition to amputating the breast and cutting out lymph nodes, Le Cat removed part of the pectoralis major muscle, a procedure recommended by Jean Louis Petit, director of the French Academy. All three surgeons also believed the disease was hereditary. In Avignon, Le Dran was asked to treat a nineteen-year-old nun suffering from a breast tumor. He suggested surgery but the nun refused, telling him that so many of her relatives had died of the disease that she was already doomed as well. He rejected out of hand other treatments, insisting that pastes, salves, and external potions were useless, as were internal pharmacological remedies. In 1758 Le Dran's memoirs appeared in English translation. By the time Rush got to Paris in 1769, they were required reading for medical students.[14]

Mastectomies were well known at the time in Philadelphia, Boston, and New York. In 1728 Dr. Zabdiel Boylston, a Boston surgeon, had amputated Sarah Winslow's breast to remove a malignant tumor. She survived the surgery and lived another thirty-nine years, dying in 1767 of old

Bathsheba's Breast

age. Local physicians believed that the operation had achieved the cure. The Winslow case was well known among prominent American physicians, and Rush's apprenticeship at Pennsylvania Hospital no doubt included training in mastectomies. What he had acquired in Paris from Le Dran, Petit, and Le Cat was a conviction that mastectomy was the *only* effective treatment.[15]

His Grand Tour over, Rush returned to Philadelphia knowing as much about cancer as anyone in the world—which was not much. He rejected Galen's black bile theory and put no trust in the notion that breast cancer was related to the acidity of bodily fluids. He had little use for topical remedies. He had not seen any chemical, poultice, powder, cream, or salve that cured malignant tumors. In fact, he wrote that "the knife should always be preferred to the caustic. In cancerous ulcers . . . such particularly as have their seat in the neck, in the breasts of females, and in the axillary glands, it [caustic medicines] can only prolong the patient's misery."[16]

During the next twenty years, Rush practiced medicine in Philadelphia, served in the 2nd Continental Congress, signed the Declaration of Independence, and volunteered as a surgeon in the Continental Army. He corresponded regularly with European friends, securing the latest medical news. Like many others, he had concluded that cancer was not contagious. James Nooth, surgeon to the Duke of Kent and a physician in Dorchester and Bath, England, had treated hundreds of breast cancer patients, and he had not seen their nurses, sisters, or daughters come down with the disease. To make sure breast cancer was not infectious, he removed a small piece of breast carcinoma tissue from a patient and implanted the specimen into an incision in his left arm. He developed a small sore which, after several days, formed into a scab and fell off. Nooth repeated the experiment many times with the same results. In his journals he wrote: "I am convinced, that those persons who give their attendance to cancerous subjects, are not so liable to get this cruel disease by absorption, as has been too generally supposed."[17]

Other scientists repeated Nooth's experiment. Jean Louis Alibert, a physician and faculty member at the Hôpital de St. Louis in Paris, in 1808 asked his medical students to join him in the inoculations. They reluctantly cooperated. All received injections of breast cancer tissues and experienced localized inflammatory reactions as their immune systems rejected the foreign tissue. Although one student's infection also involved the axilla lymph nodes, he recovered within a few days. Breast cancer was not contagious.[18]

Rush put every alleged cancer cure to a laboratory test; his skepticism only deepened. He remained open-minded about the possibilities of finding medicinal treatments in nature. In a letter to John Foulke in 1780, Rush advised him to "converse freely with quacks of every class and sex, such as oculists, aurists, dentists, corn cutters, cancer doctors, etc. etc. You cannot conceive how much a physician with a liberal mind may profit from a few casual and secret visits to these people."[19]

Not that he ever found a cure. In 1789, when he pondered Mary Washington's condition, Rush offered no hope. When Elisha Hall asked about the effectiveness of Hugh Martin's cancer powder, Rush told him the brutal truth. Three years before, he had put Martin's tonic to the test, carefully examining the powder in his own laboratory. He told Hall, "Arsenic . . . is the basis of Dr. Martin's powder . . . . I am disposed to believe that there does not exist in the vegetable kingdom an antidote to cancers." Mastectomy was out of the question too. Mary Washington's disease was too advanced. "From your account of Mrs. Washington's breast," Rush continued, "I am afraid no great good can be expected from the use of it . . . it is not in my power to suggest a remedy for the cure of the disorder you have described in her breast."[20]

Although Rush did not realize it, he was in the midst of an intellectual revolution. The old treatments still did not work, and the new theories had little connection to biochemical reality. Nonetheless, the intellectual rebellion against Galen had altered medical thought. For two millennia, medical savants had viewed breast cancer as a systemic disease, a malady of the entire body, not just one of its appendages. A breast tumor, it was believed, was more symptom than sickness, a bellwether of more fundamental flaws in the body. The humoral imbalance could, and usually would, manifest itself in a different organ. Black bile seeped throughout the body, mushrooming into multiple tumors. Even if the tumors were removed, the destructive black bile still bubbled away, ready to produce new cancers.

But when physicians identified a blocked lymphatic vessel or a clogged lymph node as the source of cancer, they rejected systemic theories in favor of local, mechanical processes. The presence of a tumor did not necessarily imply more serious, underlying problems; confined to a single site before spreading, the cancer could be treated locally. And the sooner the better. Delay only gave the tumor time to colonize. Until well into the twentieth century, despite astonishing progress in medical technology, scientists adhered to that logic—cancer was a local disorder that, if caught and eradicated in time, could be cured. And the cure was surgery. During the course of his lifetime, Rush and the brightest physicians around the world gradually rejected every recorded medicinal treatment—external or internal—for breast cancer.

When Rush received a letter in 1811 from Abigail "Nabby" Adams, daughter of John Adams, the former president of the United States, he knew exactly what to say. She needed advice about her breast. Perhaps the disease had started out as a tiny dimple. On a man's chin it would have looked rugged and distinguished. On a woman's cheek it might have been called a "beauty mark." But it was on her left breast and Nabby wondered what it was. She had never noticed it before. Perhaps it was just another sign of age, an indicator that she was not a young woman anymore. Actually the dimple was not really the problem. Beneath the dimple, buried an inch below the skin, a small malignant tumor attached itself to surface tissues and drew them in, like a sinking ship pulling water down its own whirlpool. Nabby was forty-two years old.

At first she did not give it much thought, noticing it now and then when she bathed or dressed. Nor did she talk about it. She was a shy, somewhat withdrawn woman, quiet and cautious in her expressions, most comfortable with people who guarded their feelings. She blushed easily and rarely laughed out loud, allowing only a demure half-smile to crease her face when she was amused. She had a pleasant disposition and a mellow temperament, both endearing to family and friends. Nabby was a striking woman, with long, red hair, a round face, deep-blue eyes, and a creamy, porcelain complexion. She commanded respect, not because of an aggressive personality but simply because of the quality of her mind and her unfailing dignity.

She was born in Quincy, Massachusetts, in 1766. Her parents named her Abigail Adams, but they began calling her "Nabby" when she was still an infant. Nabby had an extraordinary childhood. Not only was her father a future president of the United States, but her mother Abigail Adams was the most prominent woman in early American society. Her younger brother John Quincy was destined to win many honors, among them the

U.S. presidency. From the time of her birth, Nabby's parents busied themselves with colonial politics, eventually playing leading roles in the American Revolution. They raised her on a steady diet of political talk about freedom, liberty, rights, despotism, and foreign policy. Nabby absorbed it all.

An only daughter, Nabby enjoyed the special attentions of her father,
who felt the need to protect and pamper her. Abigail doted on her, dressing her up in the latest fashions when she was little and counseling her
when she was an adolescent. Their relationship evolved into a deep friendship. Nabby took it all in stride, never becoming spoiled or self-indulgent.
She was even-handed, thick-skinned, and unafraid of responsibility.[21]

In 1783, when Congress appointed her father as minister to England,
Nabby was seventeen years old. The family took up residence in a house
on Grosvener Square in London. Caught up in a whirlwind of social and
political activity, they met King George III at court and other prominent
politicians at parties and banquets common to the life of an ambassador.
After a few months, Nabby became acquainted with William Smith, a
thirty-year-old veteran of the Continental Army and secretary to the
American legation in London. A dashing, handsome figure, Smith raced
around London in a two-seated carriage, the eighteenth-century equivalent of a modern sports car. He dressed well and kept company with
people in London's expatriate community, especially Latin American lib-
erals and radicals interested in securing independence from Spain. He was
bold and impetuous, inspired by courage and limited by poor judgment.
Because of his work with the U.S. legation, and his role as secretary to
Minister John Adams, he saw a great deal of the Adams family, and Nabby
fell secretly in love with him. Drawn to Nabby's beauty, grace, and intel-
ligence, he soon felt the same way about her. They married in June 1786,
after a courtship which John and Abigail felt was too short. They accepted
it, however, because "a soldier is always more expeditious in his courtships
than other men."[22]

But Colonel William Smith was a soldier without a war, a has-been
at the age of thirty, and Nabby, an innocent victim of what her brother
John Quincy called "fortune's treacherous game," faced a difficult life.
Colonel Smith was not cruel. In fact, he always loved and cared for Nabby
and their three children. With a stoicism that would have made the most
devout Puritan proud, she accepted her fate and made a life for her family
wherever Smith settled. The problem was that Smith never really settled

Bathsheba's Breast

down. He wasted his life away, winning and losing political appointments, dabbling in Latin American coups d'état, dragging Nabby and the children back and forth between New York and London in search of a new power broker or another promising deal. He spent more money than he ever earned, and Nabby worried constantly about bills and the family reputation. Early in the new century, Smith tried his hand at real estate speculation, but he lost everything. In 1809, when Nabby first noticed the lump in her breast, they were living on the edge of the frontier, on a small farm along the Chenango River in western New York, where Smith spent his days behind a walking plow and a mule.

Nabby was a well-informed woman, and breast cancer was as much a dread disease in the early 1800s as it is today. No records exist describing her initial reaction to the lump, but it is safe to say that concern about the dimple flared into gut-twisting fear. Like so many women, then and today, she tried to ignore the lump, hoping that in the busy routines of running a small farm and household she would not have time to think about it. But cancer has a way of asserting itself, finally obliterating even the most elaborate denials. Nabby was no exception. The lump grew ominously, in spite of the efforts of local healers and their potions. She wrote home to her parents in February 1811 that her doctor had discovered "a cancer in my breast." As soon as they received the letter, the Adamses wrote back urging her to come to Boston for medical advice.

In June 1811, with the lump visible to the naked eye, a desperate Nabby returned to Massachusetts, accompanied by her husband and daughter Caroline. As soon as she arrived in Quincy, she wrote to Benjamin Rush, describing her condition and seeking his advice. When Abigail first looked at her daughter's breast, she found the condition "allarming." The large tumor distended the breast into a misshapen mass. John and Abigail took Nabby to see several physicians in Boston, and they were cautiously reassuring, telling her that the situation and her general health were "so good as not to threaten any present danger." They prescribed hemlock pills to "poison the disease."[23]

Soon after those reassuring examinations, however, the family received an unsettling reply from Benjamin Rush. In her initial letter, Nabby told Rush that the tumor was large and growing, but that it was "movable"—not attached to the chest wall. Rush found the news encouraging, as would most cancer specialists today. Malignant tumors which are "movable" are better candidates for surgery, since it is more likely that the surgeon can get what is termed a "clean margin"—a border of non-cancerous tissue surrounding the tumor—reducing the odds that the cancer will recur or spread. Knowing that Nabby had already traveled from western New York to Boston to seek medical advice, Rush wrote to John and Abigail, telling them to break his news gently to Nabby:

> I shall begin my letter by replying to your daughter's. I prefer giving my opinion and advice in her case in this way. You and Mrs. Adams may communicate it gradually and in such a manner as will be least apt to distress and alarm her.
>
> After the experience of more than 50 years in cases similar to hers, I must protest against all local applications and internal medicines for relief. They now and then cure, but in 19 cases out of 20 in tumors in the breast they do harm or suspend the disease until it passes beyond that time in which the only radical remedy is ineffectual. This remedy is the knife. From her account of the moving state of the tumor, it is now in a proper situation for the operation. Should she wait till it suppurates or even inflames much, it may be too late . . . . I repeat again, let there be no delay in flying to the knife. Her time of life calls for expedition in this business . . . . I sincerely sympathize with her and with you and your dear Mrs. Adams in this family affliction, but it will be but for a few minutes if she submits to have it extirpated, and if not, it will probably be a source of distress and pain to you all for years to come. It shocks me to think of the consequences of procrastination.[24]

Mastectomy was Nabby's only chance, but first the family had to convince William Smith, who was in an advanced state of denial. When he learned of Rush's recommendation, he reacted indignantly, heading for libraries to learn whatever he could about the disease and hoping to spare her the operation. He convinced himself for a while that perhaps the tumor would just go away, that it was not so bad. Nabby's mother had more faith in Rush and wrote to Smith: "If the operation is necessary as the Dr. states it to be, and as I fear it is, the sooner it is done the better provided Mrs. Smith can bring herself along, as I hope she will consent to it." She even asked her son-in-law to be with "Nabby through the painful tryal." Smith finally agreed. They scheduled the operation for October 8, 1811.

The day before the surgery, John Warren, Boston's most skilled surgeon, met with the family in Quincy. He gave Nabby a brief physical examination and told her what to expect. His description was nightmarishly terrifying, enough to make everybody reconsider the decision. But Rush's warning—"It shocks me to think of the consequences of procrastination in her case"—stuck in their minds. Nabby had no choice if she ever hoped to live to see her grandchildren.

The surgery took place in an upstairs bedroom of the Adams home in Quincy. It was as bad as they had all feared. John Warren was assisted by his son Joseph, who was destined to become a leading physician in his own right, and several other physicians. Exact details of the operation are not available, but it was certainly typical of early-nineteenth-century surgery. Warren's surgical instruments, lying in a wooden box on a table, were quite simple—a large fork with two six-inch prongs sharpened to a needle point, a wooden-handled razor, and a pile of compress bandages. In the corner of the room a small oven, full of red-hot coals, heated a flat, thick, heavy iron spatula.

Nabby entered the room as if dressed for a Sunday service. She was a proper woman and acted the part. The doctors were professionally attired in frock coats, with shirts and ties. Modesty demanded that Nabby unbutton only the top of her dress and slip it off her left shoulder, exposing the diseased breast but little else. She remained fully clothed. Since they knew nothing of bacteria in the early 1800s, there were no gloves or surgical masks, no need for Warren to scrub his hands or disinfect Nabby's chest before the operation or cover his own hair. Warren had her sit down and lean back in a reclining chair. He belted her waist, legs, feet, and right arm to the chair and had her raise her left arm above her head so that the pectoralis major muscle would push the breast up. A physician took Nabby's raised arm by the elbow and held it, while another stood behind her, pressing her shoulders and neck to the chair.

Warren then straddled Nabby's knees, leaned over her semireclined body, and went to work. He took the two-pronged fork and thrust it deep into the breast. With his left hand, he held onto the fork and raised up on it, lifting the breast from the chest wall. He reached over for the large razor and started slicing into the base of the breast, moving from the middle of her chest toward her left side. When the breast was completely severed, Warren lifted it away from Nabby's chest with the fork. But the tumor was larger and more widespread than he had anticipated. Hard knots of tumor could be felt in the lymph nodes under her left arm. He razored in there as well and pulled out nodes and tumor. Nabby grimaced and groaned, flinching and twisting in the chair, with blood staining her dress and Warren's shirt and pants. Her hair matted in sweat. Abigail, William, and Caroline turned away from the gruesome struggle. To stop the bleeding, Warren pulled a red-hot spatula from the oven and applied it several times to the wound, cauterizing the worst bleeding points. With each touch, steamy wisps of smoke hissed into the air and filled the room with the distinct smell of burning flesh. Warren then sutured the wounds, bandaged them, stepped back from Nabby, and mercifully told her that it was over. The whole procedure had taken less than twenty-five minutes, but it took more than an hour to dress the wounds. Abigail and Caroline then helped Nabby pull her dress back over her left shoulder as modesty demanded. The four surgeons remained astonished that she had endured the pain so stoically.

Nabby had a long recovery. She did not suffer from postsurgical infections, but for months after the operation she was weak and feeble, barely able to get around. She kept her limp left arm resting in a sling. Going back to the wilds of western New York was out of the question, so she stayed in Quincy with her mother, hoping to regain strength. What sustained all of them during the ordeal was the faith that the operation had cured the cancer. Within two weeks of the surgery, Dr. Rush wrote John Adams congratulating him "in the happy issue of the operation performed upon Mrs. Smith's breast . . . her cure will be radical and durable. I consider her as rescued from a premature grave." Abigail wrote to a friend that although the operation had been a "furnace of affliction . . . what a blessing it was to have extirpated so terrible an enemy." In May 1812, seven months after the surgery, Nabby Smith felt well again. She returned home to the small farm along the Chenango River.

But she was not cured. Breast cancer patients whose tumors have already spread to the lymph nodes do not have good survival rates, even with modern surgery, radiation treatments, and chemotherapy. In Nabby's case, long before Warren performed the mastectomy, the cancer had already spread. Nabby suspected something was wrong within a few weeks of arriving home in New York. She began to complain of headaches and pain in her spine and abdomen. A local physician attributed the discomfort to rheumatism. The diagnosis relieved some of her anxiety, since she was already worried that the pain had something to do with cancer.

But it was not "the rheumatism." That became quite clear in 1813 when she suffered a local recurrence of the tumors. When Warren amputated her breast and excised tissues from her axilla, he thought he had "gotten it all." But cancer is a cellular disease, and millions of invisible, microscopically tiny malignant cancers were left behind. By the spring of 1813 some of them had grown into tumors of their own—visible in the scar where Nabby's breast had once been and on the skin as well. Her doctor in New York changed the diagnosis: the headaches and now excruciating body pains were not rheumatism. The cancer was back—everywhere.

She declined steadily in the late spring, finally telling her husband that she "wanted to die in her father's house." William Smith wrote John and Abigail in May that the cancer had returned and that Nabby wanted "to spend her state of convalescence within the vortex of your kindness and assiduities than elsewhere." The colonel was back in denial. Since the country was in the midst of the War of 1812, he told his in-laws that he had to go to Washington, D.C., for a military appointment and that he would return to Quincy as soon as Congress adjourned. John and Abigail prepared Nabby's room and waited for her arrival. The trip was unimaginably painful—more than three hundred miles in a carriage, over bumpy roads where each jolt stabbed into her. Nabby's son John drove the carriage. When they finally reached Quincy on July 26, she was suffering from grinding, constant pain. Her appearance shocked John and Abigail. She was gaunt and thin, wracked by a deep cough, and her eyes had a moist, rheumy look. She groaned and sometimes screamed with every movement. Huge, dark circles shadowed her cheeks, and a few minutes after she settled into bed, the smell of death fouled the air.

Nabby's pain was so unbearable, and her misery so unmitigated, that Abigail slipped into a depression so deep she could not stand even to visit her daughter's room. It was John Adams who ministered to their dying daughter, feeding her, cleaning her and seeing to her personal needs, combing her hair and holding her hand. He tried to administer painkillers, but nothing seemed to help. Smith returned from Washington, and the deathwatch commenced. On August 9, Nabby's breathing became shallow and the passage of time between breaths lengthened. The family gathered around her bedside. She drew her last breath early in the afternoon.

A few days later, in a letter to Thomas Jefferson, John Adams wrote: "Your Friend, my only Daughter, expired, Yesterday Morning in the Arms of Her Husband, her Son, her Daughter, her Father and Mother, her Husbands two Sisters and two of her Nieces, in the 49th Year of Age, 46 of which She was the healthiest and firmest of Us all: Since which, She has been a monument to Suffering and to Patience." Jefferson understood his friend's pain: "I know the depth of the affliction it has caused, and can sympathize with it the more sensibly, inasmuch as there is no degree of affliction produced by the loss of those dear to us, while experience has not taught me to estimate . . . time and silence are the only medicine, and these but assuage, they never can suppress, the deep drawn sigh which recollection for ever brings up, until recollection and life are extinguished together."[25]

CHAPTER THREE

William Stewart Halsted and the Radical Mastectomy

He was the best surgeon in the world, perhaps the best ever. William Stewart Halsted presided over the Johns Hopkins University surgical staff like a medieval prince, dominating those around him by virtue of intellect, technical skill, and scientific judgment. But Halsted had a secret. One morning in 1908 he was about to enter the surgical theater to operate on a woman with breast cancer. Eager observers filled the tiered rows, edging to the front of their seats in anticipation of watching the master at work. The operation he was about to perform—removal of the breast, axillary lymph nodes, and underlying chest muscles, all in a single, fluid motion—already bore his name, the Halsted radical mastectomy. The female patient was prepped and ready, an anesthetic already sending her deep into unconsciousness. The rest of the medical team surrounded the surgical table and waited for the master.

But Halsted was not feeling well as he scrubbed. Aches and pains, a light sweat, and a small, barely noticeable tremor in his hands afflicted him; he needed a little help before entering the operating suite. A dose of cocaine calmed his nerves. The aches and pains disappeared, the sweat dried on his forehead, and the tremor subsided. He sauntered into the amphitheater, acknowledged the students with the slightest of nods, positioned himself over his patient, and sliced into her chest.

The operation he performed that morning was centuries in the making. Physicians had steadily recommended more and more aggressive surgery, primarily because patients so often had new tumors sprouting on their torsos a few months or a few years after the initial operation. Removing as much tissue as possible seemed to provide the only realistic possibility of preventing recurrence. Jean Louis Petit, the renowned eighteenth-century French surgeon and director of the French Academy in Paris, wrote in the 1740s that "the roots of cancer are the enlarged lymphatic glands; that the glands should be looked for and removed and the pectoral fascia and even some fibres of muscle itself should be dissected away rather than leave any doubtful tissue. The mammary gland too should not be cut into during the operation . . . . [T]here is little hope to expect a perfect cure if they are not both clearly extricated together." In 1848 Benjamin Bell, a surgeon at the Edinburgh Royal Infirmary in Scotland, insisted that "even when only a small portion of the breast is diseased, the whole mamma should be removed. The axillary glands should be dissected by opening up the armpit."[1]

By the mid–nineteenth century, the idea of en bloc surgery—removal of the breast, chest muscles, and axilla lymph nodes in one motion, without even cutting into the tumor—was gaining ground. In 1854 Alfred-Armand Velpeau, the leading surgeon at the University of Paris, urged colleagues to treat breast cancer aggressively, cutting away the breast as well as underlying chest muscles. Glasgow surgeon Joseph Lister performed an en bloc mastectomy on his sister, Isabella Pim, in 1867. It was a qualified success, even though Lister operated on his dining room table. Isabella lived for three more years before dying of a liver metastasis. Charles Hewitt Moore, director of the cancer institute at Middlesex Hospital in England, was even more aggressive, insisting on the en bloc removal of the breast, axillary lymph nodes, underlying chest muscle, and skin, all without ever touching the tumor itself with the scalpel. Anything less, Moore insisted, was "a mistaken kindness to the patient," since the tumor was destined to return with a deadly vengeance.[2]

By the early nineteenth century, most physicians knew that surgery was the only hope, but many shied away because of the risks. Before Halsted could launch the era of the radical mastectomy in the 1890s, three problems had to be solved: how to prevent postsurgical infections, how to anesthetize patients, and how to tell the difference between benign and malignant lesions. Erysipelas, a streptococcus infection, posed the most immediate problem. Surgeons were ignorant of the killer germs they carried on their fingers and instruments. Even the most skilled were as likely to kill patients as save them.

James Syme, surgeon to the queen of Scotland and professor of clinical surgery at the University of Edinburgh, represented state-of-the-art surgery in the early 1800s. But for all of his technical abilities, he operated under filthy conditions. In 1833, for example, an older woman named Allie, with her son James, came to the hospital with a diseased right breast. John Brown, Syme's assistant, examined her and concluded immediately that she was in trouble. "What could I say?" Brown later wrote. "There it was, that had once been so soft, so shapely, so white, so gracious and bountiful, so full of all blessed conditions, [now] hard as a stone, a centre of horrid pain, making that pale face, with its gray, lucid, reasonable eyes and its sweet, resolved mouth, express the full measure of suffering overcome. Why was that gentle, modest, sweet woman, clean and lovable, condemned by God to bear such a burden?" Syme examined the woman the next day and recommended a mastectomy. "She courtesied [sic]," Brown wrote, " . . . and said: 'When?' 'Tomorrow,' said the kind surgeon, a man of few words . . . . The following day, at noon, the students came in, hurrying up the great stair . . . eager to secure good places; in they crowded, full of interest and talk." Syme, wanting to make his patient as comfortable as possible, agreed to let her pet dog Rab accompany her.

The next morning, dozens of medical students gathered in the surgical theater. But when Allie arrived—dressed in a mutch (a loose-fitting cap worn by old women or babies in Scotland), a white gown, a black bombazine petticoat, white worsted stockings, and her carpet-shoes—the medical students fell into respectful silence. Following dutifully behind her was her dog Rab, looking, in Brown's words, "perplexed and dangerous; forever cocking his ear and dropping it as fast." During the operation, Allie kept a stoical silence, but the dog "growled and gave now and then a sharp, impatient yelp; he would have liked to have done something to that man. But James had him firm . . . . It is over; she is dressed, steps gently and decently down from the table . . . then turning to the surgeon and the students, she courtesies, and in a low, clear voice, begs their pardon if she has behaved ill."[3]

It is hard to imagine a modern surgeon performing a mastectomy with the patient's pet dog barking, growling, and lunging at him. Small wonder the death rate was so high. All too often, patients who survived the operation died in a few days or weeks. In 1841, for example, missionary physicians in Hawaii urged Queen Kapiolani, a Christian convert, to undergo a mastectomy for her breast cancer. When the white doctors explained the procedure, Kapiolani hesitated, but they finally changed her mind, telling her to muster the same courage she had used in defying Pele, the volcano goddess, and being baptized. During the operation, the surgeon asked how she was doing, and Kapiolani replied, "It is painful, but I think of Christ who suffered on the cross for me and I am able to bear it." The surgery took thirty minutes, and Kapiolani did not utter a moan. She recovered quickly, but about three days later a red welt appeared on the surgical scar. It became red, tender, and sore, and she started running a very high fever. The missionary doctor recognized erysipelas, but there was nothing he could do. The infection spread, and she died deliriously on May 5, 1841, two weeks after the operation.[4]

At the time of her death, on the other side of the world, medical students at the University of Vienna struggled with the mystery of infection. There were two obstetrical divisions at the university hospital, one where doctors and medical students delivered babies and another staffed by midwives. An average of 3,500 babies were born annually in each division. The physicians' section experienced a twenty percent mortality rate. After delivery, about seven hundred women died of erysipelas—or what they described as childbed or puerperal fever. But in the midwives' domain, only sixty died. Old-timers discussed the discrepancy frequently, only to shrug their shoulders at the mystery. But in 1847 Ignac Semmelweis, a young obstetrician, figured it out. Doctors routinely performed autopsies on the dead, and then, their fingers dripping in cadaver fluids, hustled over to the maternity ward to deliver babies, without washing their hands. Semmelweis guessed that the doctors transferred some invisible ailment from the cadavers to the birthing mothers. He decided to wash his hands in a chlorine solution and instructed others to do the same. In April 1847, the last month hands were not washed, eighteen percent of the mothers died of infection. In May 1847, the infection rate, and the death rate, dropped to only one percent. Semmelweis had given birth to the notion of asepsis.[5]

Although tradition-bound veterans ridiculed hand-washing "obsessions," younger physicians in Vienna, Berlin, Paris, London, and New

Bathsheba's Breast

York converted to clean hands and clean wounds. Joseph Lister, a surgeon at the Glasgow Royal Infirmary, decided that infection occurred when an invisible, external entity—probably some vapor or humor—entered the wound. He had no idea what that entity was until he heard about Louis Pasteur's work in France. Using a microscope to study yeasts fermenting sugar into alcohol, Pasteur spied small microbes at work. When Lister learned of Pasteur's discovery, he concluded that the microbes were the invisible agents he suspected. He started washing his hands, bandages, surgical instruments, and the relevant parts of a surgical patient's body in carbolic acid—antiseptic surgery. Surgical infection rates dropped dramatically, and in 1869 he published his findings in *Lancet,* England's premier medical journal. J. Collins Warren, great-grandson of the physician who operated on Nabby Adams in 1811 and a physician himself, visited Lister in 1869 and came back to Massachusetts General Hospital to perform the first antiseptic mastectomy later in the year.[6]

The advent of aseptic and antiseptic techniques paved the way for more radical procedures. So did anesthesia. For centuries surgeons had faced wide-awake patients; radical surgeries were complicated and highly unpredictable. In 1831, for example, John Warren performed a mastectomy on Nancy Barker, a thirty-three-year-old woman from Maine. "The patient sat in a chair," Warren wrote eight years later. "The right arm was extended, raised above a horizontal line, in order to give tension to the skin, and permit access to the armpit." Warren then put his scalpel to work. "The skin on the surface of the breast, with the diseased nipple, were included in an oval incision. The breast was dissected from the pectoral muscle, and left connected with the axillary glands, while the extirpation of these glands was effected. As they adhered to the great axillary vessels, they were detached by dissection, and by insinuating the finger where the cellular substance was loose."

But the operation then spun out of control. She began to struggle with Warren and, "at the same instant," he remembered, "a bubbling or gurgling noise . . . was heard . . . the posture of the patient was changed, and she was supported by those around. Some brandy was poured down the throat, and ammonia introduced into the nostrils. The pulse, however, became less distinct than before . . . . At this moment, the livid colour of the cheeks gave place to suffusion of vermillion red—and no glow on the cheek of youthful beauty ever gave one so much pleasure as that flush."

But it was to no avail. Her breathing became more shallow and ceased. Warren opened her larynx and inserted a bellows to help her breathe, but after twenty minutes, "there was no remaining hope of the restoration of the patient to life." Her friends, who witnessed the event, did not want him to keep trying to revive her. They were in a hurry. They wanted "to take advantage of a vessel then sailing for their home."[7]

Few surgeons relished a mastectomy. Without anesthesia, patients endured horrible pain, and physicians could never be sure how they would react. More often than not, patients squirmed and grimaced, trying to fend off the scalpel, even while knowing the surgery was necessary. Lorenz Heister, an eighteenth-century German physician, warned surgeons about struggling mastectomy patients. "Many females," he wrote, "can stand the operation with the greatest courage and without hardly moaning at all. Others, however, make such a clamor that they may dishearten even the most undaunted surgeon and hinder the operation. To perform the operation, the surgeon should be steadfast and not allow himself to become discomforted by the cries of the patient." Richard Kay, a contemporary of Heister, had a cooperative patient. He had performed a radical mastectomy on a Mrs. Driver, but she soon had a recurrence and returned to his office, insisting on more surgery. She was "determined," he wrote in his diary, "to undergo a second amputation." It was a big job. Kay remembered that he "took off the Skin . . . I dissected from her . . . five hundred different distinct Schirrous knots or young Cancers."

Not surprisingly, there was a premium on speed. Patients could endure a few moments of pain, but the likelihood of their grimacing, wincing, struggling, and fighting back increased with time. Samuel de Wind, a physician-surgeon in Middleburg, The Netherlands, holds the all-time record for speed. In 1759, he performed a mastectomy on his wife, Berdina Tak. From the time he grasped her breast in a pair of amputation forceps, to the time he placed compresses on the wound, the operation took only two minutes. She died a few weeks later.[8]

Catastrophic results were not unusual. When examining a lesion, late-eighteenth-century physicians took note of the position of the nipple, since tumors beneath could sometimes pull it out of place. They manipulated the tumor with their fingers, trying to determine its hardness as well as the regularity of its surface. Hard, irregular growths were less likely than soft, regular lesions to be benign cysts. They felt for large lymph nodes in the underarm as well as in the neck and clavicle areas. They tried to determine if the tumor was movable, or if it had attached itself to the skin or chest wall. The spread of hard tumors into regional lymph nodes made for a death sentence. Surgeons hated operating on such lesions, not only because the procedures were difficult and time-consuming, but also because the patients eventually died anyway. Hendrik Ulhoorn, an Amsterdam surgeon, remembered the case of Mrs. Jacob Klinge of Zwolle, The Netherlands, in 1741. Suffering from a large tumor which had spread to the underarm lymph nodes and attached itself to the wall of her chest, Klinge insisted on a mastectomy, even though eight surgeons in Amsterdam refused to operate. She finally found a doctor to perform the surgery, but it was a disaster. He cut away the breast but kept encountering more and more tumor, as he carved deeper and deeper into her body, into the lymph nodes under her arm and collarbone, and tried to scrape diseased tissue off the chest wall and dig it out from between her ribs—all this with Klinge fully awake and screaming in pain.[9]

Even under the best of circumstances, pre-anesthesia mastectomies traumatized patients and surgeons alike. Fanny Burney's case is the best known. A native of England, she wrote her first novel, *Evelina*, in 1778; its critical acclaim gained her access to England's most important literary circles. She wrote *Cecelia*, her second novel, in 1786. Burney married Alexandre d'Arblay, a French royalist living in exile in London, and they lived off her royalties. Her novel *Camille* appeared in 1796. In 1802, with Napoleon firmly in power in France, Madame d'Arblay and her husband moved to Paris.

Soon after arriving, she wrote in her diary that she was suffering from "a very strong menace of inflammation upon the breast." In 1806 the condition returned and lingered. The pain became so acute in August 1811 that she went to Antoine DuBois, a prominent Paris physician. DuBois brought Baron Dominique-Jean Larrey, Napoleon's surgeon, in for a consultation, and they both decided that Burney needed a mastectomy. They scheduled the operation for September 30, 1811, in her home. On the morning of the operation, Burney wrote that she "finished my breakfast, not with much appetite, you will believe! Forced down a crust of bread." She spent some time preparing the salon and writing a "few words to M. d'A [Alexandre d'Arblay] in case of a fatal result."

That afternoon, DuBois and Larrey, accompanied by five other physicians, all dressed in black, showed up at her home and ordered her to a bed. "Astonished," she wrote, "I turned to Dr. Larrey who had promised that an arm chair would suffice; but he hung his head and would not look at me. I now began to tremble violently, more with distaste and horror of the preparations than of the pain . . . . I looked at the door, the windows—I felt desperate—but it was only a moment, my reason then took over and my fears and feelings struggled vainly against it." Over Burney's protests, DuBois ordered the nurses and maids from the room, and she lamented, "Ah, then, how did I think of my Sisters!—not one, at so dreadful an instant, at hand to protect . . . and guard me."

The physicians were nervous—DuBois in a state of agitation and Larrey "ashen-faced with tears in his eyes." She climbed onto the bed and the surgery began. Burney wrote that DuBois "placed me upon the mattress and spread a cambric handkerchief upon my face. It was transparent, however, and I saw, throughout it, that the bed was instantly surrounded by seven men . . . . I refused to be held, but when, bright through the cambric, I saw the glitter of polished steel, I closed my eyes . . . . A silence the most profound ensued, which lasted for some minutes . . . . Again through the cambric, I saw DuBois's hand move up, while his finger first described a straight line from top to bottom of the breast, second, a cross, and third, a circle; intimating that the WHOLE was to be taken off." Burney sat up in bed, took off the handkerchief and protested, wondering why the whole breast had to come off when the pain seemed isolated to one spot. DuBois pushed her back down. "Hopeless . . . I closed once more my eyes, relinquishing all watching, all resistance, all interference, and sadly resolute to be wholly resigned."

The cutting began, with Larrey wielding the knife. "When the dreadful steel was plunged into the breast—cutting through veins—arteries—flesh—nerves—I needed no injunctions not to restrain my cries. I began a scream that lasted unintermittingly during the whole time of the incision . . . . When the wound was made and the instrument was withdrawn, the pain seemed undiminished . . . . But when again I felt the instrument—describing a curve—cutting against the grain . . . while the flesh resisted in a manner so forcible as to oppose and tire the hand of the operator, who was forced to change from the right to the left—then, indeed, I must have expired . . . . The instrument this second time withdrawn, I concluded the operation over."

But it was not over. When DuBois and Larrey tried to lift the breast off the chest wall, the tumor adhered to the underlying muscles. She went on in her journal: "Presently the terrible cutting was renewed—and worse than ever, to separate the bottom, the foundation of this dreadful gland from the parts to which it adhered . . . . Oh heaven! I then felt the knife rackling against the breast bone—scraping it! I . . . remained in utterly speechless torture." Larrey asked the other surgeons if the task was completed, but DuBois saw something he did not like, and he redirected. "Again began the scraping," Burney wrote. "And after this, Dr. Moreau thought he discerned a peccant atom—and still and still, DuBois demanded atom after atom . . . the evil was so profound, the case so delicate, and the precautions necessary for preventing a return so numerous, that the operation, including the treatment and the dressing, lasted twenty minutes! A time, for sufferings so acute, that was hardly supportable."

When the operation was finally concluded, the doctors removed the handkerchief from Burney's face. The room looked like wartime surgery, with soiled sheets and bloody bandages everywhere. Burney opened her eyes and surveyed the carnage. "I saw my good Dr. Larrey," she recorded in her journal, "pale nearly as myself, his faced streaked with blood, and its expression depicting grief, apprehension, and almost horror." A few days later, Larrey departed for the eastern front, where Napoleon's troops were fighting Russians. At the Battle of Borodino, he must have set some kind of record. During one twenty-four-hour period, he amputated two hundred legs from wounded French soldiers. Many survived. So did Fanny Burney. The mastectomy was successful; she lived until 1840, dying at the age of eighty-eight.[10]

Such horrors began to end after October 16, 1846, when at Massachusetts General Hospital in Boston, William Thomas Green Morton, using ether, kept a patient unconscious while John C. Warren, a physician and grandson of Nabby Adams's surgeon, removed a facial tumor. Morton, a Boston dentist, used ether to put patients to sleep during extractions. After months of experimenting on dogs and cats, he administered the drug to several patients, putting them under for the one or two minutes it took to take out a bad tooth. Assisting Warren, Morton kept the patient unconscious for nearly thirty minutes, dripping ether periodically into a gauze bandage. Years later, Warren recalled the moment: "A new era has opened on the operating surgeon. His visitations on the most delicate parts are performed, not only without the agonizing screams he has been accustomed to hear, but sometimes in a state of perfect insensibility, and, occasionally, even with an expression of pleasure on the part of the patient."[11]

But the existence of anesthesia and its availability were two very different issues. The technology collided with cultural assumptions about women and pain. Sentimentalists had long celebrated the pain of childbirth as a prerequisite to the development of maternal instincts. One mid-century New York obstetrician concluded, "The very suffering which a woman undergoes in labor is one of the strongest elements in the love she bears for her offspring." Others believed that pain developed a heroic character. Samuel Gregory of the Boston Female Medical College rejected anesthetics because "this suffering one's self to avoid a trifling pain is no mark of prudence or courage." Augustus Gardner, a New York City gynecologist, argued in 1872 that the blessings of pain "are not limited to the mere physical strengthening of other facilities . . . this baptism of pain and privation has regenerated the individual's whole nature . . . by the chastening made but a little lower than the angels." Some prescriptions for female pain bordered on sadism. In 1850 Benjamin Hill, a Boston surgeon, tried to get breast cancer patients to accept cauterizations of their tumors without anesthetics: "I have not unfrequently had patients, after submitting, perhaps for an hour, to this 'burning alive,' without flinching or groaning, open their mouths for the first time, after I had got through, to express their fears that the operation had been not carried far enough, because they had felt it so much less than I had given them reason to expect." Hill went on to extol the virtues of "pain as moral medication."

But even surgeons prepared to use anesthesia could be burdened by a host of prejudices. Most Americans believed that older women were not as subject to pain as younger women because time had diminished their sensitivities. Poor women were considered oblivious to pain. "Country women," argued Dr. William Dewees in 1806, "are more obnoxious to it [pain], than those of the cities." J. Marion Sims, the father of American gynecology, regularly performed experimental operations on slave women because "white women are too sensitive to pain." The *London Medical and Chirugical Review* claimed in 1817 that "negresses will bear cutting with nearly, if not quite, as much impunity as dogs and rabbits." Surgeons often limited anesthesia to well-to-do white women who "needed" to be protected from pain. It was not until the 1890s that most surgeons became willing to use anesthesia on every patient.[12]

The third stage in the development of the Halsted radical mastectomy took place under a microscope. Throughout medical history, unnecessary surgeries were common because physicians could not tell the difference between benign and malignant tumors. They often removed entire breasts to get rid of what were only benign lumps. They were dealing with a bewildering variety of breast diseases, some benign, others malignant, without the benefit of cellular pathology. The most common type of breast cancer is infiltrating ductal carcinoma, found in about seventy percent of breast malignancies. But there are other tumors as well, including papillary carcinomas, infiltrating papillary carcinomas, comedo carcinomas, medullary carcinomas, tubular carcinomas, mucinous or colloid carcinomas, intracystic papillary carcinomas, lobular carcinomas, invasive lobular carcinomas, Paget's disease of the breast, inflammatory breast cancer, adenocystic carcinoma, carcinosarcomas, lipid-rich carcinomas, and metaplastic carcinomas.

Doctors also confronted a range of benign breast diseases, such as lactational mastitis, nonlactational mastitis, chronic subareolar abscesses, intraductal papillomas, intraductal papillomatosis, cytosarcoma phylloides, fibroadenomas, and pseudolumps caused by clumps of dead fat cells, protruding ribs, or simply denser tissues in the breast. The best an early nineteenth century physician could do was look at a tumor and, based on its gross appearance, decide if it was dangerous or not. Prudence and caution forced them, when confused, to decide in favor of malignancy and treat it accordingly. In 1839 John Warren wrote, "All tumours of this organ [breast] are in danger of being considered to be cancers, and treated accordingly . . . every tumour in the breast must be esteemed suspicious, and worthy of careful attention."[13]

Margaret Moffette Lea is a case in point. In 1840, at the age of twenty-two, she married forty-seven-year-old Sam Houston, the hero of Texas independence. Anxious to please his young bride, he surrendered to her teetotaling ways, cutting down on alcohol, much to the surprise of his closest associates. Political duties kept him away for weeks and months at a time, but they nurtured their relationship with daily letters. Their first child, Sam Houston, Jr., was born on May 25, 1843. Before the birth, Margaret Lea, as Texans remember her, complained of tenderness in her right breast, and the condition persisted for several years. In February 1847, while Sam was in Washington, D.C., serving as a U.S. senator, she wrote him a worrisome letter: "I have suffered two or three mails to pass without writing to you for the reason that my breast was in such condition that I could not write without detriment to myself. It has risen three times and the last time presented such an angry appearance that Brother Charles prevailed on us to send for Dr. Smith."

Ashbel Smith, a physician and leading figure in the movement for Texas independence, traveled to East Texas and examined Margaret. He decided not to operate, especially with Sam so far away. The tumor did not resemble other breast cancers Smith had seen, so he recommended a topical treatment and went home. Within days, however, she asked him to return. The tumor had flared up, causing great discomfort. Smith examined her and scheduled surgery for the first week of March, advising her to stop breastfeeding the baby so that she could "dry up the breast." He also assured her that "the operation will be a mere trifle and easily performed in two minutes." Smith left, planning to come back in two weeks for the operation, but Margaret's mother begged him to come back sooner because "we think the cancer is advancing more rapidly than usual."

Smith agreed, bringing whiskey to dull her senses during the operation. A teetotaler and temperance advocate, she refused the alcohol. After a lifetime condemning "demon rum" and eight years getting her husband off the bottle, she was not about to succumb. Crises tested faith, and she would not fail her test. Instead of swallowing the whiskey, she clenched a silver coin between her teeth, closed her eyes, and let Smith amputate much of her right breast. In a letter to Sam written later in the day, Smith said: "It was with some anxiety that I undertook so serious an operation in your absence, but an operation offered the only possible cure and its necessity was urgent. It is useless to mention to you that Mrs. H. bore the pain with great fortitude."

Two weeks later, the wound became infected and Sam, who had arrived home from Washington, wrote to Smith again: "From immediately below the wound, there is diagonally across the stomach, bearing the left side, something like a cord or tendon, which is quite sore, and she is fearful that it may be a root of the Cancer." Another physician treated her and the inflammation soon disappeared. She was cured and lived another twenty years, dying of yellow fever on December 3, 1867, in Independence, Texas.[14]

What Margaret Lea Houston called cancer was probably mastitis, a painful but benign inflammation affecting nursing mothers. The ability to distinguish between benign and malignant diseases, and to perform mastectomies only for malignant tumors, depended on the development of cellular pathology, a scientific discipline that emerged in Germany, just when Ashbel Smith was operating on Margaret. Joseph Jackson Lister, a wine merchant in England, developed a reliable microscope in 1826, and by the 1840s similar instruments were being widely manufactured throughout Europe. German physicians first used microscopes to study normal and pathological tissues.[15]

In 1838 Matthias Jakob Schleiden, a German botanist at the University of Jena, discovered the cellular structure of plant tissues. A year later, in Berlin, Theodore Schwann wrote *Mikroskopische Untersuchungen*, portraying the cell as the basic unit of animal tissues. Johannes Müller, a comparative anatomist in Berlin, argued in 1839 that cells were the building blocks of all living tissues. He also claimed that cytosarcoma phylloides, a large breast tumor which for years had been considered malignant, was benign. Benjamin Brodie, a physician at St. George's Hospital in London, described benign cystic lesions of the breast in 1844 and noted the differences between them and deadly malignancies. With each new tool for distinguishing benign from malignant tissues, surgeons reduced the number of unnecessary mastectomies.[16]

The real founder of cellular pathology, however, was Rudolf Virchow, a Prussian-born student of Johannes Müller. A child prodigy, Virchow was fluent in Latin by the age of twelve. In 1839, he entered the Friedrich-Wilhelms Institute of the University of Berlin, where Müller introduced students to the wonders of cellular pathology. While other students suffered under a rigid curriculum that kept them in class sixty hours a week and in the laboratory and library the rest of the time, Virchow's intellect left him time to study medicine, French, Italian, Greek, Hebrew, Arabic, archaeology, and politics. He wrote home to his father that all he wanted to do was acquire "a universal knowledge of nature from the Godhead down to the stone." Müller quickly recognized Virchow's talent.

Virchow soon surpassed his mentor. He received the M.D. in 1843 and then interned at the Charite Hospital in Berlin. The young physician discovered leukemia in 1845 and described the nature of thrombosis in 1846. In 1847, he founded *Virchows Archiv*, a pathology journal still being published. In his laboratory, modern pathology was born, sending to the scrap heap of history all earlier theories about the nature of disease. He argued that all cells grow from similar cells, that all living tissues have a single cellular ancestor in the ooze of the primordial past. He studied the cellular physiology of normal and abnormal tissues. Disease, he concluded, was the result of cellular disorders—biochemical malfunctions within cells that could only be cured biochemically by restoring the cells to normal or eradicating them altogether.

Virchow spent the rest of his life expanding the frontiers of cellular pathology. He explained the nature of carcinomas—tumors erupting in a bed of epithelial tissues—and malignant sarcomas of bone and connective tissues. Inside the membranes of cancer cells, he analyzed the disheveled nuclei until he could distinguish one type of tissue from another and one type of cancer from another. He took note of cellular differentiation and the wild, unbridled multiplication of malignant cells, their penchant to grow and expand. When Virchow died in 1902, surgeons had more reliable techniques for distinguishing benign lesions from malignant ones and, in terms of breast diseases, the ability to make rational choices about mastectomies.[17]

Asepsis, anesthesia, and cellular pathology made radical mastectomies possible. William Stewart Halsted made it a reality. He was born on September 23, 1852. His roots reached back to Long Island's Puritan aristocracy, but the family fortune was all nineteenth century, the product of a successful importing business. He enjoyed a privileged childhood in a luxurious townhouse on 14th Street and Fifth Avenue in Manhattan and a country estate in Irvington, New York. He attended Andover and Yale, where he "majored" in football, baseball, crew, and parties, managing to graduate without crossing the library doorsill. In 1874, after a dissipating summer at the beach, Halsted enrolled as a medical student at the College of Physicians and Surgeons in New York City. His father was a member of the board of directors.[18]

Halsted surprised everybody. He proved to be an ideal student, winning honors in clinics and in basic sciences. He interned at Bellevue Hospital and worked for several months as house physician at the New York

Hospital. Like Benjamin Rush a century before, he embarked on a European tour, but instead of spending two years in London and Paris, Halsted traveled farther east—to Vienna, Leipzig, and Berlin—where Germans had elevated medicine to new heights. He studied anatomy and surgical technique under Theodor Billroth, the father of modern surgery, and cellular pathology under associates of Rudolf Virchow. He also observed Richard Volkmann, the talented surgeon at the University of Leipzig, who in 1865 argued that in cases of breast cancer, surgeons were obligated to remove the fibrous covering of the chest muscles in order to minimize recurrence. Halsted returned to New York in 1880 as visiting physician to Charity Hospital, and within a few years he was also on the staffs of Bellevue, Presbyterian, New York State Emigrant, and Chambers Street hospitals.

During the mid-1880s, Halsted earned a reputation as the country's most gifted surgeon. A proponent of aseptic techniques, he insisted, fanatically some colleagues thought, on a germ-free surgical environment, even going so far as building at Bellevue his own operating room under a tent outdoors because he found the surgical suites filthy. He pioneered the use of rubber gloves to protect patients and surgeons alike, and he was the first surgeon to transfuse blood and to employ intravenous infusions of salt solutions. He wrote dozens of articles for scientific journals and began the systematic training of surgeons that eventually evolved into today's residency system.

At the same time, he became a drug addict. Early in the 1880s, several German physicians began experimenting with cocaine as a surgical anesthetic, and Halsted took up the pursuit, trying to find ways of using the drug as a general anesthetic and as a local to block major nerve trunks. Along with several colleagues, he toyed with the drug personally, enjoying its exhilarating effects though innocent of its addictive powers. His behavior soon became erratic. He missed work for days and sometimes weeks, appeared late for operations, gave rambling lectures, mumbled to himself, and wrote articles with hopelessly confused syntax. Colleagues passed off his behavior as the idiosyncrasies of genius, but he suffered a complete breakdown in 1886, one even they could not conceal. When a friend arranged for Halsted to take a long vacation cruise, the good doctor took along his own supply of cocaine. When it ran out with two weeks left at sea, he broke into the ship's pharmacy to get more.

Halsted knew he was in trouble, and he checked himself into Butler Hospital, a psychiatric facility in Providence, Rhode Island. After several months there, he accepted a faculty position at the Johns Hopkins University Medical School. In November 1886 he moved to Baltimore, but within a few weeks he was back on cocaine. Halsted returned to Butler in April 1887 and remained there until January 1888. He succeeded in weaning himself away from the narcotic, but the cure was expensive. He replaced one drug with another, and Halsted never got the monkey off his back. Still, he managed the addiction well. During the next thirty years, he became the leading surgeon in the world, pioneering a whole range of new techniques. The pre-anesthesia surgery of the past, based so much on speed of movement, gave way to deliberate precision in which the surgeon excised diseased tissue so that normal physiological processes could be restored. During his years at Charity, he experimented with breast cancer and, over the course of the next fifteen years, developed what became known as the Halsted radical mastectomy, an operation that dominated breast cancer treatment for two generations.

Early in the 1880s, when he was still working in New York, he searched for a way to reduce the recurrences of the disease which so commonly afflicted patients within a year of their initial surgery. During his stay in Europe, Halsted learned that Theodor Billroth's mastectomy patients had an 82 percent chance of developing new tumors on their chest walls. Richard von Volkmann, who routinely excised the fascia of the chest muscles along with the breast and the axilla, enjoyed more success, with "only" 60 percent of his patients suffering recurrence. Halsted wanted to improve on those rates.

It was not a simple challenge. Women usually did not visit physicians in the early stages of the disease. They procrastinated, hoping that the lump was not a cancer, that they there not destined for a horrible death. What Halsted and other surgeons encountered was advanced, inoperable disease. In 1905, for example, he examined a woman whose tumor measured eight by seven centimeters, quite large by contemporary standards, but Halsted described it as a "*small* [author's emphasis] infiltrating scirrhus with metastases to the axilla." Most breast cancer patients showed up with larger tumors, and their surgeons had told them to go home to die, that there was nothing to be done. But Halsted wanted to help even advanced breast cancer patients.[19]

Bathsheba's Breast

In 1890 he wrote, "About eight years ago I began not only to typically clean out the axilla in all cases of cancer of the breast but also to excise in almost every case the pectoralis major muscle . . . and to give the tumor on all sides an exceedingly wide berth." Halsted felt he had no choice, since "it is impossible to determine with the naked eye whether or not the disease has extended into the pectoral muscle." Across town, at New York Hospital, Willie Meyer was moving in the same direction. In 1894 he published his own clinical experience: "In the great majority of cases of cancer of the breast the pectoralis muscle is also involved by the disease, and that, if left in place, the growth is more liable to recur, it has become . . . the duty of the surgeon always to remove this muscle with the breast and the axillary contents."[20]

But removing the breast, axilla, and pectoralis muscle was not enough for Halsted. He knew that cancer was a cellular disease, and he worried about his own role in spreading it. A careless surgeon who cut into the tumor with the scalpel, lifted the breast away with his hands, then moved into the axilla and scooped out lymph nodes with his fingers probably scattered tumor cells all over. Instead, Halsted called for a radical mastectomy—removal of the breast, axillary nodes, and both chest muscles—in a single en bloc procedure. The surgeon cut widely around the tumor, removing all the tissue in one piece, making sure that the "glands and fat should not be pulled out with the finger, as advised, I am sorry to say, in modern textbooks and as practiced very often by operators."[21]

He reported the results of his own radical mastectomies regularly at medical conferences and in professional journals during the 1890s and 1900s and became a medical celebrity. He offered an alternative, a choice, a possibility for breast cancer patients in a surgical world bereft of hope. Before Halsted, the recurrence rate of the breast cancer in the vicinity of the original tumor was so great that in spite of the surgery, women usually underwent brutally painful deaths, succumbing to their cancers as Anne of Austria had done two centuries before, with huge, draining, ulcerative tumors pocking the torso, neck, and armpit. In an 1894 article, Halsted reported, "Most of us have heard our teachers in surgery admit that they have never cured a cancer of the breast . . . . We rarely meet [even today] a physician or surgeon who can testify to a single instance of a positive cure of breast cancer."[22]

Halsted offered patients and surgeons the possibility of a cure, or if

William Stewart Halsted and the Radical Mastectomy   61

not a cure, at least palliative treatment in which patients never suffered through raging damages of untreated breast cancer. The cancer spread to internal organs or bones, eventually taking the patient's life, but death from breast carcinoma, after a successful Halsted mastectomy, was not the horror it had been for so many centuries. He presented a paper at the 1898 meeting in New Orleans of the American Surgical Association, reporting on a series of 133 patients. Of them, seventy-six were more than three years out from the initial surgery, and 52 percent were disease-free, with no sign of tumors in the chest area or symptoms of systemic disease. For the assembled surgeons, the report was breathtaking, particularly since so many of his patients had initially sought treatment with advanced tumors. When Halsted finished, a panel member stood up and made sure the audience realized the significance of what they had just heard: "In Dr. Halsted's series are included cases once regarded as absolutely unfit for operation, and even in these [cases] lives have been prolonged by surgical interference and rendered more comfortable. Best of all, in some very serious cases the disease has not returned after a lapse of years. [Halsted] deserves and has our grateful acknowledgments for the brilliant light which he has thrown upon these dark places of surgery."[23]

During the next two decades, Halsted performed hundreds of radical mastectomies, and his students and colleagues in the surgical establishment did tens of thousands more. In the process, he learned more about the behavior of the disease. He continued to accumulate data on the efficacy of the operation and on the results of 210 radical mastectomies he had performed. The database was now large enough for Halsted to attempt to determine the seriousness of a tumor—"staging" it—and make a prognosis. The article's title proclaimed hope—"The Results of Radical Operations for the Cure of Carcinoma of the Breast." Of the 210 women he treated, sixty of them, when they first presented themselves, had breast carcinomas without lymph node involvement. More than 85 percent were still alive three years later. For women with positive lymph nodes, the prognosis was not nearly so good. Of those 110 women, only thirty-one percent survived for three years. It was even worse for the forty patients with metastasis to the supraclavicular lymph nodes. Only 10 percent had a three-year survival rate. Halsted's conclusion was simple and clear: women who received a radical mastectomy before the tumor spread

Bathsheba's Breast

to regional lymph nodes had excellent odds. Women who delayed treatment were doomed.[24]

In fact, what Halsted recommended soon materialized in Baltimore. Word spread that a woman with breast cancer who received the Halsted operation had a chance to be cured. In the 1880s and 1890s, when he pioneered the operation, Halsted saw only advanced breast cancer patients. All fifty of the women in his original 1894 study suffered from advanced tumors with lymph node involvement. By 1907, Halsted reported, "Women are now presenting themselves more promptly for examination, realizing that a cure of breast cancer is not only possible, but if operated upon early, quite probable. Hence, the surgeon is seeing smaller, still smaller tumors, cancers which give not one of the cardinal signs." He even ventured a prognosis for breast cancer patients: "The prognosis is quite good in the early stage of breast cancer, two in three being cured, and bad, three in four succumbing, when the axillary glands are demonstrably involved."[25]

While Halsted developed the radical mastectomy, American medicine was finishing a virtual revolution in gender relationships. At the beginning of the nineteenth century, treatment for most ailments was largely the domain of women, because the family was the center of social and economic life. In an essentially domestic economy, women assumed responsibility for the care of the sick, and they drew on networks of other women and a reservoir of medicinal herbs and folk traditions. Midwives and homeopaths dominated the medicine of the common people. Sick women were usually treated by women healers. Professional medicine existed in urban centers, but its impact was confined to an elite few.

But as the century progressed and the Industrial Revolution destroyed the traditional domestic economy, the distance between domestic and professional medicine widened. Medicine relied more and more on rigorous scientific knowledge, and the training of physicians became institutionalized. Like law and theology, medicine became a profession. Law schools and seminaries had long been closed to women, and professional medicine imposed similar restrictions. Not allowed to go to college, except to train as teachers, or to pursue postgraduate professional training, women disappeared from the ranks of physicians. Even when they managed to beat the odds and secure formal training, professional medical societies denied them membership. Medicine became the exclusive domain of men.

Sick women were now treated by men. They were also increasingly treated by men they did not know, especially if they suffered from breast cancer. At Johns Hopkins University, and at a number of other university medical centers, female cancer patients were referred to male surgeons anxious to push the survival envelope a little more each year. Academic surgeons were also scientists bent on proving the efficacy of treatments, and progress became synonymous with longer survival time. The university setting depersonalized medicine. Women with breast cancer became scientific objects as well as patients, subject to the whims of male physicians afflicted with gender biases and scientific detachment. The rise of radical surgery in the late nineteenth century rested on the twin pillars of male dominance and scientific objectivity.[26]

CHAPTER FOUR

Superradicals and
the Medicine of Mutilation

The doctor fidgeted uncomfortably. He was about to break bad news to a prominent patient. In 1891 Alexander Clark sat at the pinnacle of his profession, monitoring the health of William Ewart Gladstone, leader of the Liberal Party and former prime minister of Great Britain. British doctors hailed Clark as one of the best, and London's elite approached him regularly with their aches and pains. Alice James, who lived in a London town home, was one of them. She had ignored the lump in her breast for months, but when it finally caused some pain, friends urged her to consult Clark. He arrived at her bedside within hours of receiving the message. It did not take more than a glance and a few probes of the breast and the armpit to confirm, in his own mind, the horror she was about to face.

After covering the diseased breast with her nightgown, Clark stuttered briefly, cleared his throat, and cautiously told Alice James that she suffered from inoperable, terminal breast cancer. But she then surprised him. She did not gasp at the news, or cry, whimper, scream, or yell. She was neither stoical nor cynical. Instead, the prospects of dying from breast cancer flooded her with waves of sweet relief, washing away a lifetime of self-doubt and frustration. Clark had delivered death sentences many times before, but her sigh of thanksgiving caught him off-guard; she shook his hand, graciously thanking him for the report.

She was a curious woman, the younger sister of America's most brilliant intellectuals—psychologist William James and novelist Henry James. Gender had doomed her intellect to obscurity. She was analytically brilliant, politically radical, hilariously funny, and frustrated because society never let her talents flower like those of her brothers. She spent a lifetime fighting a depression that masqueraded as neurasthenia, neuralgia, spinal neurosis, and hysteria, the vague, ill-defined women's diseases of the nineteenth century. Her father showered the boys with time and attention, nurturing their intellects, praising their early forays into literary criticism, and investing much time, money, and energy to make their triumphs possible.

He all but ignored Alice. Henry James loved and trivialized Alice. He expected her to marry well—perhaps a New England industrialist or a merchant—raise a family, and disappear into history as a footnote to her siblings. Sickness became her revenge. From the time she was a little girl, she repeatedly "took to her bed," periodically knocking at death's door only to rally again, leaving family members frustrated even while they worried and doted over her. Only in sickness could she attract her father's attention.

And now, at the age of fifty, she really was sick. After a lifetime of being sick without knowing why, Alice James exulted in the diagnosis. In her diary, she wrote: "Ever since I have been ill, I have longed for some palpable disease, no matter how conventionally dreadful a label it might have . . . . To any one who has not been there, it will be hard to understand the enormous relief of Sir A. C.'s uncompromising verdict, lifting us out of the formless vague . . . . One would naturally not choose such an ugly and gruesome method of progression down the dark Valley of the Shadow of Death, and of course many of the moral sinews will snap by the way, but we shall gird up our loins and the blessed peace of the end will have no shadow cast upon it."

Gird them up she did. Clark supplied her with enough opium to dull the pain, and Alice faced death with aplomb, welcoming a real battle with a real enemy, relishing the chance to experience something her brothers had never felt. Late in 1891 she wrote to William: "I count it as the greatest good fortune to have these few months so full of interest and instruction in the knowledge of my approaching death. It is as simple in one's own person as any fact of nature, the fall of a leaf or the blooming of a rose, and I have a delicious consciousness, ever present, of wide spaces close at hand, and whisperings of release in the air." She fought the good fight. The tumor spread to her liver and lungs, and she died on March 4, 1892. Henry was at her side. "Her face," he recorded in his journal, then seemed "in a strange, dim, touching way, to become clearer. I went to the window to let in a little more of the afternoon light . . . and when I came back to the bed she had drawn the breath that was not succeeded by another."[1]

Had she been at Johns Hopkins that year, Halsted would have operated. Had she come down with the tumor ten years later, in 1902, a British surgeon would have performed the operation. The radical mastectomy would not have saved her life, but it might have bought more time and made her demise more comfortable. During the first four decades of the twentieth century, the radical mastectomy dominated breast cancer treatment. The operation had extended life and cured many, and its palliative effects for those who did not survive were considerable. By 1920, nearly thirty years after Halsted pioneered the technique, cure rates held steady. Of the women who came to Johns Hopkins for breast cancer treatment, approximately one-third had Stage I disease—breast tumors but no spread to the axilla lymph nodes. Nearly 85 percent of them were alive five years after the operation. Half of the women Halsted examined already had tumor involvement in the axilla. Of those, only a third survived for five years. Finally, one out of six of Halsted's patients had tumors in the axilla and in the supraclavicular nodes near the neck. Their five-year survival rate was only 10 percent.

The radical mastectomy, however, was not an unmixed blessing. Even in the hands of such skilled surgeons as Halsted, some patients did not survive the operation. The rate of surgical mortality steadily declined during the early 1900s, but the risks were still quite real. Some women opted for a few more years of life rather than taking a chance on the surgery. Others avoided the radical mastectomy because the operation would leave them permanently wounded and disfigured, with side effects that lasted a lifetime. After the operation, women had to deal with a deformed chest wall, hollow voids under the collarbone and in the armpit, chronic pain, and lymphedema, or swelling in the arm because the removed underarm lymph nodes could no longer process circulatory fluids efficiently. More than a few women concluded that the cure was worse than the disease.

Still, the Halsted mastectomy altered the medical landscape, giving women a ray of hope and inspiring a new public health movement—the crusade for early detection. In 1904, E. S. Judd of the Mayo Clinic wrote, "The point I wish to emphasize . . . is that the surgeon can provide a definite cure in the majority of cases where the patients present themselves for treatment on the appearance of the first symptoms."[2]

The American Society for the Control of Cancer (ASCC), forerunner of the American Cancer Society, directed the public health campaign to convince women to see their doctors about any breast lumps. Founded in 1913 to educate the public, the ASCC was dominated by surgeons who promoted, with the zeal of Bible-belt circuit riders, the conviction that only in the scalpel could women find relief. One ASCC pamphlet preached the following message: "How a wise woman won the battle against cancer. She had faith in her physician. He had confidence in his power. Lose no time . . . Medical cancer cures are bogus. Barring the use of radium or similar means for the small affairs of the skin, surgical operation is the only cure for cancer."[3]

Established cancer therapy had become the domain of surgeons, since no other therapies worked. Samuel Hopkins Adams, a prominent muckraking journalist for the New York *Sun* and *McClure's Magazine* who exposed the patent medicine business, wrote in 1913, "No cancer is hopeless when discovered early. Most cancer, discovered early, is curable. The only cure is the knife." ASCC waxed even more eloquent, telling women that "in regard to tumors . . . lynch law is by far the better procedure than 'due process.'" The analogy was disturbingly accurate, given the direction breast cancer would take in the next several decades.[4]

By the 1920s, the ASCC campaign for early detection and surgery, as well as more systematic training of surgeons in medical schools around the world, dramatically affected breast cancer treatment. Because of the spread of surgical residencies as postgraduate training, which Halsted had pioneered at Johns Hopkins, young physicians in teaching hospitals throughout the United States and Europe learned how to perform the radical mastectomy. The number of breast operations steadily increased between 1905 and 1925. In 1927, the *Journal of the American Medical Association,* in a special study of cancer treatment in nineteen American cities, revealed that operations for breast cancer outnumbered all other cancer surgeries by four to one. Approximately fourteen thousand women died of breast cancer in the United States in 1925, but there were more than twenty thousand breast cancer operations that year. Some were second and third operations for local recurrences, and others were lumpectomies to remove benign tumors. The development of frozen tissue slides in the early 1900s allowed surgeons to remove suspicious lumps, have pathologists evaluate the tissue immediately, and decide then and there whether to perform a radical mastectomy or just remove the benign lump, giving rise to the new subdiscipline of surgical pathology. The Halsted mastectomy became the most common major surgical procedure in the world.[5]

Improving on Halsted soon inspired the best surgeons. In spite of their technical skills and creative innovations, however, they all functioned within a fixed intellectual paradigm. Three ideas dominated the medical consensus. Ever since the 1760s, scientists had been fanatically loyal to the notion that cancer was a local disorder which, if caught and eradicated in time, could be cured. In 1907 Halsted made clear his intellectual commitment to that notion: "Though the area of the disease extends from cranium to knee, breast cancer in the broad sense is a local affliction." Pathologists reinforced prevailing assumptions by identifying tumors according to their origins in different organs of the body. Anatomists argued that tumors remained confined to a local site for an extended period of time, during which surgeons could eradicate them. But if tumors went untreated for too long, malignant cells eventually, at a rather precise moment, disengaged from the tumor and spread in a centrifugal pattern away from the original site, becoming regional in their destructiveness rather than local. Finally, physicians accepted Rudolf Virchow's theory about the metastasis, or spread, of tumors to distant locations. In 1863, he wrote that the lymph nodes act as filters, serving as a barrier to the dissemination of tumor cells throughout the body. By dissecting infiltrated lymph nodes, surgeons could prevent the spread of the disease to distant locations.[6]

In 1906, William Handley, Hunterian Professor of Surgery and Pathology at the Royal College of Surgeons in London, provided a theory of tumor metastasis that explained Halsted's success. Ever since leaving medical school, Handley had combined surgery and pathology, with breast cancer his speciality. He spent his days in surgical theaters, pathology labs, and autopsy rooms, operating on living women, studying the cellular structures of their tumors, and then bringing all of his forensic skills to bear on their cadavers during postmortem examinations. Tumor recurrence and tumor metastasis intrigued him.

Physicians had speculated for centuries about metastasis—how and why cancer spreads from its original site to distant locations—but even into the early twentieth century, no consensus emerged. Ancients believed that black bile spawned systemic tumors, and even when the humoral theory gave way to cellular pathology, its remnants survived. As late as 1900, Rudolf Virchow believed that tumors emitted "morbid juices" which spread through the bloodstream, infected a new site, and erupted into a secondary tumor. He did not believe that individual cells migrated and evolved into new tumors. Joseph Coats, on the other hand, was convinced that tumor cells moved through the bloodstream and lymphatic system. A physician in Glasgow in the late 1800s, Coats viewed each cancer cell as a potential new tumor if it managed to relocate. At the same time, Julius Cohnheim, a student of Virchow and a pathologist at the University of Leipzig, argued that tumors originated in immature embryonic cells that had been left behind in tissues, and that metastatic tumors had colonized new locations through the circulatory system.[7]

Handley had his own ideas about metastasis. In 1906 he wrote *Cancer of the Breast and Its Operative Treatment,* providing cancer specialists with a scientific rationale for aggressive surgery. He proposed a "cancer permeation" hypothesis—cancer spreads in a centrifugal pattern, along the plane of deep fascia tissues beneath the skin and along lymphatic vessels. Metastasis is a physically contiguous process, expanding from one cell to another, outward from the original tumor. If, for example, breast cancer spreads to the brain, it does so contiguously via the meningeal artery. If it makes its way to organs of the abdominal cavity, it does so by permeating the rectus sheath. If tumor becomes deposited in the bones of the spine or pelvis, it did so by physically extending itself through various tissue levels. Cancer does not, he claimed, except in the rarest of circumstances, spread through the bloodstream. Handley's theory became gospel in the new field of oncology. And for the next seventy-five years, most physicians incorrectly assumed that cancer was a local, not a systemic disease.[8]

Handley provided a generation of surgeons with a scientific rationale consistent with the surgery they were already performing. Tumor spread, as far as Halsted was concerned, was "a definite more or less interrupted or quite uninterrupted connection between the original focus and all the outlying deposits of cancer . . . the centrifugal spread annexing by continuity—a very large area in some cases." In 1907, when he first read Handley's book, Halsted bought the theory immediately. "Although it undoubtedly occurs, I am not sure that I have observed . . . metastasis which seemed definitely to have been conveyed by way of the blood-vessels; and my views as to the dissemination of carcinoma of the breast accord so fully with Handley's that I may, in justice to him . . . quote now and again from his admirable chapters."[9]

More radical surgery was the logical extension of Handley's theory. Inadequate surgery explained recurrences after a mastectomy; tumor cells had already expanded beyond the tissues removed in the original mastectomy. To prevent such recurrences, surgeons must be more extensive, removing as much tissue as possible. Halsted urged surgeons to be more aggressive:

> We must remove not only a very large amount of skin and a much larger area of subcutaneous fat and fascia, but also strip the sheaths from the upper part of the rectus, the serratus magnus, the subscapularis, and at times from parts of the latissimus dorsi and the teres major. Both pectoral muscles are, of course, removed. A part of the chest wall should, I believe, be excised in certain cases, the surgeon bearing in mind always that he is dealing with lymphatic and not blood metastases and that the slightest inattention to detail, or attempts to hasten convalescence by such plastic operations as are feasible only when a restricted amount of skin is removed, may sacrifice his patient.

In autopsies, pathologists found that the tumors had spread to other lymph nodes besides the axilla—to the supraclavicular nodes under the collarbone and to the internal mammary nodes under the breasts and inside the chest cavity. If surgeons removed all tumor cells in the vicinity before they had spread, so the logic went, cures were possible. Because of their convictions that breast cancer was local, physicians pondered surgical procedures even more aggressive than Halsted's. Anesthesia, asepsis, antisepsis, and blood transfusions provided the luxury of considering more extensive operations. The only way to stop breast cancer from recurring and spreading, they concluded, was to remove even more tissue during the initial surgery.[10]

Halsted was one of the first to try. By the late 1890s, he was already experimenting with an operation that removed the breast, axilla nodes, chest muscles, and supraclavicular nodes in one procedure. Although he worried about long-term side effects—poor lymphatic drainage and accompanying swelling of the arm and torso, limited range of motion for the arm and neck, and the cosmetic problems of a virtually concave chest wall—he dismissed them as necessary evils. "After all, disability," he wrote in 1891, "is a matter of very little importance as compared with the life of the patient. Furthermore, these patients are old. Their average age is nearly fifty-five years. They are no longer very active members of society." Although he did not pursue the idea, he gave some thought to a shoulder amputation along with the radical mastectomy. "It must be our endeavor," he wrote, "to trace more definitely the routes traveled in the metastases to bone, particularly to the humerus, for it is even possible . . . that amputation of the shoulder joint plus a proper removal of the soft parts might eradicate the disease." Amsterdam surgeon C. W. G. Westerman did in 1910 what Halsted only contemplated, performing a radical mastectomy, cutting out three ribs, and then amputating a woman's shoulder near her neck, pulling out many of the supraclavicular nodes with portions of the rib cage and collarbone.[11]

But such experiments were just that until the late 1920s and 1930s. Halsted eventually abandoned dissections of the supraclavicular and internal mammary lymph nodes, confining his breast surgeries to the classic operation he had pioneered. Being more aggressive was easier said than done. The development of cellular pathology, anesthesia, and antiseptic medicine permitted more aggressive operations and transformed surgery into the only curative treatment for cancer. No longer burdened by the physical struggle of agitated, pain-wracked, wide-awake patients, Halsted created a science out of surgery. But moving surgery beyond Halsted required new scientific and technological developments, the modern equivalents of the nineteenth-century advances. When surgeons in the 1920s and 1930s performed massive, complicated operations, they encountered two insurmountable problems: serious blood loss and severe infection. Mortality rates were too high to justify the operations.

Both problems were solved by the late 1940s. In extensive surgical procedures which consumed several hours and involved cutting through large amounts of tissue, blood loss was usually severe. Patients could be sent into shock or suffer brain damage from lack of oxygen. The problem

Bathsheba's Breast

was daunting enough to make even the most aggressive surgeons conservative. Experiments in blood transfusion had been going on for centuries, but clotting and rejection were all too common. In 1900, however, Karl Landsteiner of the University of Vienna discovered the basic blood groups and established criteria for typing them. Patients could be matched for type and receive blood their bodies would accept. The solution to the clotting problem appeared in 1915 when Richard Lewison, a New York surgeon, discovered that sodium citrate retarded clotting. By 1917, Allied army surgeons, using sodium citrate as an anticoagulant, regularly transfused wounded soldiers during surgery. Finally, Oswold Robertson, a Canadian army physician, developed the technique of adding glucose to donated blood and storing it in a cold "blood bank," providing surgeons with a reliable blood supply. In 1937, during the Spanish Civil War, cold-stored blood was used widely for the first time in surgical transfusions. Able to overcome the effects of blood loss, surgeons contemplated more aggressive procedures.[12]

But even the most careful surgeon, practicing aseptic and antiseptic techniques and enjoying modern blood transfusion techniques, often shied away from massive procedures involving the removal of large amounts of tissue because of the threat of infection. The wider the surgical field and the longer the procedure took, the higher the odds of postoperative infection. The discovery of antibiotics solved the problem. In September 1928, Alexander Fleming was a bacteriologist at St. Mary's Hospital in London studying the staphylococcus bacterium. One evening, his assistant filled several petri dishes with a staphylococci-loaded broth and incubated them at body temperature. Fleming had instructed lab assistants to keep the dishes covered to avoid contamination, but one forgot that evening and left a dish uncovered. During the night an airborne fungus infected it. The next morning, Fleming noticed that the staph germs flourished in all the covered dishes, but the uncovered petri dish sprouted a fungus but no staph germs. The fungus had killed them. For several weeks, he tested the fungus against other germs—streptococci, gonococci, diphtheria, bacilli, tetanus, anthrax, actinomycetes, and syphilis—and found it equally effective. He had discovered penicillin, and over the course of the next fifteen years bacteriologists perfected other antibiotics. Liberated from the risks of infection and hemorrhage shock, surgeons were ready to launch the era of the superradicals.[13]

Younger surgeons assumed the challenge of improving on Halsted. They had long chafed at the lack of progress in improving long-term outcomes. By the end of World War II, a half century had passed since Halsted perfected the radical mastectomy, with the master himself in his grave for a generation. Yet even the best surgeons still relied on his procedures, and survival rates held steady. The Mayo Clinic proudly announced in 1957 that the overall five-year survival rate for all of its 1947 and 1948 radical mastectomy patients was 61 percent. Most surgeons, however, knew that breast cancer patients could not really feel safe for ten years, and when ten-year periods were analyzed, the cure rate fell to not much above where it had been when Halsted worked the surgical theaters at Johns Hopkins. Mayo emphasized that all patients survived the operation; operative mortality had become virtually nonexistent.[14]

A few of the best and most aggressive surgeons, hoping to improve survival rates, decided to push the Halsted-Handley logic to its limits. At the University of Copenhagen in the 1930s, Erling Dahl-Iversen experimented with extrapleural dissections of the internal mammary lymph nodes, as did Mario Margottini in Rome and S. A. Kholdin in Moscow. At the University of Minnesota, Owen Wagensteen performed radical mastectomies that included removal of the supraclavicular and mediastinal nodes. The Wagensteen approach involved a typical Halsted radical mastectomy, then splitting the patient's sternum and moving into the chest cavity to scoop out the internal mammary nodes and supraclavicular nodes. Before operating on women, Wagensteen biopsied their regional lymph nodes to make sure there was no tumor spread there. He eventually performed hundreds of the surgeries, but his operative mortality was very high—more than thirteen percent. Critics would later charge Wagensteen with recklessness—taking women with small breast tumors and no lymph node spread, and then killing nearly one out of seven in the operating room. Many argued about the cost of progress.[15]

Although the discovery of antibiotics and the development of new methods for transfusing blood made more radical surgery possible, the intellectual climate of World War II and the postwar years made it far more likely. A generation of young surgeons, trained in the United States medical schools but tested in the mobile field hospitals of Europe and the Pacific, found themselves employing extraordinary surgical techniques to treat horrific battlefield wounds and, astonishingly, seeing many soldiers survive. Faith in the efficacy of surgery deepened. At the same time, a consensus emerged about the future of science and technology. The success of the Manhattan Project—the crash U.S. government program to develop an atomic bomb—convinced most Americans that scientists, physicians, and surgeons could tackle any medical challenge. The late 1940s and 1950s witnessed the advent of superradical surgical procedures to treat cancer, including total gastrectomies, which removed the stomach, spleen, and pancreas, en bloc, and then connected the small intestine to the esophagus; interscapulothoracic amputations, which removed a patient's arm, shoulder blade, and collarbone; hemipelvectomies, which took off a leg and the attached pelvic bone; and semicorporectomies, which took off the lower half of the body.

In the world of breast cancer, the superradical mastectomy appeared, and its chief architect was Jerome Andrew Urban. A surgical oncologist in the best sense of the word, Urban possessed the physical skills and coordination of a gifted athlete, but he was not, like so many surgeons of the past, just a journeyman meatcutter. A keen, scientific intellect drove his work. Born in Brooklyn in 1914, Urban took a bachelor's degree at Andrew College and his M.D. at Columbia. After interning at Lenox Hill Hospital in New York City, he did a residency in surgical oncology during World War II at Memorial Sloan-Kettering, just when the hospital was acquiring its reputation as the best cancer center in the world. Urban studied there under the tutelage of George T. Pack, the most radical of the radical surgeons, a man whose ego, surgical technique, and fearlessness earned him the nickname "Pack the Knife." Pack performed interscapulothoracic amputations and hemipelvectomies like other surgeons did appendectomies and tonsillectomies. His self-confidence was matched only by his speed, and his commitment to excising every cancer cell knew no bounds. Urban took his surgical cue from Pack but specialized in breast cancer.

A half-century had passed since Halsted first announced the radical mastectomy, and breast cancer survival rates had improved. Women were more likely to visit a physician in the early stages of their illness, when tumors were small and more confined; the radical mastectomy reduced local recurrence rates and increased long-term survival. But for Jerome Urban, a half century was too long. It was time to replace Halsted and lift surgical oncology to a new level.

In 1949, he pioneered a new mastectomy. Like Halsted before him, Urban functioned in the intellectual shadow of William Handley. Handley's son, R. S. Handley, extended his father's logic, showing in 1949 that for women with tumors in the medial portion of the breast, a strong likelihood exists that tumors will metastasize to the axilla lymph nodes and to the internal mammary nodes behind the sternum and rib cage. The only way to improve survival rates was to extend the radical mastectomy, to remove the breast, the axillary nodes, the chest muscles, and the internal mammary nodes in a single procedure. A few months after Handley published his report, Urban performed a superradical mastectomy. His logic was simple: "We should increase our salvage of early operable cases over the present results obtained with the usual radical mastectomy, which completely neglects the internal mammary lymphatic chain."[16]

Urban carefully selected patients. He avoided women with advanced tumors, in whom metastases had probably already become widely disseminated, since they would not provide any reliable sense of how successful he was in improving survival rates. Urban wanted women whose tumors were small, either without palpable axilla involvement or axilla tumors movable to the touch. Several of his forty patients had tumors less than one centimeter in size—tiny even by today's staging standards. In Urban's innovative experiment, they underwent massive surgery to cure a breast tumor the size of a pea.

It was a difficult, complex procedure, requiring up to five hours and consuming three pints of blood. He started with a long, elliptical incision, reaching from the armpit across the chest to the sternum, then down the sternum toward the navel. He then lifted the breast, axilla lymph nodes, and pectoralis major and minor muscles away from the torso, exposing the rib cage and sternum. To remove the internal mammary lymph nodes, Urban sawed lengthwise through much of the sternum, then moved two to three inches away from the sternum, cutting out an equal portion of several ribs and lifting out the internal mammary nodes with them. He then finished the operation, removing the breast, axilla, and chest muscles, fashioning a graft to cover the hole in the chest wall, pulling the other breast toward the center of the torso to help cover and protect the gap in the chest wall, and then suturing the wound closed. The operation often left patients with one breast sitting like a target near the middle of their chests. Urban was more than a little sanguine about side effects. "At present," he wrote in 1952, "forty patients have undergone this operation with no fatalities and no increase in postoperative disability . . . . We now know it is possible to perform such a procedure without adding to the operative mortality, morbidity, or the patient's postoperative discomfort and disability."[17]

The so-called superradical mastectomy, however, was not the only heroic surgical procedure breast cancer patients endured in the mid-twentieth century. They also often found themselves at the receiving end of operations to cut off estrogen production. During the nineteenth century, the idea prevailed in most scientific circles that the uterus, and later the ovaries, were dominant organs in women, controlling not only physical health but mood and behavior as well. Rudolf Virchow best captured the consensus when he wrote, "Woman is a pair of ovaries with a human being attached; whereas man is a human being furnished with a pair of testes." Not surprisingly, some physicians looked toward the ovaries for an explanation of breast cancer's elusive mysteries.[18]

It was common knowledge, and had been for decades, that younger women with breast cancer had a decidedly worse prognosis than postmenopausal women. Physicians had also observed, without understanding, the erratic behavior of breast tissues in premenopausal women. Sometimes benign tumors increased in size before a woman's period and then subsided after. Finally, physicians knew that after menopause, many women experienced a gradual decline in the volume of breast tissue. By the time women entered old age, their breasts were much smaller in size than they had been during childbearing years. All these observations left the distinct impression that breast tumors, normal breast tissue, and ovulation were intimately, but mysteriously, connected.

In 1889, Albert S. Schinzinger, professor of surgery at the University of Freiburg, made a startling proposal to the German Surgical Society. At the time he was sixty-one years old. His stiff bearing, thick mustache, and oversized goatee hid an easygoing nature. A pleasant, practical bent marked his personality and his surgery. Troubled by the high death rate of premenopausal breast cancer patients, he asked his colleagues whether they "should not undertake the somewhat unpleasant task of making the ladies prematurely old by removing their ovaries, thus making the mammary glands atrophy sooner and giving rise to the possibility that cancer nodes might become demarcated in the shrinking tissue." He went on to suggest the possibility of removing a patient's ovaries before the mastectomy as a way of getting at more tumor tissue, giving birth to surgical castration as a breast cancer treatment.[19]

He was not the only physician intrigued by the relationship between tumors, breasts, and menstruation. George Beatson, a surgeon in Glasgow, had pondered the problem ever since medical school. Born in Trincomalee, Scotland, in 1844 to a military family, he was an unusually tall, athletic child, possessed of a congenial personality and dogged determination. Handsome and charismatic, Beatson succeeded at everything he tried, especially medical school. He received a medical degree in 1878, having studied surgery at the Royal Infirmary under Joseph Lister. Beatson became a well known, talented physician in Edinburgh, and in 1895 was appointed to the staff of the recently established Glasgow Cancer Hospital.

In 1874, anxious to get to work on the thesis required for the medical degree, but needing financial support and time for data collection, he volunteered to supervise a well-to-do psychiatric patient for several months. He lived at the man's estate in western Scotland. There Beatson decided to write about lactation in animals. The abundance of sheep and cattle in the region offered an opportunity for practical research.

Lactation fascinated him. From his own analyses, he concluded that during lactation, epithelial cells in the breast undergo a fatty degeneration, producing milk for a sucking child. In the farms of western Scotland, he also noticed that the removal of the ovaries from cows which had recently calved stimulated milk production, or, in his mind, accelerated the degeneration of the epithelial cells. During walks over the heathered hills, he wondered if removal of the ovaries in women with breast cancer might induce a similar degeneration of the tumor cells. Although he had no clear conception of the role of hormones in tissue behavior, he was certain that "we are perhaps in error in assigning to the nervous system the entire regulation of the metabolic change in the tissues of the body. I am satisfied that in the ovary of the female and the testicle of the male we have organs that send out influences more subtle . . . and more mysterious than those emanating from the nervous system, but possibly much more potent than the latter for good or ill as regards the nutrition of the body."[20]

During the next twenty years, Beatson experimented by removing ovaries from rabbits, sheep, and cows and studying resulting tissue changes. In June 1895, he was ready to try his theories out on a human

Bathsheba's Breast

being. He selected a young woman whose recurrent breast tumor was inoperable and metastatic. He removed both her ovaries and then waited to see what happened. Within weeks, her tumors shrank. Two months after the operation, he took some cancer tissue from the woman and looked at it under a microscope; the cells appeared to be undergoing a fatty degeneration. Six months later, the woman seemed to be free of disease. Convinced that he had come upon a new treatment for breast cancer, Beatson reported his findings in May 1896 to a medical society in Edinburgh.

The report electrified the audience. Beatson's theory was not based on any knowledge of endocrine function. Modern oncologists know that the malignant cells in some breast cancers possess estrogen receptors, latching on to the estrogen which the ovaries have released. Beatson erroneously located the source of all breast cancer in the ovaries, arguing that somehow the ovaries were the primary site of disease, and that by removing them the malignant cells would, somehow, starve or break down. Critics told Beatson of patients who developed breast cancer after hysterectomy. What about them? Or what about women whose breast cancer appeared long after menopause? He listened, but he disregarded their arguments—at least for a while.

Other surgeons in Great Britain and the continent began performing the procedure on patients with inoperable disease. German and Austrian physicians used the term "castration" to describe the operation, but Beatson and the British, with typical English reserve, preferred the more sexually neutral and scientific "oophorectomy." Beatson continued with the operation, but he too soon developed doubts. For many women, the operation had little effect at all; their tumors did not even subside. Early in 1899, his first patient relapsed, with both local recurrences on the torso and metastatic lesions. The woman died in April, having survived for forty-six months. None of his other patients enjoyed such long remissions. By 1902 they were all dead.

Beatson was more surgeon than scientist. It was James Stanley Boyd of England who compiled the first reliable statistics on removal of the ovaries. Boyd received his medical degree at University College, London, and eventually headed the department of surgery at Charing Cross Hospital in London. One contemporary called him the "high priest of aseptic and antiseptic surgery, he was the first of the Charing Cross surgeons to give up operating in a frock coat." He performed his first oophorectomy in 1896, just months after listening to Beatson. During the next four years, he collected case studies on fifty-four other patients and reported that nineteen had benefitted from the surgery. An editorial in the *British Medical Journal* concluded, "The operation influences cancer of the breast favorably but not permanently."[21]

Early in May 1897, Boyd examined a young woman with advanced breast cancer. Her extensive tumors ruled out a Halsted radical mastectomy. He thought about the problem for several weeks and decided that the woman might benefit from a "prophylactic" oophorectomy. Perhaps removal of the ovaries might shrink the tumor, making possible a radical mastectomy. The young woman agreed, and Boyd's supposition worked. Her tumors regressed enough to make the radical mastectomy feasible, although she died a year later. Boyd began performing the procedure in conjunction with radical mastectomies. His logic was more consistent with contemporary opinion than Beatson's. Boyd disputed the notion that the ovaries were the primary site of breast cancer; instead, he argued that the ovaries secrete a substance that regulates ovulation and menstruation, and that in some cases stimulates tumor growth. He concluded that the operation was only temporarily successful in some patients because the body, in the absence of ovaries, compensates for the loss of the secretion. At that point in the disease cycle, the tumors started growing again.[22]

Combining radical mastectomies with bilateral oophorectomies did not last long. The operations were debilitating and the results unpredictable, since physicians had no way of determining which tumors possessed estrogen receptors. In 1902, at the annual meeting of the British Medical Association, Henry Morris of Middlesex Hospital raised serious questions about the double procedure. He urged ovary removal only for inoperable tumors, where the radical mastectomy was useless. When the radical mastectomy was indicated, he wanted the oophorectomy held back until after a recurrence. If the recurrence never happened, the patient would not have to deal with the hormonal consequences of losing her ovaries. If a recurrence took place after mastectomy, physicians would still have another option. At the meetings, Morris argued, "To perform oophorectomy at the same time as primary excision of the growth seems to be a wasteful expenditure of a resource which, if held in reserve, may be of great value at a later period should local recurrence take place."[23]

By the early 1900s, prominent physicians in Great Britain, the United

States, and Western Europe regularly employed oophorectomies to treat breast cancer. They abandoned simultaneous radical mastectomies and oophorectomies, holding in reserve the option of removing ovaries if the initial surgery failed to eliminate the disease. After 1915, however, oophorectomies became less common. Scientific understanding of the endocrine system was still in its infancy, and physicians could not tell which women might benefit from the operation. Many hesitated to perform the surgery randomly since only 20 percent of patients would experience any remission at all. Even when successful, the benefits were temporary, usually lasting for a matter of months before the tumors returned. Only a handful of women enjoyed longer remissions. The potential benefits did not compensate for the costs and risks. By 1920, most surgeons employed oophorectomy only as a last resort.[24]

What they did not understand was the body's capacity to adjust to an oophorectomy. The endocrine system could at least partially compensate for removal of the ovaries. In the absence of ovaries, the adrenal glands secreted androstenedione, a hormone the body converts into estrone, which stimulated estrogen-based tumor cells, providing them hormonal stimulation. In the first few months after losing ovarian function, many breast cancer patients experienced temporary shrinkage or remission of their tumors. As the adrenal glands assumed some of that function, however, the estrone-fed tumors proliferated and spread again, eventually killing the patient.[25]

But in the 1930s, when scientific understanding of the endocrine system improved, new surgical possibilities materialized. Charles Huggins of the University of Chicago pioneered the new treatment. Born in Nova Scotia in 1901, Huggins earned his medical degree at Harvard and completed a surgical residency at the University of Michigan. Specializing in urology, he concentrated his research efforts on prostate cancer in men. The existence of a functional connection between the prostate gland and the testes had been known since 1837, when two French surgeons accidentally removed a man's testicles while performing a hernia operation. They subsequently noticed a shrinkage in the size of his prostate gland. In 1941 Huggins established a link between testosterone and prostatic carcinoma. He developed the theory of androgen deprivation—cutting off the supply of male hormones to the prostate gland. In 1941, Huggins performed the first bilateral orchiectomy—castration—to treat a man whose prostate cancer had spread to his spine. The patient experienced a three-year remission of his disease.[26]

But orchiectomy no more cured prostate cancer than oophorectomy cured breast cancer. Although two-thirds of men with prostate cancer experienced a temporary remission, the tumors soon returned. Huggins guessed that the adrenal glands might be taking over for absent testicles. He was right. In 1945 he performed a bilateral adrenalectomy on a prostate cancer patient who had previously been castrated. The tumors shrank, just as they had two years before after the man's orchiectomy. Aware of the literature on hormones and breast cancer, and the development of the oophorectomy, he guessed that a similar process worked in women: when the ovaries were removed, the adrenal glands picked up some hormonal production. In 1952, the same year Jerome Urban reported on the super-radical mastectomy, Huggins began performing bilateral adrenalectomies on women who had previously undergone radical mastectomies and oophorectomies. The surgery involved cutting into the abdominal cavity and removing the adrenal glands off both kidneys. The operation succeeded. Many of the women saw a regression in their tumors.[27]

The recent development of hormone replacement drugs, particularly cortisone, had paved the way for the adrenalectomy. Huggins had the tools for helping adrenalectomy patients maintain some endocrine function, but the therapy was crude. Patients might experience a temporary remission, but severe side effects debilitated many of them. The adrenal glands serve two basic functions—supplying glucocorticoids and mineralocorticoids to the body. In the absence of glucocorticoids, patients often suffer from low blood sugar, obesity, fatigue, and depression. The side effects of insufficient mineralocorticoids include low sodium levels, high potassium levels, fatigue, and dizziness. Even though surgeons performing adrenalectomies tried to offset side effects with cortisone replacements, the substitutes were still in a crude state of pharmaceutical development and the surgeons had difficulty adjusting individual dosages.

Worse, the Huggins adrenalectomy was not a cure. The vast majority of women undergoing the operation eventually succumbed to breast cancer. Their tumors returned, sooner or later, and it did not take much imagination to conclude that the body was still compensating, still managing to generate hormones even in the absence of ovaries and adrenal glands. In November 1952, Rolf Luft and Herbert Olivecrona of the Uni-

Bathsheba's Breast

versity of Stockholm presented their theory at the Mayo Clinic. They argued that when the ovaries and adrenal glands are removed, the pituitary gland assumes their functions, secreting biochemicals which other body tissues convert into estrone. Eliminating the source of the hormones appeared to be the only way of addressing the problem; cutting off the flow of those hormones meant more surgery, this time in the brain—a hypophysectomy to remove the pituitary gland.

Ever since the early 1900s, surgeons had performed hypophysectomies to treat pituitary tumors. Luft and Olivecrona, and then a number of other prominent neurosurgeons, adopted the procedure to treat breast cancer patients whose tumors had recurred in spite of radical mastectomies, oophorectomies, and adrenalectomies. In terms of risks and side effects, the hypophysectomy posed more danger than oophorectomies and adrenalectomies. Before the more recent use of the transphenoidal approach through the nose, surgeons took a transfrontal route, boring into the skull through the forehead, just above the nose. The pituitary rests at the junction of the optic nerves, just under the brain's frontal lobe. Surgeons performing hypophysectomies flirted with disaster. Often the operation was uneventful, but many women left the hospital with permanently impaired vision, personality changes, and cognitive difficulties. Even then, their tumors usually returned to kill them.[28]

By the mid-1950s—with superradical mastectomies, oophorectomies, adrenalectomies, and hypophysectomies—faith in the medical establishment peaked. The development of highly elaborate, technically intricate medical procedures was not simply a product of scientific progress. Patients had to be willing to submit to such extraordinary operations, and that was as much a cultural phenomenon as a scientific one. Until the twentieth century, only the finest of lines separated doctors from quacks and science from superstition. Patients were more likely to die from medical treatment than from the disease. It was not until 1910 in the United States that, as one historian has written, "a random patient, with a random disease, consulting a doctor chosen at random, had a better than fifty percent chance of profiting from the encounter." Just as physicians developed heroic surgical procedures for treating breast cancer, women became more and more willing to submit to them.[29]

But early in the twentieth century, a revolution in public attitudes occurred. Anesthesia eliminated most surgical pain while aseptic and antiseptic methods reduced postoperative infections. The Industrial Revolution and advent of rapid technological change generated a new faith in science. Doctors had labored diligently during the previous fifty years to incorporate the latest scientific advances, raising the standards of medical training, and rationalizing licensing standards. They scored stunning victories over scourges of the past. In 1901 physicians traced the source of yellow fever to mosquitoes. They identified the bacterial agent behind whooping cough in 1906, and in 1908 developed a successful serum for treating spinal meningitis. In 1908 lice were identified as the culprits behind typhus epidemics, and Paul Ehrlich discovered the drug Salvarsan to treat syphilis. Public health campaigns limited outbreaks of killers of the past—yellow fever, smallpox, typhus, and cholera. Biochemists treated diabetes with insulin in the 1920s, and the first antibiotics all but eliminated the dangers of many infectious diseases. Early in the 1950s, the polio vaccine offered protection against that crippling epidemic. With doctors winning the fight against many diseases, breast cancer patients, hoping for the same progress against their afflictions, submitted to radical surgery.[30]

They are a nameless sorority of several hundred women today, forgotten by all but their families, their illnesses buried in microfilmed case reports filed systematically within the medical records section of the world's greatest hospitals. With middle- and upper-class resources, they enjoyed access to the best medicine money could buy, trekking to places like Memorial Sloan-Kettering in New York, the Roswell Park Memorial Institute in Buffalo, the Mayo Clinic in Minnesota, or the Dana-Farber Cancer Institute in Boston, hoping to find the holy grail of long-term survival. Desperate to see their children grow up, determined not to let breast cancer put them in early graves, they placed themselves, literally, on the cutting edge of surgical technology.

They consulted the finest surgeons in the world, men anxious to win a battle against breast cancer, to do for their generation what William Stewart Halsted had done for his. And in the late 1940s and early 1950s, those men carried out a no-holds-barred war against the disease. The women became a sisterhood of guinea pigs, living objects of new surgical protocols. They were the chosen few who experienced it all. When they first reported to Erling Dahl-Iversen, Jerome Urban, Owen Wagensteen, and Mario Margottini, they suffered from Stage 1 and Stage 2 disease, breast tumors that were relatively small in size and without axillary metas-

Bathsheba's Breast

tases, or small tumors with limited axillary involvement. They received su-perradical mastectomies, losing their breast, chest muscles, and the axil-lary internal mammary, and sometimes supraclavicular lymph nodes. Those whose tumors recurred after the surgery sometimes underwent oophorectomy. Within months, when it became clear that removal of the ovaries provided only a temporary benefit, surgeons cut out both of their adrenal glands to stop the production of estrogen precursors. When that was not enough, they bored into skulls to cut out the pituitary gland. Sev-eral decades before, when surgeons first started trying to improve on Hal-sted, one specialist posed the following recommendation for breast cancer patients: "It may be accepted as a safe rule, that when in doubt about symp-toms in patients at the cancer stage: *Don't wait, explore!*" Explore they did.[31]

CHAPTER FIVE

New Beginnings

ASSAULT ON THE RADICAL MASTECTOMY

In the wake of World War II, and the success of the Manhattan Project in developing an atomic bomb, faith in science and technology spiked in American culture, and hope for a cure for cancer waxed just as strong. In what twenty-twenty hindsight sees as egregious hyperbole, news magazines and even some oncologists spoke of America's cancer-free future. According to a 1950 issue of *U.S. News and World Report*, "Millions of dollars, hundreds of scientists, and careful planning are being used in what authorities regard as medicine's counterpart of the wartime atom bomb project." In 1958, John Heller, head of the National Cancer Institute, remarked, "I've spent many years in cancer research. Now I believe that I will see the end of it." Such confidence, if unwarranted, was nevertheless rooted in real science and technology. Ever since Galen, surgery had been the only cancer treatment that had stood the test of time, but the advent of radiotherapy and chemotherapy had added real weapons to oncology's arsenal.[1]

On the evening of March 29, 1896, Rose Lee approached the entrance of a darkened factory. She was about to become radiotherapy's first guinea pig. Emile Grubbe, a German immigrant who worked there, greeted her at the door and escorted her upstairs. An 1894 mastectomy had failed to cure her; surgeons had excised several recurrences in 1895. When the tumor returned again, she made an appointment at the Hahnemann Medical College in Philadelphia. She had four children to raise and wanted to live long enough to finish the job. The news was not good. Professor Richard Ludlum informed Lee that her tumor was inoperable. Nothing could be done. When she pleaded, begging for something, anything, to treat the tumor, he referred her to Grubbe, a second-year medical student.

Grubbe financed his medical education working nights at a plant that manufactured Crookes tubes. William Crookes, a London physicist, had invented the tube—a sealed glass container with air vacuumed out of it—which allowed electricity to pass from a negative wire to a positive wire in the form of a ray. The tube glowed and gave off heat as "cathode rays" bounced off the glass. In November 1895, at the University of Würzburg, Professor Wilhelm Roentgen wanted to find out if cathode rays ever got outside the glass tube. He covered a Crookes tube with cardboard, switched on the electricity, and soon noticed a faint green light appearing on a metal screen about three feet away. The glow surprised him, since he knew the cathode ray, even if it penetrated the glass and cardboard, could not be more than a fraction of an inch in length. The green glow was a ray of some kind, but not a cathode ray.

He tinkered with the phenomenon for several weeks, discovering that the rays, soon to be called x-rays, penetrated soft tissues and could be used to photograph body parts. Not everyone viewed his experiments with scientific detachment. When he x-rayed his wife's hands and showed her the bones and her wedding rings, she panicked and scurried out of the laboratory. Roentgen reported his findings to the Physical Society of Würzburg and distributed copies of the paper to prominent physicists all over Europe, giving birth, in the process, to the modern medical discipline of diagnostic radiology. The news raced through the medical world. Richard Ludlum had read about it in February 1896.[2]

Grubbe had complained about swelling, redness, pain, hair loss, and dermatitis on his hands after working with Crookes tubes. Guessing that the invisible x-rays might be destroying skin cells, Ludlum took a long shot and told Rose Lee that perhaps they could also destroy her breast tumors. At the factory, Grubbe hooked up a Crookes tube to an electrical outlet, rummaged through a Chinese tea box for lead foil, surrounded Lee's breast with the foil, and then situated the lighted tube over her breast for an hour. He repeated the treatment eighteen nights in a row. A few weeks later, Ludlum noted that the tumors had shrunk and her pain had subsided. By then, however, she was complaining of headaches, listlessness, and spinal pain, and her complexion had assumed a jaundiced hue. Ludlum knew the end was near. Rose Lee died two months later, but she was the first woman in history to receive radiation treatments for breast cancer. Other physicians at leading hospitals in Europe and the United States immediately began to experiment with such treatments.[3]

In Paris, Marie Curie soon provided another treatment. A genius, Marie had spoken in full sentences at age two and could read at three. She had the memory of a savant. Her sister Bronia was almost as bright. The two young women made a deal to their mutual advantage. Bronia went to Paris first, lived off her sister's earnings as a teacher and governess, and received her medical degree in 1891. Marie arrived in Paris a few months later. Bronia financed her sister's physics major at the Sorbonne. In 1895, Marie married physicist Pierre Curie.

Theirs was an extraordinary collaboration. Working closely with Henri Becquerel, another Sorbonne physicist, Marie Curie discovered polonium, radium, and the principle of radioactivity. During the next several years, she worked with Sorbonne chemists and produced pure radium in the metallic state. In 1903 she received the Nobel Prize in physics, shared with Becquerel and her husband, for discovering radioactivity, and in 1911 she won the Nobel Prize in chemistry for isolating radium crystals. In spite of being the only person ever to win Nobel Prizes in different disciplines, she failed in her bid for election to the all-male French Academy of Science. Undaunted, Curie spent the rest of her career at the Radium Institute, investigating the chemical properties of radioactive substances.[4]

Radium's medicinal possibilities had dawned on Becquerel in 1901 when he noticed dermatitis and first-degree burns on his left hip. He had no trouble isolating the source of the problem, since he regularly carried small vials of radium around in his lab pocket. The crystals obviously damaged the outer layer of skin cells. Pierre Curie experimented on his own hand, with the same results. Within a few years, physicians in major teaching hospitals treated a variety of tumors by exposing them to radioactivity, either externally or by inserting radium-filled glass or metal tubes directly into the malignant tissues. In many cases, they noticed a temporary regression of the tumors.[5]

They had no idea why radium adversely affected tumors. Radioactive elements are unstable, spontaneously disintegrating at the atomic level and emitting alpha, gamma, and beta rays. When human cells—normal as well as malignant—are exposed to those rays, they are ionized, becoming unstable. The rays bombard atomic structures, dislodging electrons and disheveling genetic material, and killing the cell during mitosis, or the division cycle. Because cancer cells divide so rapidly, they exist more frequently in a state of mitosis and are more vulnerable. They tend to die before normal cells. Exact dosage is key. Physicists must supply enough alpha, beta, and gamma rays to kill the cancer, but not enough to destroy normal cells. For the first time, doctors did not have to rely on surgery alone.

It was in Great Britain, rather than in the United States, that the radioactive attack on the radical mastectomy began. Geoffrey Keynes of St. Bartholomew's Hospital in London led the assault. He was born in Cambridge on March 25, 1887, to John and Florence Keynes. His older brother, John Maynard, was destined to become the most influential economist of the twentieth century. At Cambridge, Geoffrey stayed away from the "dismal science," preferring the more predictable world of physics and chemistry. After graduating, he studied medicine and surgery at St. Bartholomew's. One year after earning a surgical degree in 1913, he found himself with the Royal Artillery in France, practicing surgery on the shattered bodies of young men. The carnage of World War I changed him forever. He later remarked, "I saw enough disconnected hands, legs, feet, arms, and heads to last a lifetime." Keynes came away from the war an expert in field surgery but with an aversion to unnecessary mutilation. After years of putting maimed bodies back together, he became obsessed with conservative surgery—doing as little damage as possible to a patient's body. He specialized in gastrointestinal, thyroid, and breast surgery. Keynes did not like the Halsted mastectomy. Removal of the breast, axilla, and chest muscles left women with concave torsos, rib cages covered by only a thin layer of skin, severe edema, chronic pain, and limited motion. There had to be a better way. While most surgeons in the 1920s and 1930s contemplated more extensive surgery to improve survival rates, Keynes thought about preserving, or even improving, the existing survival rates with less debilitating procedures.

After the war, he returned to St. Bartholomew's and wondered if radium treatments might replace radical surgery for breast cancer. Keynes experimented first with women whose tumors were inoperable, exposing their breasts to radium crystals. Upon witnessing some regression in larger tumors, he speculated about employing radiation on women with operable tumors. "Having satisfied myself that radium could be used successfully when the disease was beyond surgery," he wrote, "I began to wonder whether it might not be used, perhaps in combination with conservative surgery, for treating cancer of the breast in its earlier stages." Beginning in 1924, he categorized the Halsted radical mastectomy as unnecessarily aggressive. Less radical procedures could achieve similar survival rates when combined with radium treatments, without inflicting anywhere near the same damage. Keynes began performing lumpectomies on women with operable breast cancers, following up with interstitial radiation—implanting tubes filled with radium crystals—in the breast and the axilla. Because eight percent of his patients experienced local recurrences, a figure Keynes found too high, he became somewhat more aggressive early in the 1930s, preferring a wide lumpectomy or modified mastectomy—removal of the breast and axilla nodes, while leaving the chest muscles in place.

In 1935 he compiled five-year survival records for patients receiving modified mastectomies and radiation, and he compared them with Halsted's. The results were all but identical and remained so at ten years and fifteen years. Of six hundred patients treated for breast cancer at St. Bartholomew's between 1930 and 1935, the overall fifteen-year survival rate for those receiving radical mastectomies was 42 percent. Exactly 42 percent of the women undergoing simple mastectomy and radiation treatments were also alive fifteen years later. Keynes claimed success, and, late in the 1940s, just when the superradical mastectomy appeared, he preached to anyone who would listen the need to abandon radical mastectomies in favor of conservative surgery and radiation. Most surgeons scoffed at his claims, and for years he was a lone voice in a medical wilderness.[6]

During the 1930s and 1940s, radiotherapy evolved and became more powerful. Keynes employed interstitial radiation to treat his patients, but physicists gave doctors the option of external beam radiation by increasing the voltage of x-ray machines, which gradually permitted the treatment of deep-seated tumors. The first Crookes tubes produced 50,000 to 100,000 volts of electricity, only enough to treat superficial lesions. Any attempt to apply such weak radiation sources to deeper tumors failed because they severely damaged skin. The Coolidge hot cathode tube, invented in 1913, generated 140,000 volts, and in 1922 an improvement on the Coolidge tube produced 200,000 volts. Each voltage increase permitted radiation to reach deeper tumors without inflicting so much damage on surface tissues. The California Institute of Technology bragged about its 750,000-volt x-ray tube in 1930, and four years later Mercy Hospital in Chicago topped that with an 800,000-volt radiotherapy contraption. In the years after World War II, physicists developed megavoltage linear accelerators exceeding 100,000,000 volts.[7]

In addition to more powerful machines, physicists experimented with radiation doses. During the first two decades of the twentieth century, they simply exposed tumors to large, single doses, but they could never give "tumorcidal" doses because they killed normal tissues as well. For example, 6,500 "rads" of radiotherapy will kill many solid tumors, but if given in one dose on one day, they will also destroy all normal tissues near the tumor. The problem physicists faced, and still face, was how to deliver a deadly dose of radiation to tumors without killing other organs. At the Radium Institute in Paris, Marie Curie and her associates developed "fractionated" treatment—delivering "tumorcidal" doses of radiation over the course of several days or weeks. Gradually, over the next several decades, scientists came to understand the biophysics of radiation. By the 1990s, for example, radiotherapists might attack a solid tumor by exposing it to 180 rads of radiation daily for six weeks, eventually giving the tumor a cumulative, deadly dose. Too little radiation did not destroy the cancer. Just the right amount killed cancer cells without inflicting too much damage on surrounding tissues. Too much radiation killed everything. Ironically, Marie Curie herself eventually got too much of the radiation. She died of radium-induced leukemia in 1934.[8]

Early in the 1930s, Robert McWhirter, an Edinburgh radiotherapist who worked closely with Keynes at St. Bart's, took advantage of the new technologies. Brilliant as well as politic, McWhirter returned to Edinburgh in the mid-1930s and managed, in what must be the most successful sales blitz in medical history, to convince his surgical colleagues to abandon the Halsted mastectomy in favor of simple mastectomy and radiotherapy. During the next decade, as physicists developed more powerful machines to deliver external doses of radiation, he used them to treat breast cancer patients. For women with operable tumors, McWhirter had a surgeon perform lumpectomies, or "tylectomies" as he called them, on very small lesions and simple mastectomies on larger ones. He then radiated the surgical area as well as the axilla, supraclavicular, and internal mammary lymph nodes. In 1948, he published ten-year survival rates of his patients, which mirrored those of radical mastectomies at the best teaching hospitals in the United States. Keynes had his first convert.[9]

Keynes also convinced David Patey of the Middlesex Hospital to scuttle Halsted, except in cases where tumor had actually invaded the chest muscles, and to develop a more conservative approach. He decided to preserve the pectoralis minor muscle in what he termed a "modified radical mastectomy." "With elevation of the arm," he wrote, "retraction of the pectoralis major and removal of the pectoralis minor, it is easy to do a complete clearance of the axillary glands and fatty tissue right up to the apex of the axilla." In 1948 Patey reported the results of radical versus modified radical mastectomies he had performed between 1930 and 1943. Survival and recurrence rates were the same.[10]

By the late 1940s, Keynes, McWhirter, Patey, and a few others urged the abandonment of radical mastectomies in favor of modified radical mastectomies, simple mastectomies, and lumpectomies combined with radiotherapy. A few years later, early in the 1950s, when they heard about superradical mastectomies for early stage breast cancer patients, they were incredulous. If the Halsted radical mastectomy was no longer warranted, the superradical mastectomy constituted criminal assault on a woman's body. "My God," Keynes sighed to a colleague at St. Bartholomew's, "how can they really believe that such carnage is necessary?" Keynes had had enough. He retired from medicine and spent his remaining days studying English literature.

Patey felt a sense of resignation. Science had produced radicals, modified radicals, superradicals, simples, and lumpectomies, sometimes combined with radiotherapy and sometimes not, but he was not convinced they had made much progress against the disease. Along with Keynes and McWhirter, Patey had devoted his career to the idea that less was better, that although physicians were not much better than Halsted at curing breast cancer, they were doing less damage to women. He was prophetic in his understanding of the future of breast cancer oncology, for he believed passionately that the disease was systemic in nature, not local at all. "Until an efficient general agent for the treatment of carcinoma of the breast is developed," he wrote in 1948, "a high proportion of cases are doomed to die of the disease whatever combination of local treatment by surgery and irradiation is used, because in such a high proportion of cases

Bathsheba's Breast

the disease has passed outside the field of local attack when the patient first comes for treatment."[11]

The search for such a "general agent" was already under way. Back in the 1600s, Fabricius Hildinus of the University of Berlin had mixed a unique brew for one of his breast cancer patients: "Take suckling puppies, put them in wine and distill it half off. Then take the puppies out and boil them in sufficient quantity of goldenrod water or common water with goldenrod in it. When the decoction is made, add the water that was distilled off the young dogs and boil them together til the flesh comes off the bones. Distill them all together, keep the water for use, wet dry clothes or rags in this and apply it to the ulcerous carcinoma . . . it heals the sore by cleansing and drying." Serious chemotherapy, however, with its treatments grounded in scientific logic and tested in clinical trials, had to wait for the twentieth century.[12]

Dr. Eduard Bloch of Linz, Austria, hoped he had come upon a chemical that could help one of his patients—Klara Hitler. When Alois Schicklgruber Hitler was forty-eight years old, he married Klara Polzl, his twenty-five-year-old niece. He was a notorious philanderer, and his first wife divorced him when she learned of his affair with their maid, Fannie Matzelberger. He married Fannie two years later, but when she developed a severe case of tuberculosis, Alois invited his niece Klara to move in and help care for his wife and two small children. Klara performed more than simple household duties. When Fannie died in 1884, Klara was already pregnant with Alois's child. He married her in January 1885, and Gustave was born several months later. Ida was born in 1886, and Otto in 1887. The infant Otto died two weeks later, and diphtheria killed Gustav and Ida early in 1888. Klara was devastated and went into a deep depression. Her fourth child, Adolf, was born on April 20, 1889.

She lavished the new baby with love and protection, breast-feeding him into his fifth year, an unusually long time even for nineteenth-century Austria. Women regularly nursed their babies for about two years, simply because nursing often suppressed ovulation and new pregnancies. But while Klara showered Adolf with attention, Alois administered abuse masked as discipline. He beat the boy regularly and daily meted out vicious attacks on the family dog. Adolf despised his father. When the old man died in 1903, the fourteen-year-old secretly celebrated. The ordeal had bonded mother and son. He confided in her, shared his ideas about life, and listened to her counsel. She was everything his father was not—kind, patient, thoughtful, and forgiving. Her death in 1907 shocked him into a deep depression.

Klara Hitler first noticed the lump in her breast in 1905, but she ignored the warning, not mentioning it to her physician until January 1907, when chest pains kept her awake at night. Eduard Bloch, a Jew and for years the Hitler family doctor, examined her and diagnosed advanced breast cancer. He said nothing to Klara, preferring to let Adolf inform his mother. The next day, when Bloch broke the news, Adolf started to cry, pleading with the doctor, "Does my mother have no chance at all?" "Only then," Bloch recalled thirty years later, "did I realize the magnitude of the attachment that existed between mother and son. I explained that she did have a chance, but a small one. Even this shred of hope gave him some comfort." Bloch advised a radical mastectomy. "She accepted the verdict as I was sure she would—with fortitude. Deeply religious, she assumed that her fate was God's will. It would never occur to her to complain. She would submit to the operation as soon as I could make the preparations."

Bloch referred her to Dr. Karl Urban, chief of surgery at the Hospital of the Sisters of St. Mercy in Linz, Austria. Also a Jew, Urban was widely regarded as the best surgeon in Upper Austria. After examining Klara Hitler, he agreed that she needed the operation. Several days later, he performed the mastectomy. Tumors appeared to have invaded the chest wall, and he came away from the operation decidedly pessimistic. Bloch went immediately to the Hitler home at 9 Bluetenstrasse and informed the children. "The girls received the word I brought with calm and reserve. The face of the boy was streaked with tears, and his eyes were tired and red. He listened until I had finished speaking. He had but one question: 'Does my mother suffer?'"

Urban was right. The tumors had already spread to the pleural tissues of her chest. Halsted's procedure would not be enough. By the time she had recovered from the surgery, the metastases were already draining her energy and stealing her weight. Hitler dutifully attended his mother for several months, sleeping in an alcove off her bedroom and waking up at her every whimper. In October, Klara's decline accelerated, and Adolf approached Bloch again, begging him to try something, anything, to save her life. Bloch warned Hitler that his mother was gravely ill, and that her only chance was a painful, experimental chemotherapy treatment. It involved reopening the mastectomy scars and applying massive doses of iodoform, an iodine-based medicine, with gauze to the open wounds. The chemical burned its way into the tissues, with Klara screaming and writhing through the treatment and whimpering afterward for hours. The iodoform paralyzed her throat so that she could barely swallow. Bloch performed the treatment for forty-six consecutive days in November and early December. Adolf was beside himself, watching his mother suffer. She died on December 21, 1907.

Hitler was inconsolable. Two days later he visited Bloch to settle the bill. The young man wore a dark suit and a loosely-knotted cravat. He shook Bloch's hand, and said, "I shall be grateful to you forever." Hitler then bowed formally and paid him in full—359 kronen, a considerable sum. For several years, he wrote to Bloch, remembering him on holidays with some of his own hand-painted postcards, sent from Vienna. Bloch kept most of them.

Thirty years later, after Germany's peaceful conquest of Austria in the *anschluss* of 1938, the postcards came in handy. Gestapo agents began harassing Austrian Jews, and Bloch started dropping names—actually one name—to protect himself. Local Gestapo officials examined the postcards and authenticated them. Bloch secretly got word to Klara Hitler, the Führer's younger sister, that he wanted to emigrate to the United States. She passed the news to the Führer. Within weeks Bloch had the necessary visa documents, travel permits, ration cards, and an exemption from having to wear a "J" on his clothes. In November 1938, as he crossed the Austrian border into Switzerland, Bloch penned a note to Hitler: "Your Excellency: Before passing the border I want to express my thanks for the protection which I have received." It was a curious irony: While Hitler contemplated the liquidation of millions of Jews, he made sure one escaped. Consciously, he was thankful for Bloch's treatment of his mother. But perhaps subconsciously, he remembered the daily horrible iodoform treatments. Perhaps, in a warped inner vision, he remembered a Jew torturing his mother.[13]

Actually, Bloch's experiments with iodoform, though unsuccessful, were part of that quest. Iodoform was not really chemotherapy in a modern sense. Bloch used it as a caustic to destroy the cancer cells still lingering in Klara's chest. It was a local treatment, different in kind but not in philosophy from the hemlock and arsenic pastes of the past. The modern era of chemotherapy was a post–World War II phenomenon, when oncologists began to view breast cancer as a systemic disease needing systemic as well as local treatments.

Indirectly, Adolf Hitler was present at the dawn of the modern age of chemotherapy. In August 1914, when World War I erupted in Europe, he crossed the Austrian frontier into Bavaria and joined the German army to fight for the Fatherland. He proved to be an excellent soldier—courageous, long-suffering, and more than willing to carry his fair share. Although wounded several times, he remained with his unit, insisting again and again that he was fit for duty. Four days after receiving the Iron Cross for valor in October 1918, he was caught in an Allied attack when canisters filled with mustard gas exploded near his position, temporarily blinding him and sending him into a coma for several weeks. Thousands of other soldiers on both sides also suffered chemical warfare wounds. The aftereffects on survivors were severe. Victims suffered from compromised immune systems, gastrointestinal disorders, anemia, hair loss, blindness, weight loss, and chronic fatigue.[14]

After the war, forensic pathologists studied the gas survivors and performed autopsies on the dead. Scientific journals on both sides of the Atlantic noted high levels of bone marrow aplasia, degeneration of lymphoid tissues, and severe ulceration of the gastrointestinal tract. During the interwar period, the U.S. army continued its studies of nitrogen mustard, and when Germany invaded France in 1940, the army's biological warfare division signed contracts with Louis Goodman and Alfred Gilman of Yale University to develop antidotes for gas attacks. Both men had already made the connection between the chemical's impact on lymphatic tissues and its possible impact on lymphatic cancers and leukemia.[15]

A 1943 naval battle jump-started their research. On December 2, German aircraft attacked Allied ships in the port of Bari, Italy. Sixteen ships were sunk and eight others badly damaged. Several of the ships were on a top-secret mission—delivering mustard gas for possible use against the German army. When the ships exploded, tons of the gas clouded the harbor, and torrents of liquid gas poured into the water. Panic-stricken sailors abandoned ship into a toxic soup of burning oil and seawater bubbling with nitrogen mustard. More than one thousand American sailors died from exposure to the gas, as did several thousand Italian civilians.

The army assigned Colonel Steward F. Alexander to investigate the incident and evaluate the effects of nitrogen mustard. He was astonished to learn that the blood cells of some who died in the attack had disappeared and lymphatic tissues had all but melted away. He later recalled, "I remember thinking that if nitrogen mustard could do this, what could it do for a person's leukemia or lymphosarcoma?" He forwarded his report to Yale, where Goodman and Gilman began administering nitrogen mustard—an alkylating agent—to lymphoma patients. The results were immediate; a significant number of participants in the study enjoyed temporary remission of their tumors. On the eve of World War I, a physician at the General Memorial Hospital in New York (to become the Memorial Sloan-Kettering Cancer Center) had remarked, "Throughout the centuries the sufferers of this disease [cancer] have been the subject of almost every conceivable form of experimentation. The fields and forests, the apothecary shop and temple have been ransacked for some successful means of relief from this intractable malady. Hardly any animal has escaped making its contribution in hide or hair, tooth or toenail, thymus or thyroid, liver or spleen in the vain search of a means of relief." But now, a medicine possessed at least some certifiable capacity to kill cancer cells. A military disaster in the Mediterranean had given birth to chemotherapy.

During the next decade, oncologists developed other anticancer drugs. Nitrogen mustard, and a whole series of other alkylating agents with tongue-twisting names—sarcolysin, chlorambucil, triethylenethiophosphoramide, cyclophosphamide, triethylenemelamine, melphalan, and busulfan—exhibited powerful anticancer properties, especially on lymphomas and lymphosarcomas. In Boston late in the 1940s, Sidney Farber produced folic acid drugs, which brought temporary remissions in cases of acute leukemia. The first cancer ever to be cured through chemotherapy was the choriocarcinoma—cancer of the placenta in pregnant women. In 1956, Min Chiu Li and Roy Hertz of the National Cancer Institute used methotrexate, another folate antagonist, to treat the tumor. Most women receiving treatment were cured. The victory against choriocarcinoma stimulated tremendous interest in chemotherapy. The National Cancer Institute established the Cancer Chemotherapy National Service Center to develop permanent relationships between major pharmaceutical companies, the federal government, and research universities to develop new drugs.[16]

The late 1940s and early 1950s were heady days in the cancer war. Radiotherapy and chemotherapy had great promise, but supporters exaggerated their potential, raising the hopes of breast cancer patients around the world. The Manhattan Project's success in developing an atomic bomb raised public consciousness about the power, for good and evil, of atomic energy. Cancer treatment was a beneficial side effect. A 1944 article in *Reader's Digest* hailed radiotherapy as "one of the most fantastic events in human history." Lauding the radiotherapy facilities of the Chicago Tumor Institute, the writer, with more than a little hyperbole, claimed, "If there were tumor institutes like Chicago's in every American city, the fight against cancer would soon be nearly one third won." Robert Hutchins, chancellor of the University of Chicago, enlisted in the campaign rhetoric, announcing in 1949, "We can be sure that atomic energy in its various forms will contribute heavily to the final victory," which would come, he confidently prophesied, "by 1956." The excitement was infectious, at least for a while.[17]

Chemotherapists were guilty of equal hyperbole. The chief evangelist for chemotherapy in the United States was Cornelius Rhoads, who took over Memorial (formerly General Memorial) in 1939. Trained as a pathologist, "Dusty" Rhoads headed up the Army Chemical Warfare Division during World War II and became thoroughly acquainted with alkylating agents. Convinced that medicine had entered a golden age, he preached a medical gospel of confidence and optimism. The future of oncology was in the pharmacy, not the operating room. In 1953, like a booster describing his town to outside investors, Rhoads proclaimed: "Inevitably, as I see it, we can look forward to something like a penicillin for cancer, and I hope within the next decade."[18]

But it was not to be. For breast cancer patients, progress was slow, even torturous. Chemical agents, like radiation, damage and then destroy cancer cells during mitosis. The fastest growing cancer cells—white blood cells in children, testicular cells in young men, and placenta cells in pregnant women—were the most vulnerable to chemical agents. Solid tumors, including breast cancer, grow more slowly, and with their cells dividing less rapidly, they are less vulnerable. Although oncologists hoped that they would be able to find a chemical treatment for breast cancer as successful as methotrexate had been for choriocarcinoma, cures proved elusive. Some of the alkylating agents, as well as folate antagonists like aminopterin and methotrexate, had a modest impact on some breast tumors, but there was no magic bullet.[19]

In spite of all the progress, physicians were not much better in 1950 at curing breast cancer than they had been in 1900. The debates among surgeons and radiotherapists had nothing to do with cures. They revolved instead around just how much physical damage was required to treat the disease. Patients were not much better off than they had been under William Stewart Halsted's scalpel. They also faced an array of difficult treatment possibilities, enough to stress even the most self-confident, decisive woman.

In 1950, when Maude Louis Gilpatric learned she had breast cancer, the medical debate could not have been more polarized. Maude was the wife of John Guy Gilpatric, a popular novelist and short story writer whose work had appeared in the *Saturday Evening Post* since the late 1920s. John Gilpatric was best known for creating "Muster" Colin Glencannon, chief engineer on the "S. S. Inchcliffe Castle," a freighter regularly plying the world's oceans. He wrote dozens of Glencannon adventure novels and short stories, earning a good living as a freelancer. John and Maude met in college and married in 1920. An unusually devoted couple, the Gilpatrics made their home in Santa Barbara, California.

Maude ignored a lump in her right breast for more than a year before visiting a surgeon in Santa Barbara. Early in July, he biopsied the lesion. During the next several days, while waiting for the pathologist's tissue report, the Gilpatrics pondered the "what ifs" and explored options with a number of physicians. They heard about mastectomies, radical mastectomies, superradical mastectomies, oophorectomies, adrenalectomies, hypophysectomies, and combinations of all these with radiotherapy. They were told there might even be an experimental chemical they could try. The range of opinions, and their inability to find a consensus, troubled them. So did the possible outcome, since their surgeon, with a headshaking sigh, told them they had probably waited too long before seeking treatment. On July 9, the pathology report was in: the tumor was malignant. The Gilpatrics had already made their decision. They had a nice meal at a favorite restaurant, went home and put on their pajamas, and wrote a note to friends and family about being treated by "mercy bullets," not "magic bullets." John Gilpatric loaded two "mercy bullets" into a .32-caliber pistol and shot one of them, lovingly, into the back of Maude's head, then turned the gun on himself. There were just too many choices.[20]

CHAPTER SIX

Beauty and the Breast

THE GREAT AMERICAN OBSESSION

Breast cancer did what nothing else could do: it silenced Alice Roosevelt Longworth. For more than half a century, she held forth as Washington, D.C.'s unofficial satirist, pillorying everybody in town every chance she got. Born in 1884 to Theodore and Alice Lee Roosevelt, she spent her teenage years in the White House. Her wedding in 1906 to Nicholas Longworth was the social event of the decade. The marriage quickly soured, spoiled by Longworth's womanizing and Alice's self-centered personality. She came to loathe him. Two days after his funeral in 1931, she showed up at a Washington party with none of the trappings of a grieving widow. She drank, laughed, and told stories to anyone who would listen. A partygoer remembered, "Never have I seen such a relieved widow in all my life . . . . I have a feeling she hated him." In a final act of defiance, Alice took her husband's beloved Stradivarius violin and burned it in the fireplace.

She became the most self-sufficient, self-contained woman in Washington. She thrived on gossip—the more salacious the better—and kept on the sofa a pillow bearing a crocheted homily: "If you can't say something good about someone, sit right here by me." She valued controversy for controversy's sake, humiliation for humiliation's sake. Few of Washington's movers and shakers escaped her barbs. Woodrow Wilson was dubbed "our pedantic, professorial, Presbyterian President." When she learned of President Warren Harding's sexual escapades on White House desktops, she laughed uproariously and then spread the news around Washington that "we have a president . . . who doesn't even know beds were invented—and his campaign slogan was 'Back to Normalcy.'" Calvin Coolidge's mother, she claimed, "must have weaned him on a pickle." A die-hard Republican, Alice was crazy with rage at fifth cousin Franklin Roosevelt's victory in the election of 1932. "My poor cousin," she remarked a year later, "he suffered from polio so he was put in a brace; and now he wants to put the entire U.S. into a brace, as if it were a crippled country— that is all the New Deal is about." Her description of Thomas Dewey, the Republican presidential candidate in 1944 and 1948, all but ruined him politically: With his "waxworks mustache and bland features," she remarked, "he looks like the little man on the wedding cake."

But in 1956, Alice Roosevelt Longworth confronted something she could not and would not talk about. She contracted breast cancer and underwent a radical mastectomy. The stigma of losing a breast was profound enough in the 1950s to silence the one woman in America who feared nothing. She swore her physician and nurses to secrecy, threatening to ruin them if they breathed a word about the operation. The conspiracy of silence worked. Neither the Washington newspapers nor her closest relatives knew about the disease. In the 1950s, Americans did not talk about breast cancer.[1]

While Alice Roosevelt Longworth was having a mastectomy in Washington, Erling Dahl-Iversen was approaching retirement at the University of Copenhagen. He was no longer a rebellious young surgical Turk. More than thirty years had passed since medical school, and he had become part of the establishment, a good old boy at the university hospital. Age caught up with him, replacing the naive faith of youth with an elderly skepticism. For twenty years, he had put patients under his superradical scalpel, cutting away pounds of tissue in what he thought was the best means of prolonging life. Over the years, however, doubts eroded his confidence. He had often vacationed at Mon Klint, a small island off Denmark's southern Baltic Sea coast, where he enjoyed setting up an easel near the four-hundred-foot cliffs that overlooked the ocean, and painting the hours away. While he composed landscapes there, he fretted about the number of his superradical patients who eventually died anyway. According to the logic of metastasis—that cancer was a local disease confined for a considerable period to its original site and neighboring lymph nodes— aggressive surgery should have saved many of them.

But it had not. During the late 1950s, as long-term data accumulated, Dahl-Iversen realized, with more than a few pangs of guilt, that the superradical mastectomy had been an elaborate blunder. He had mutilated hundreds of women. In a 1959 interview, he admitted as much: "As to your question," he wrote to an American surgeon, "I may say that in my clinic we have, since January 1959, ceased carrying out my extended operation, realizing that the results after extended radical operation and after Halsted's operation followed by roentgen treatment were identical." Richard Handley, the London surgeon who first demonstrated the nature of metastasis to the internal mammary nodes, also abandoned the superradical in 1959: "I have rather given up a full intercostal [the ribs] section because it seemed to me that the cases I did did not do so well as the ordinary radicals."[2]

Others came around more slowly. Jerome Urban, the famous American proponent of the superradical, presented preliminary findings in 1958, nine years after he invented his procedure. He possessed data on three hundred women, 61 percent of whom were free of disease at five years— a better result, he thought, than the 48 percent rate expected for women "treated by radical mastectomy and postoperative x-ray therapy." He concluded that the superradical mastectomy was especially beneficial for women whose "primary lesions arise in the medial and central portions of the breast." Five years later, however, he was less sanguine. With each passing year, more patients relapsed. By 1963 the ten-year rates were in, and only half of the women were disease free. "Unfortunately," Urban wrote, "the extended operative procedures do not represent a major breakthrough in the treatment of breast cancer." Other superradical surgeons—such as Owen Wagensteen in Minnesota and Mario Margottini in Rome—soon arrived at the same conclusion. The superradical mastectomy was dead.[3]

Advocates of the superradical returned to Halsted; meanwhile, other European surgeons stepped back from the radical mastectomy as well, converting to the gospel of Geoffrey Keynes, Robert McWhirter, and David Patey—less extensive procedures would be just as successful. Evidence mounted in their favor. In 1960, François Baclesse led a team of surgeons and radiotherapists at the Curie Foundation in Paris. Between 1937 and 1953, they had treated one hundred women with simple excision of the tumor and radiation. Most of the patients had either refused mastectomies, or their doctors had originally performed lumpectomies under the mistaken impression that the lesions were benign. When subsequent pathological studies revealed malignancies, the women decided against mastectomies and opted for radiotherapy instead. The five-year survival rates startled American surgeons; nearly two-thirds of the women were disease-free, a result identical to what they could have expected from the Halsted.[4]

The advent of "staging" systems raised more questions about the value of radical surgery. During the 1920s, German pathologist D. P. von Hansemann and Boston surgeon Robert P. Greenough argued that breast cancer cells could be microscopically classified by degree of malignancy. Class I tumor cells, with low levels of malignancy and aggressiveness, were eminently curable. Class II cells were more aggressive and less curable; and Class III malignancies, which were highly aggressive, were incurable, regardless of treatment. In addition to pathological classification, German surgeons in the early 1900s had staged tumors anatomically. Small tumors, confined locally to the breast, became known as Stage 1 disease. Stage 1 patients enjoyed excellent long-term survival rates. Stage 2 disease indicated larger tumors in the breast with cancer spread to the axillary lymph nodes under the arm. Survival rates were not as good. Patients with Stage 3 disease—tumor involvement of the breast, the axilla, and surrounding tissues—had even worse outcomes.

By the 1930s, in Germany and Scandinavia, surgeons were abandoning radical surgery for Class III and Stage 3 patients. Surgeons in the United States proved slower to accept staging systems, but in the late 1940s and early 1950s, Cushman D. Haagensen and Arthur Purdy of Columbia-Presbyterian Medical Center in New York City developed what became known as the Columbia Clinical Classification System, which staged breast cancers from A to D. Haagensen and Purdy insisted that only stages A and B were operable. Hugh Auchincloss, a surgeon at Columbia-Presbyterian, converted to the modified radical mastectomy in the early 1960s because he had concluded that mastectomy patients with fewer than five cancerous lymph nodes had good chances of long-term survival, while those with more positive nodes had dimmer outcomes. In either case, radical mastectomy was unnecessary. Women with fewer than five positive nodes did not need it, nor did the women with five or more. Slowly but surely, the modified radical mastectomy gained more traction in the American surgical establishment.

Some physicians even postulated heresy, arguing that for most breast cancer patients, their outcome was predetermined, a product of the biological imperatives of their own cancer cells, regardless of the treatment course they adopted. Ian MacDonald, a Canadian-trained surgical pathologist who worked at St. Vincent's Hospital in Los Angeles, argued in a controversial 1951 article that early detection was hardly a cure-all and might even be completely irrelevant. The size of the tumor was less significant than its biology—the aggressiveness of its cellular structure and its likelihood to metastasize. At the same time, Neil E. MacKinnon, a Canadian biometrician, posed a similar argument, claiming that in most cases, small lumps were small because they were slow-growing in the first place and less likely to metastasize. A few other iconoclasts joined the tiny bandwagon in the 1950s and early 1960s, claiming that most of the time, radical surgery "cured" tumors that were, for all intents and purposes, nonlethal anyway. Such notions had revolutionary potential, undermining a treatment paradigm that rested on the twin pillars of early detection and swift treatment with radical surgery.

A 1963 international study illustrated the confusion. Physicians at Grace Hospital in Detroit, Barnes Hospital in St. Louis, Middlesex and St. Bartholomew's hospitals in London, the Radium Center in Copenhagen, and Memorial Sloan-Kettering Hospital in New York constructed a retrospective study. Among women with Stage 1 disease, the superradical mastectomy achieved a 77 percent five-year survival rate. Surgeons employing conservative mastectomy—removal of the breast, axilla, and pectoralis minor muscle but not the pectoralis major—cured 75 percent of patients. Five-year survival rates for women receiving the Halsted mastectomy were 76 percent. Over 70 percent of women receiving a simple mastectomy, without axilla removal, and radiation doses in excess of four thousand rads were alive five years later. For women with Stage 2 disease, survival rates were lower. The women receiving the superradical enjoyed five-year survival rates of 48 percent. The Halsted mastectomy also achieved 48 percent. A simple mastectomy combined with radiation, without removal of the axilla, achieved 50 percent. More than a few surgeons wondered if any procedure really mattered.[5]

With scientific opinion so muddled, some surgeons turned conservative. The merits of limited surgery and radiotherapy seemed more evident to Europeans than to Americans. Treating breast cancer with combinations of surgery and radiotherapy became common in France, Germany, Austria, and Scandinavia. During the 1950s, the number of European surgeons routinely performing the Halsted procedure dropped sharply. A 1969 survey of British surgeons demonstrated that only one in five still did radical mastectomies, except in the most advanced cases. Instead, they had taken up the standard of Geoffrey Keynes, relying on less radical operations and radiotherapy. In 1952, Keynes commented on the shift: "Orthodoxy has been greatly shocked by this subversive tendency—but history cannot be denied."[6]

It was a different story in the United States. While European surgeons scuttled the radical mastectomy, nearly three out of four American surgeons still regarded it as the treatment of choice. American surgeons enjoyed far more prestige and power in the pecking order of medical respectability than their European counterparts. In Europe, teaching hospitals existed long before surgery gained any respect as a discipline. For centuries, physicians viewed barber-surgeons as dim-witted but dexterous meat-cutters to whom they shuttled the dirty work of medicine. In the twentieth century, surgeons still occupied a lower rung on the European ladder of medical prestige. But in the United States, the development of hospitals in the late nineteenth century as centers of healing coincided with the rise of surgery as a medical discipline. Surgeons dominated hospitals and controlled the anticancer crusade. Working-class culture also held surgeons in high regard. Everyday citizens could not fathom the intricacies of physicists touting megavoltage rays or chemists concocting killer brews. Surgery was more understandable. Bold men with skilled hands cut out disease, like slicing brown spots out of apples, making the fruit wholesome again. The surgeons themselves, jealously guarding their turf, viewed radiotherapists and their invisible rays with hostility and suspicion.[7]

Gender also slowed the movement toward less radical protocols. In 1970, less than seven percent of America's 300,000 physicians were women. Only 3 percent of general surgeons and less than 1 percent of surgical oncologists were women. Most female physicians in the United States worked in family practice or as psychiatrists or pediatricians, specialties that did not enjoy much prestige in the medical community. In

1975 every member of the American Cancer Society's Breast Cancer Advisory Committee was male. In Europe, on the other hand, the percentage of women physicians was substantially higher, and in many major hospitals gender parity characterized breast cancer sections. At the Oncology Institute in Moscow, most of the medical staff directing breast cancer treatment were women. The same was true in the late 1960s at the Royal Infirmary in Edinburgh, Guy's Hospital and Royal Marsden Hospital in London, and Karolinska Institute in Stockholm. Where women physicians possessed a voice in treatment protocols, conservative surgery was far more common. Rose Kushner, a breast cancer patient advocate, wrote in 1975, "Knowing a breast must be amputated is terrifying. Having physicians who can empathize and sympathize because they, too, have breasts must be very supportive."[8]

Economic incentives also encouraged performance of radical mastectomies. There was more money for surgeons in radical mastectomies than in more conservative procedures. In 1974 the California Relative Value Scale, used by health insurance companies throughout the country to determine surgical fees, gave a Halsted radical a total of seventy points but only fifteen for a lumpectomy and thirty for a modified radical mastectomy. Insurance companies paid less than half as much for modified radical mastectomies as they did for radicals.[9]

Even as the scientific evidence mounted in the 1960s, most American surgeons remained skeptical. There were, however, a few rebels, many of whom, not surprisingly, were women. Ruth Guttman, a radiologist at Francis Delafield Hospital, the breast cancer unit of Columbia-Presbyterian Medical Center in New York, knew of Geoffrey Keynes and opposed the superradical mastectomy. The operation constituted, in her mind, unnecessary violence against women. To prove her point, she launched a remarkable clinical trial. One prerequisite for the superradical mastectomy had been negative axilla and internal mammary lymph nodes. Surgeons biopsied all prospective patients and excluded from the operation every woman whose lymph nodes held cancer cells. Guttman brought those "rejects" into her clinic, where she offered lumpectomies followed up by radiation. She aimed the radiation beam as if it were a superradical operation, covering the breast, the axilla lymph nodes, the mediasternal nodes, the internal mammary nodes, and the chest muscles. In 1962 she published an article in *Cancer* claiming that her patients enjoyed survival rates equal to those of similarly afflicted women undergoing radical and superradical mastectomies, and that her patients still had their breasts and chest muscles.[10]

Vera Peters, an oncologist at Princess Margaret Hospital in Toronto, provided new ammunition to conservative surgeons and radiotherapists. One of the few female surgeons in North America, she had followed Keynes's research with keen interest, launching a clinical trial of her own in 1939. She selected 184 women whose breast tumors had been small, with no lymph node involvement, and treated them with a "wedge resection" or "quadrantectomy," leaving most of the breast intact, and then following up with radiotherapy. She also included in the study 552 women who had received radical mastectomies. Peters then performed a matched pair analysis—three of the radical patients to one of the quadrantectomy patients—and compared results based on age, size of tumor, and year of treatment. In 1963, she published her results in the *Journal of the American Medical Association*. Survival rates for the quadrantectomy patients at five and ten years were as good as those for patients receiving the superradical and radical mastectomies.[11]

The most well-known American iconoclast was George Crile, a surgeon at the Cleveland Clinic in Ohio. Known as "Barnie" to close friends, he was a Harvard-trained physician whose cherubic countenance and gentle demeanor inspired confidence. He started questioning the logic of radical mastectomies soon after his residency, and during the early 1950s the doubts deepened. In 1955 his book *Cancer and Common Sense* upset the American surgical establishment. Crile rejected the consensus that cancer was simply a local disease, arguing that some cancers "are incurable long before [they] can be recognized, no matter how often or how thoroughly the patient is examined . . . because they spread into the bloodstream long before they are ever detectable . . . . The natural course of this type of cancer could not be affected even by the most perfect diagnosis and treatment." He also condemned the "rush to surgery" mentality. Physicians should encourage patients to take enough time to evaluate treatment options. "There is no clear evidence that immediate treatment is any more effective than treatment given a little later . . . the factor of time has been so overemphasized . . . that it takes courage for a doctor to refuse to operate immediately." Crile was unique because he questioned the efficacy of many protocols. While admitting that surgery "is, in many cases, the best weapon we have . . . we should recognize [its] value without exaggerating it." He condemned "ultraradical surgery" because it inflicted too much damage on patients without yielding improved survival rates. Such operations, he suspected, somehow compromised the body's defenses and often led to distant metastases. In the field of oncology, Crile argued, "the frontier is no longer surgery."

Most of Crile's arguments would stand the test of time, but in 1955 he was considered a dangerous extremist. He had a few allies, such as Oliver Cope of Harvard and William A. Nolan of Minnesota, but the surgical establishment generally waxed shrill in its condemnation. Elmer Hess, president of the American Medical Association, accused Crile of offering "a dangerous, fatalistic philosophy of cancer. We fear it may lead readers . . . to reject steps they can take for their own protection." John R. Heller, head of the National Cancer Institute, claimed that Crile's thesis is "contrary to the teaching of the country's 81 medical schools and to the experience of physicians and surgeons." To Alfred Blalock, president of the American College of Surgeons, Crile "has made certain statements which can be misconstrued by the public and which may actually do great harm." Enthusiastic proclamations of innovative European and Canadian surgeons changed few minds among their American counterparts, who discarded the news as the hyperbolic exaggerations of socialist foreigners. American surgeons still scalpeled off the breast, axilla nodes, and both chest muscles, even for the tiniest of lesions. Stubbornly refusing to consider other options, they remained dogmatically faithful to Halsted's ghost. Crile did not endear himself when he stated unequivocally that greed was the real reason behind the staying power of the Halsted mastectomy. "Partial mastectomies that remove the affected part of the breast and reconstruct the rest," he wrote, "are not only more time-consuming and more difficult to perform, but medical insurance plans pay surgeons less for doing them than for removing the breast. In short, the surgeon is paid 2 to 3 times as much for performing a mutilating operation than for performing one that leaves the woman relatively intact."[12]

Transforming the prevailing mind-set would take more, much more, than data, statistics, and refereed articles in scientific journals. American surgeons did not come around for years, not until the sexual revolution and modern feminism altered the cultural and political landscape, changing forever American attitudes about power, eroticism, and physical beauty. An ironic conjunction of scientific evidence, soft-core pornography, gender politics, and rampant sexism spawned a fresh intellectual milieu in which male surgeons and female patients confronted each other. Squeezed between the *Playboy*-shaped libidos of American men and the increasingly strident demands of American women, surgeons took a new look at the female breast and gradually became more amenable to its preservation.

Beginning in the 1950s, an unprecedented fetish of the female breast surfaced in American popular culture. The erotic nature of the breast is hardly an American phenomenon; it is deeply rooted in the evolutionary past. In lower mammals, where the sense of smell is critical to survival, the olfactory system plays the key role in sexual arousal. During the estrous cycle, when females are instinctively attractive and receptive to males, they emit hormonal secretions and odors which males find irresistible. But the sense of smell has lost much of its potency in human beings. Human evolution selected in favor of vision, not smell, so large-brained creatures could more successfully manipulate their environment.

At the same time, the forces of sexual attraction came to rely more on sight than smell. Among such primates as chimpanzees, gibbons, and mountain gorillas, the external genitalia of females engorge with blood during estrous, swelling into readily visible organs and often displaying a variety of rich colors. Males may still detect the smell of hormones, but it is the visual stimulus that lets them know the female is fertile and ready to mate.

As tens of thousands of generations appeared, human beings left behind their four-footed ancestors and stood upright, ready to use their hands and opposable thumbs to control the world around them. The act of standing up, however, changed the nature of sexual arousal. It was still visual, since the sense of vision is so important to human beings, but female genitals had become less visually accessible. According to some anthropologists, breasts assumed the role of letting men know that females were hormonally mature and ready to reproduce. Only in human beings do female breasts appear during puberty instead of with the first pregnancy. Breast development constitutes an external, visual sign of puberty, and its role in sexual arousal and reproduction is deeply embedded in the genes of human beings.[13]

The breast also occupies center stage as an erotic symbol in art history. In fact, as long as human beings have produced art, the female breast has been portrayed as a mechanism of fertility and arousal. The ancient Venus of Willendorf, cast by Central European tribesmen more than fifteen thousand years ago, personifies fertility, her engorged breasts resting on a round abdomen ready to give birth. In 2600 BCE, an Egyptian sculptor immortalized Prince Rahoty and his princess Nofret, exposing her beauty in a V-necked, cleavage-revealing gown complete with the visible protrusion of nipples. Greek sculptors, such as the artist who carved *Dying Niobid* from marble in 450 BCE, glorified the naked female form. *Snake Goddess,* a Minoan piece sculpted around 1600 BCE on the island of Crete, features a young woman dressed in a floor-length gown with long sleeves, high tunic, and completely exposed breasts.[14]

But American society in the last half of the twentieth century glorified the erotic nature of the female breast. Fashion designers exposed more flesh to public view and, in the process, created idealized images of body parts formerly camouflaged by clothing. Body hair, for example, became a new problem. Women felt no need to shave their calves until hemlines climbed up from the ankle early in the 1900s. Shaving underarms was not obligatory until the 1920s when sleeveless gowns revealed armpits to the world. Men had body hair; women were not supposed to have it. So they did not, employing razors, depilatories, and electrolysis to give their bodies the soft hairlessness of a baby. Men's magazines escalated the game in the 1960s, airbrushing away all signs of pubic hair. Bikini-cut bathing suits in the 1980s and 1990s then brought on new tortures, forcing many women to shave the pubic area.

Body hair was only one dimension of the straitjacket modern fashion wrapped around women. Women had long purchased cosmetics to cover facial blemishes and enhance the appearance of the eyes, nose, and lips, but as the twentieth century went on, society demanded more and more perfection. Each new square inch of exposed skin came under public scrutiny. Perfection's critical eye hated scars, blemishes, moles, freckles, birthmarks, blood vessels, fat dimples, stretch marks, hair follicles, pores, pimples, and rashes. With their bodies on display, American women became increasingly preoccupied with weight control, not so much for health as for appearance. No longer protected by full-length dresses with long sleeves and high necks, millions of women worried about the appearance of individual body parts. Most came to despise something about their bodies and yearned for a remedy. Fleshy thighs, long noses, thin lips, knock-knees, fat tummies, flat buttocks, wide hips, and cellulite suddenly became social problems. Whole industries, responding to a multibillion-dollar market, "shaped," "toned," "sculptured," and "smoothed out" women's bodies. "Infomercials" promising perfection became staples of late-night and early-morning television. Cosmetic lines included powders, creams, and blushes for women to use on their legs, arms, hands, necks, chests, and upper backs. Tanning creams and tanning salons sprouted to color white skin and give the appearance of health and beauty. Some women even worried about protruding belly buttons, a concern unknown to an earlier generation innocent of *Playboy* magazine and bikini bathing suits.

Of all the body parts, women's breasts emerged as the physical icons of American popular culture, the sina qua non of eroticism and beauty. The sexual revolution was a cultural earthquake whose first tremors rattled America in 1949, when Norma Jean Baker, soon to be known as Marilyn Monroe, posed nude for Tom Kelley, a friend and photographer. She was a redhead then, but her beguiling combination of innocent vulnerability and powder-keg sexuality exploded off the photograph. Three years later, with Monroe a budding young starlet at Twentieth Century Fox, the photo adorned calendars in gas stations, garages, barber shops, and boys' bedrooms all over America.

In 1953 Hugh Hefner, a young entrepreneur convinced that America was ready for a glossy men's magazine, paid $500 for the rights to the photograph. At the last minute, before the printer ran sixty thousand copies of the magazine, he changed its name from *Stag Party* to *Playboy*. With Marilyn Monroe his first centerfold, he sold 53,000 copies. One year later, *Playboy*'s circulation topped 100,000, and by December 1956, after only three years in publication, it hit 600,000. Hefner was a rich man, and the *Playboy* empire—complete with mansions, clubs, and nude, willing women —was born.

Hefner carefully selected the *Playboy* models. He had a particular look in mind—young, wholesome, and innocent, women without trashy lines or tawdry looks, not really virgins but not too sexually experienced either. Rebelling against his Calvinist upbringing, he marketed sex and pleasure as positive pursuits, not dirty or even inappropriate. Compared to the sleazy, nasty competition in the market of men's magazines, *Playboy* seemed almost wholesome to American men, a vehicle for the unencumbered expression of their fantasies.[15]

Hefner's favorite "Playmate" was Barbie Benton, whose big, bouncing breasts soon became the standard. Over time, under the leering eyes of tens of millions of American men, the breasts of Hefner's "bunnies" and playmates ballooned in size, becoming larger, rounder, and firmer, sometimes achieving gargantuan, gravity-defying proportions, spilling out of the largest DD-cups in a cornucopia of fleshy excess. Small-breasted women fell out of favor in soft-core's glossy inner pages. Sex symbols from Mamie Van Doren and Jayne Mansfield in the 1950s to Dolly Parton in the 1990s needed more than platinum blonde hair to arouse lust.

Playboy was the first and most successful product in the soft-core industry. Dozens of imitators entered the prurient market, sporting such suggestive names as *Penthouse, Swank, Gent, Hustler, Velvet, Chic, Club, International, Genesis, Gallery, Mayfair, Whoppers, Dude,* and *Topps.* By the 1980s, once plastic surgery had become an art form, many models sported huge, manufactured, larger-than-life breasts. The centerfolds stepped onto a freak show merry-go-round of appearances in men's magazines, gentlemen's clubs, hard- and soft-core films, and talk shows, promoting the virtues of freedom, sexuality, and large breasts. Although none of the *Playboy* clones came close to Hefner's peak monthly circulation of six million copies, they collectively purveyed images of big breasts to tens of millions of American men. In the process, they created, and reinforced on a monthly basis, a new tyranny—a cultural expectation that large breasts were beautiful breasts and that, to be considered sexy, an American woman needed them.

The cult of the breast produced its first caricature in June 1964. Carol Doda, a platinum blonde dancer and waitress at the Condor Club in San Francisco's "Tenderloin," discovered an infallible technique for increasing her tips. On a slack evening in July, she peeled off her bikini top and burlesqued for patrons, establishing a new industry and introducing the word "topless" into the vocabulary. Within days, Doda headlined the Condor Club's entertainment marquee, dancing topless on a raised platform, rocking back and forth on a swing roped to the ceiling, and selling an ocean of booze to mostly white, middle-class men. After a few months, Condor regulars noticed a bizarre, other-worldly quality to her breasts. When she danced, they did not jiggle. As she glided back and forth on the swing, they did not sag or flatten. Carol Doda's remarkable breasts possessed a life, indeed a superstructure, of their own.

Curious reporters inquired about their scientific properties. After months of disclaimers, the topless queen fessed up. She was the proud owner of silicone-enhanced breasts. Still in its infancy, the technology was crude. Doda regularly visited a physician who repeatedly spot-injected her breasts with twenty cc of liquid silicone until they were ready to burst. In subsequent years, her silicone would break up into freakish, wandering clumps of gel, but in 1965 she possessed the firmest breasts on the planet.

Topless clubs proliferated in the 1960s and 1970s, invading small towns as well as large cities and sometimes renaming themselves "gentlemen's clubs." Every few years religious and women's groups unleashed crusades to ban them, but federal courts usually defined "topless" enterprises as legitimate, if tasteless, forms of free expression protected by the First Amendment. In 1972, when California restricted topless dancing by prohibiting nudity in businesses with state liquor licenses, bar owners successfully appealed to the federal courts. With the litigation still in progress, a reporter asked Carol Doda if she worried about losing her job. A bar patron laughed and said, "They could serve fruits and nuts and these guys would still show up. They don't come for the booze."[16]

Few escaped the fantasy. It seduced many women, convincing them of the need to evaluate their own breasts for size, shape, and firmness. The vast majority of women came up short, at least compared to the monthly playmates their husbands and boyfriends ogled. Late in the 1950s, taking advantage of the obsession, women's magazines ran more and more articles about breasts, especially the ins and outs of enhancing their "beauty." *Redbook* regularly published a feature section entitled "Beauty and the Breast," informing readers of the latest gimmicks—falsies, push-up bras, chest muscle exercises, hormone creams, and cosmetics—to make their breasts more attractive, that is, larger and firmer. In 1959 *Vogue* promised "Bosom Perfection" to women, because "the woman who feels a need for a change here is involved with the very idea of herself as a woman." A 1968 *Vogue* essay prescribed forty separate exercises to provide perfect breasts—"high and firm." *Seventeen* reminded teenage readers in 1966 that "some of the world's most beautiful actresses have larger-than-average bosoms . . . . (And don't they look great in their clothes?)." Tabloid classifieds had long included "I must, I must, I must improve my bust" promotions, but now they had exited back-page newsprint for the glossy mainstream.[17]

Soft-core pornography was not the only wrinkle on the breast obsession. In 1956 two young mothers, after pushing their new babies in strollers to a park in suburban Chicago, sat on a bench to nurse the infants. Passersby twisted their faces in Victorian disgust, giving Marian Thompson and Mary White a cause. The two women founded La Leche League several weeks later, taking the name of their new organization from a Spanish title for the Virgin Mother: *Nuestra Señora de la Leche y Buen Parto* (Our Lady of Milk and Good Delivery). Victorian prudery had closeted breastfeeding into an all but invisible activity or eradicated it outright among middle- and upper-class women. Rebelling against the recent decline in breastfeeding, Thompson and White organized chapters in more than six hundred cities, selling the gospel of nursing infants. They touted the healthy virtues of breastfeeding and trained women how to do it modestly in any social setting.

Leaguers concerned themselves with the breasts as functional entities, not as the sexual objects of a mammary-obsessed society. To those who objected to breastfeeding in public, Leaguers reacted quickly, "It's their problem, not mine." For women and men who worried that breastfeeding might sag or distend the breasts, Leaguers retorted, "God created breasts to feed babies, not to titillate men." But no less than bra burners, pornographers, and silicone-squirting plastic surgeons, La Leche League aggressively projected breasts into the public consciousness. They even marketed a bit of breast cancer insurance, emphasizing epidemiological evidence that women who breastfed had a lower incidence of the disease. Recent findings confirm at least some of that claim, demonstrating that there is a small, but nevertheless significant, correlation between breastfeeding and lower breast carcinoma rates in premenopausal women. The reason seemed obvious, at least to La Leche Leaguers. God or two million years of evolution, take your pick, had designed women to breastfeed. Industrial society gave women a new option, but it could be a deadly one. Breasts without function might very well be breasts without futures.[18]

The mystique of the breast absorbed millions of American men and women, affecting how they viewed themselves and their partners. William H. Masters and Virginia E. Johnson, who became household words in the 1970s for their academic study of American sexual behavior, became

Bathsheba's Breast

alarmed at its impact. "As the big-breasted female has become the all-American sex symbol," they wrote in 1974, "the image used to promote everything from car sales to X-rated films, men and women have been bombarded on a daily basis with the not-very-subtle suggestions that it is a definite advantage to a woman to have large breasts." The booming plastic surgery business, they argued, was no coincidence: "The small breasted woman may reach the point where she feels she must resort to plastic surgery in order to have a body that is sexually . . . acceptable."[19]

Democratic culture, especially in the United States, in theory abhors elites, including the new elite of big-breasted women. If science could bestow such gifts on Carol Doda, there was no reason why every woman could not order up breasts of choice. What had been an exotic procedure in the 1960s became common among well-heeled women in the 1970s and 1980s. Plastic surgeons turned breast enhancement into a growth industry, first injecting silicone gels into women and then implanting silicone bags of various sizes. Breast enhancement was the most popular operation; no statistic better illustrates the power of the big breast mania than the fact that by 2000 more than 2.5 million American women had undergone what Carol Doda had pioneered thirty-five years before.[20]

Big breasts had become big business, and they had assumed an aura of cultural power as well. For millions of Americans, breasts and physical beauty have almost become synonymous. Society placed a new value on breasts because of their erotic appeal. Many women with small breasts wanted to enhance them, while women with breast cancer wanted to preserve them. Mastectomies, which annihilated breasts, constituted threats to beauty, sexuality, and femininity. It was no accident that the number of breast reconstruction surgeries increased dramatically in the 1960s and 1970s. Technology evolves according to perceived needs, and what modern America wanted was breasts. Men, women, and physicians became more amenable to alternative treatment for breast cancer. The days of the Halsted radical mastectomy in the United States were numbered.

Breast reconstruction surgery delivered another blow to the Halsted radical mastectomy. A few surgeons had experimented with reconstructing breasts since 1895, when Vincent Czerny of the University of Heidelberg in Germany fashioned transplants from fatty tissue in the patient's abdomen or hip. His results were crude approximations, as were all the others until 1942, when Sir Harold Gilles, today acknowledged as the father of plastic breast surgery in Great Britain, developed a reconstruction procedure using transplanted fat and skin flaps. The problem with the Gilles reconstruction was its complexity; the procedure required six separate operations over the course of more than a year, an ordeal few patients wanted to endure.[21]

In 1960 Thomas D. Cronin, a Houston physician, began working with Dow Corning Corporation to develop a silicone-filled sac that could be implanted in women unhappy with their breasts. It was a success, and by 1964 breast enhancement surgery featuring silicone gel implants was available in most major cities. The technology opened a new era in breast reconstruction. Initially targeted at women who wanted larger breasts, implants proved to be a boon to breast reconstruction, since the surgeon had access to a variety of sizes to match the remaining breast, and because the gel possessed a texture and density somewhat consistent with those of the other breast. Such women's magazines as *Redbook, Ladies' Home Journal, McCall's, Good Housekeeping,* and *Cosmopolitan* published favorable articles on breast reconstruction in 1964, and the procedure's frequency increased throughout the late 1960s and 1970s. Surgeons refined the operation, learning to match the reconstructed breast perfectly with the companion breast and to reconstruct nipple and areola tissues.[22]

As middle- and upper-class breast cancer patients became aware of the option, they inquired more frequently about breast reconstruction, forcing surgeons to address the issue. In 1971, *Look* magazine told the story of Sheila O'Connor, a forty-two-year-old mother of three who suffered from benign fibrocystic disease. Between 1963 and 1969, she went under the knife five times for biopsies of suspicious lumps. Each time, the pathology report was benign, but she worried incessantly about breast cancer because her mother, maternal aunt, and sister had all had the disease. One surgeon treating her said, "I needn't spell it out that she was, quite properly, scared to death." He referred her to Dr. Harvey A. Zarem, who performed a "subcutaneous mastectomy," replacing most of her breast tissue with the silicone prosthesis but preserving breast skin and the nipple. During the 1970s and 1980s, articles on breast reconstruction became staples in women's magazines, exposing tens of millions of Americans to the information.[23]

Well-informed women posed a real challenge for surgeons wedded to the Halsted mastectomy. Because the operation removed both chest muscles and a great deal of skin, the patient was left with a badly deformed, concave torso—stretched skin alone covering the upper rib cage—without a foundation on which to place an implant. Surgeons found themselves telling patients that breast reconstruction was not an option after the Halsted mastectomy, and more and more women shopped around for a physician willing to treat their breast cancers in a way that would at least preserve the opportunity for reconstruction. Although subsequent progress in breast reconstruction made it possible even after radical mastectomy, those refinements did not materialize until the late 1970s and early 1980s, by which time the radical mastectomy was rapidly falling out of favor. Between 1965 and 1992, nearly 500,000 women had breast reconstruction after cancer surgery. Halsted was history.

In addition to an accumulating mass of scientific evidence and the American breast fetish, the decline of the Halsted mastectomy was accelerated by the women's movement. Modern feminism traces its origins to Betty Friedan's 1963 bestseller *The Feminine Mystique,* in which she attributed the emotional malaise afflicting so many women to society's insistence that they subordinate individual aspirations to the needs of their husbands and children. She turned that notion upside down, arguing that women could best satisfy the needs of their own families by fulfilling personal dreams first. Energized by a sense of self-worth and achievement, they would then possess the psychological and physical resources to minister to the needs of others.

Feminists initially set their sights on several goals. They wanted to transform a culture conditioning women to believe that only in housework and motherhood could they find happiness. The essential element in ending the political, legal, and economic subordination of women, feminists believed, was to raise consciousness, to shatter the stereotype of domesticity and encourage women to seek their happiness in every area of human endeavor. As long as women narrowed career choices to teaching and nursing, and as long as they acquiesced to social pressures limiting their expectations and confining their dreams to childrearing, they would never break out of their cultural bondage. Only in rejecting subordination and demanding opportunity could women achieve equality.

In addition to changing the cultural climate, feminists attacked legal restrictions based on gender. Feminism became another dimension of the larger civil rights movement. In a number of states in the 1960s and 1970s, women could still not serve on juries, purchase and dispose of property, enter into legal contracts, enjoy equal pay for equal work, gain access to a wide variety of jobs and professions, or secure their own credit lines for the purchase of homes and consumer goods. Feminists campaigned against all de jure forms of discrimination against women.

Finally, feminists promoted "reproductive freedom." The right of a woman to control her own reproductive life—participating in sex, practicing birth control, and giving birth—enjoyed the protection of the Fourth and Fifth Amendments to the Constitution, feminists claimed, by protecting individual privacy. Birth control, homosexuality, and abortion henceforth were to be treated as intensely personal, not public, concerns, free from the intervention of the state or other individuals and groups. While feminists ultimately failed to secure ratification of the Equal Rights Amendment, the Supreme Court's decision in *Roe v. Wade* (1973) upheld the right to seek an abortion up to the third trimester of pregnancy.

The media, ever anxious for a metaphor, found its symbol of feminism at the 1968 Miss America pageant. Robin Morgan, a veteran actress in television's *I Remember Mama* series, spent an hour before the pageant in her Atlantic City hotel room stringing a dozen brassieres into a train. As founder of Women's International Terrorist Conspiracy from Hell (WITCH), she intended to make a bold statement sure to be picked up by television and newspapers. Pouring some lighter fluid on the bras, Morgan ignited them and marched into the pageant, shouting for an end to sexual discrimination. She also provided a "freedom trash can" for the disposal of "old bras, girdles, high-heeled shoes, curlers, and other instruments of torture to women." As a final insult, WITCH crowned their own Miss America— a sheep. Hugh Hefner reacted predictably to the display, writing later to his staff that women's liberation threatened America, that "these chicks are our natural enemy. It's time to do battle with them. They are unalterably opposed to the romantic boy-girl society *Playboy* promotes."[24]

Feminists did not reject bra burning's symbolic imagery; it seemed an appropriate way for some women to expound their point of view. But mainstream feminists resented how the media exaggerated bra burning, acting as if an incendiary bra was a flag for the women's movement to rally around. Susan Brownmiller recalled, "No one in the women's movement ever burned a bra in public protest, yet as soon as feminists began to march, the myth of bra burners spread like wildfire." Of course, the flames were fanned by male journalists caught up in their own breast fantasies. Bra burning was just too powerful a metaphor for them to ignore or even put in proper perspective.

Feminists assaulted the American obsession with breasts. Taking on the breast mystique posed a daunting challenge, particularly given Madison Avenue's image factories that equated large breasts with sensuality and then mass-produced the stereotypes in magazines, newspapers, billboards, and television. The women's movement challenged the notion that some breasts were sexy and others were not, that some were "best" and others "worst." Breasts were just breasts, nothing more, nothing less. Large or small, round or narrow, firm or flat, they were all the same, neither beautiful nor ugly. Ruth Bell, in *Changing Bodies, Changing Lives,* told teenaged girls, "Breasts come in all shapes and sizes. There's nothing much you can do about what yours look like . . . . It would be fine if *Playboy* magazine and Madison Avenue didn't produce endless images of 'perfect busts.'" But Madison Avenue did, and women paid a heavy price. Brownmiller described its toll: "Who wants to dwell on the thought that breasts can look like udders, that breasts are udders, dry, full, swollen, dripping with milk, squeezed, sucked on, raw, tender, in pain—and ultimately used up and withered. No, we're Marilyn Monroe in her calendar pose. We're Friday-night entries in a college town wet-T-shirt contest. We float down the avenue in a Maidenform bra and the nipples don't show." Feminists claimed that media-produced breast stereotypes played an important role in gender subordination. At any given moment, just a few women possessed breasts matching the image; everyone else was lacking. And even those with "good" breasts were destined to have them only temporarily. Time and gravity soon disqualified every breast from the great American beauty contest.

Early on, some feminists took great exception to the value of breast reconstruction surgery, equating it with a pathetic need to fulfill male-driven stereotypes of female beauty. Audre Lorde, an African-American lesbian poet who underwent a mastectomy in 1978, mourned the loss of her breast but considered breast reconstruction an "atrocity" rooted in a cultural obsession for women to remain sexually attractive to men. She rejected the "path of prosthesis, of silence and invisibility of [wishing] to be the same as before." For feminist writer Kathryn Pauly Morgan, breast reconstruction constituted a setback in the movement. "Rather than as-

The Great American Obsession

piring to self-determination and woman-centered ideals of health or integrity," she wrote, "women's attractiveness is defined as attractive to men." Most breast cancer patients, however, rejected the feminist critique. Between 1965 and 2000, more than 700,000 women opted for breast reconstruction.[25]

Feminists also targeted the world of medicine as an important arena in the struggle for equality. They sought to redefine the relationship between physicians and patients. By the 1970s, the medical establishment basked in unprecedented prestige. Success in treating infectious diseases, as well as the increasingly technical scientific foundation of modern medicine, gave physicians an aura of infallibility, allowing them to dispense sophisticated cures to grateful, if ignorant, patients. Gender assumptions reinforced that power. Women had long occupied subordinate positions to men, and what was true for society was true for medicine, especially for breast cancer. The vast majority of physicians were men and almost all of the patients were women. Most physicians expected female patients to accept their counsel unquestioningly, even if the counsel required mutilating surgery.

Terese Lasser played an important role in changing the map of surgeon-patient relations. In 1952, after feeling devastated by a radical mastectomy at Memorial Sloan-Kettering, she founded Reach to Recovery, a support group of mastectomy survivors dedicated to assisting women who had recently undergone the surgery. Lasser began visiting mastectomy patients while they were still in the hospital, discussing the whole range of emotional and physical issues with them, including sexuality, breast prostheses, fashion, and exercises to reduce the swelling from lymphedema. Some surgeons banned Lasser from the halls of Memorial, but she defied them, showing up unannounced. On more than one occasion security police had to escort her from the hospital. At M. D. Anderson Hospital in Houston in 1956, one surgeon complained: "Keep those women off the floor! They are interfering with the physician-patient relationship, and I'll not have it!" But Reach to Recovery—women talking to women about breasts, sexuality, and cancer—was an organization whose time had come, and chapters sprouted throughout the United States. In 1969, the American Cancer Society officially assumed direction of Reach to Recovery, and by the 1980s three of four mastectomy patients were receiving visits.

Bathsheba's Breast

Modern feminism could not tolerate subordination of any kind, especially in the medical arena, where the right of an individual woman to control her own body was held inviolate. The male physician–female patient connection was among the most paternalistic of all relationships. The 1971 best-selling *Our Bodies, Ourselves,* compiled by the Boston Women's Health Book Collective, warned women that "doctors are not gods, but human beings with serious problems, both as people and as professionals. But so, of course, are we all. The uncomfortable difference is that the system has taught the doctor never to reveal his problems and weaknesses to us, to present himself as perfect and all wise, whereas the essence of patienthood is that we must reveal all of our doubts and vulnerabilities to him . . . . The myth still persists that we meet one another as parent and child, and that you as patient must both obey and pay money for the privilege." The antidote was simple. Women should discard their illusions of physicians as demigods and act as independent consumers of professional services. "Don't let yourself be stampeded into any sudden decisions," the Boston Women's Health Collective warned, "or forced to accept any medications or procedures you don't understand or want. It's your body." California feminist Dorothy Shinder was even more blunt, demanding an end to the "medieval maltreatment, atrocities, and discriminatory [medical] acts committed against women."

Over time, the women's movement developed a "Bill of Rights" to govern the doctor-patient relationship. Included was the right to be informed of "the pros and cons of particular treatments in the opinion of other experts, as well as the doctor's own preference and the reasons for it." Patients were also entitled to answers to any of their "questions about any examination or procedure . . . in advance of or at any time during the performance of it. Stopping any examination or procedure at any moment, at your request." Finally, the best physician would display a ready "willingness to accept and wait for a second medical opinion before performing any elective surgery which involves alteration or removal of any organ or body part."[26]

Just as the women's movement escalated the debate over gender and power, news of the medical controversy over the Halsted mastectomy left academic ivory towers and burst into the popular press, providing millions of women with enough information to question doctors recommending radical surgery. Until 1970, the feuding among American surgeons over the merits of the Halsted mastectomy remained cloistered in medical journals and professional meetings. Occasionally, the debate surfaced in the larger scientific community, making its way into such general science periodicals as *Science Digest* and *Science Newsletter*, only to submerge again into the murky depths of academe. The debate entered public consciousness in 1970, however, when George Crile announced at the American College of Surgeons meeting that since the late 1950s he had followed the lead of Europeans and opted for limited surgery—lumpectomies or quadrantectomies—for localized tumors, followed up by breast reconstruction surgery. Even without radiation treatments, he claimed cure rates at least as good as Halsted's. He also cited the work of Geoffrey Keynes and Robert McWhirter, as well as the more recent findings of Sakari Mustakallio of Helsinki, Finland, and Vera Peters in Toronto, all of whom concluded that lumpectomies and radiation were just as effective as the radical mastectomy in curing early stage disease.[27]

His presentation ignited a firestorm of controversy. Appalled at the notion that conservative surgery might be as good as the radical mastectomy, Jerome Urban accused the reformers of endangering patients, "serving only to confuse and mislead" women and creating "shopping mall medicine" where desperate patients searched for whatever treatment satisfied their preconceived notions. Urban's critique rang hollow; his confidence two decades before in the superradical mastectomy had ended up being nothing more than scientific hype. The American Medical Association also issued a statement, arguing that "large gains in the saving of lives have been achieved by the use of mastectomy, often supplemented by radiation therapy and other treatment. Pending clear proof that equally good results can be achieved by doing less . . . the public should not be stampeded into accepting less proven methods." But Crile, irascible as ever, was not about to back down. Intent on making sure that more women were aware of their options, in 1973 he wrote *What Women Should Know about the Breast Cancer Controversy*.[28]

Although treatment options continued to raise controversy, one theory about breast cancer was gaining credibility. Halsted's assumption that breast cancer was a local disease seemed increasingly tenuous. Radical surgeons had long argued that tumors remained confined to a specific site for an extended period of time. If they remained untreated too long, malignant cells, at a rather precise moment, disengaged from the larger mass and spread centrifugally away from the original site, becoming regional in their destructiveness rather than local. Lymph nodes, they believed, acted as filters, a barrier to the widespread dissemination of tumor cells. Early surgery, by removing the tumor and adjacent lymph nodes, prevented the spread of the disease to distant locations. Such was the logical foundation of surgical oncology.

By the 1960s, the logic seemed badly flawed, and the controversy over radical versus conservative surgery exposed its liabilities. Back in 1948 David Patey, pioneer of the modified radical mastectomy, had concluded that there was not much anybody could do for breast cancer patients, since "in such a high proportion of cases the disease has passed outside the field of local attack when the patient first comes for treatment." Even Jerome Urban had come to the same conclusion. "The obvious failing of all current methods of primary treatment," he wrote in 1963, "is the fact that they comprise local attacks which cannot affect pre-existing systemic spread. While all efforts should be made to combine early diagnosis with prompt and aggressive therapy, this combined effort can be expected to increase our salvage rate only moderately." Just as Hippocrates had believed two millennia before, breast cancer was a systemic disease from the very beginning, and the cures for systemic diseases had to be systemic as well.[29]

But some things had changed. In 1970, Alice Roosevelt Longworth developed cancer again, this time in her other breast. She was eighty-six years old. At first, she insisted on secrecy, explaining away her hospital stay with the quip, "I'm like an old car going in for an overhaul." Surgeons performed another mastectomy. But Alice soon wore her double mastectomies like a badge. The mood of the country had changed since 1956. America was awash in talk about breasts, and feminists had created a new discourse about women's bodies and health issues. She was no longer self-conscious or ashamed that her breasts were gone. Taking a cue from Carol Doda and the nude dancing craze, Alice proudly claimed, "I am America's only topless octogenarian." Breast cancer was about to come out of the closet.[30]

CHAPTER SEVEN

Out of the Closet

BREAST CANCER IN THE 1970S

When Neil Armstrong stepped onto the surface of the moon on July 20, 1969, Americans celebrated the triumph of technology. They had won the space race, upstaged the Soviet Union, and finished a Cold War battle that had begun in May 1961 when President John F. Kennedy stood before Congress and challenged his countrymen: "I believe that this nation should commit itself to achieving the goal, before this decade is out, of landing a man on the moon and returning him safely to earth." Eight years and $25 billion later, *Apollo 11* made good on that commitment. More astronauts soon visited the moon, driving on the dusty surface in a "moonmobile," collecting rock samples, and taking seismic readings. When Alan Shepard, whose suborbital Mercury flight in 1961 made him the first American to fly in space, finally got to the moon in *Apollo 17,* he wielded a club and drove a golf ball over the lunar horizon.

But Americans soon grew complacent about space. Critics questioned the value of the investment—whether billions spent "shooting the moon" had yielded lasting dividends. They often chastised administration officials—Democrats and Republicans—for throwing money at the moon while ignoring serious problems on earth. Politicians searched for another technological sweepstakes, but any new scientific crusade had to show tangible rewards. It also needed to be free of political controversy. Curing cancer seemed ideal. More than 200,000 Americans died of the disease each year. R. Lee Clark, president of the M. D. Anderson Hospital in Houston and a leading oncologist, picked up the space race analogy, claiming that if Congress "would appropriate a billion dollars a year for ten years we could lick cancer." Ann Landers concurred in an April 1971 column, claiming that "if the United States can place a man on the moon, surely we can find the money and technology to cure cancer." The column struck a responsive chord, prompting a million letters and telegrams to Congress. Several congressional secretaries, responsible for answering constituent requests and buried by correspondence, placed "Impeach Ann Landers" placards on their walls.

President Richard Nixon wanted a piece of the action. The cancer crusade played into the hands of Senator Edward Kennedy, who had long since staked out cancer and health care as personal turf. Concerned that Kennedy was considering a run for the presidency in 1972, Nixon wanted to neutralize the cancer issue by making it his own. In his January 1971 State of the Union message, he launched the war on cancer, telling his countrymen, "The time has come when the same kind of concentrated effort that split the atom and took man to the moon should be turned toward conquering this dread disease." Fighting cancer was like supporting motherhood and apple pie. Every American had a friend or relative who had died of cancer, and few politicians were prepared to stall or block Nixon's recommendation for giving the National Cancer Institute independent status and billions of dollars. Congress passed the legislation later in 1971. What neither Ann Landers nor Richard Nixon realized, however, was that compared to finding a cure for cancer, the splitting of the atom and the race to the moon were child's play.[1]

Throughout history, breast cancer had occupied center stage in the cancer drama, but in the 1970s the disease acquired a new public profile. Its demystification began on October 1, 1971, when Senator Birch Bayh of Indiana hastily convened a press conference in the Caucus Room of the Senate Office Building. He told a hushed crowd of reporters and cameramen that he would not seek the 1972 Democratic presidential nomination. His wife, Marvella, had just undergone a mastectomy. "I must put first things first," he told them. "During this time I want to be at her side. Her well-being and rapid recovery are more important to me than seeking the presidency."

Marvella Bayh's ordeal began early in 1970 when she "just began to be aware of my right breast . . . . I began to have these fleeting sensations, maybe two or three times a day." Her surgeon could find no lumps, however, nor did a mammogram reveal a tumor. Relieved, she resumed her normal schedule, but six months later, the sensations returned. "They didn't bother me," she recalled. "I was simply aware of that part of my body." Another physical and mammogram followed. No lumps showed up, but her surgeon noticed a slight discoloration of skin just below the nipple. He also detected a lack of mobility in underlying tissue. Marvella Bayh had a biopsy five days later, and pathologists discovered malignant cells. She underwent a modified radical mastectomy.[2]

After the surgery and her husband's withdrawal from the campaign, Marvella received thousands of letters of support, but the popular press did little with the story. It was not until a middle-aged, former child star openly discussed her battle with the disease that breast cancer began to lose its stigma and become a cause celebre among American women. Shirley Temple had charmed a nation in the worst of times, singing and dancing her way into the hearts of millions during the Great Depression. The sparkling blue eyes, the bouncing curls, the impish, dimpled smile, and the unsullied innocence beguiled a generation anxious to escape its problems. She became the hottest property in Hollywood; her name on the theater marqee guaranteed a full house, and between 1935 and 1938 Temple became the most popular film star in the United States.

Puberty changed everything. Temple was an adorable child and grew up to become a beautiful woman, but in between her eleventh and sixteenth birthdays she had a fluffy, ungainly look. The baby fat lingered a bit too long, as did the ringlets. The charming adolescent became an awkward teenager, and Hollywood image makers pulled Temple out of the spotlight. In 1939, Twentieth Century Fox and later MGM cut her back to one picture a year. She married John Agar, a young actor, in 1946, and had a baby in 1948, but they divorced in 1949. She made her last film, *A Kiss for Corliss,* that year. Temple married Charles Black, a naval officer, in 1950, and they built a happy life for themselves. An active Republican, she became involved in a number of environmental causes before they were politically fashionable. In 1969 President Nixon appointed her U.S. representative to the 24th General Assembly of the United Nations.[3]

Three years later, after decades out of the limelight, she once again

Bathsheba's Breast

won the heart of America. Even though the story originated with the tiny Redwood City (California) *Tribune,* the wire services picked it up and radio, television, and newspapers reported it throughout the country. In a society where breast cancer remained confined to a hidden corner of the national closet, the story was electrifying. Shirley Temple Black had lost a breast to cancer, and she was willing to talk about it, "for all of my sisters who have lost a breast, for all of my sisters who fear that they may." Breast cancer came into the daylight.

Early in September 1972, Shirley was methodically examining her breasts, a routine she regularly performed. "I would kind of run my fingers over my breasts, especially after my menstrual period," she wrote in *McCall's.* "There it was. A lump." Her physician decided, after a physical examination and mammogram, that it was probably a benign cyst. Just to be cautious, he urged her to have a biopsy. Already scheduled to go to Moscow for a Soviet-American conference on the global environment, she postponed the biopsy until November. In the intervening six weeks, "the lump did not . . . grow any larger—at least not to the touch. It did begin to hurt [and] occasionally I was awakened by a burning sensation in my breast."

In the interim, Black carefully reviewed some literature on breast cancer. She rejected out of hand the typical approach. Women routinely entered hospitals for biopsies, signed waivers giving surgeons permission to amputate the breast if the lump proved malignant, and then woke up from the operation wondering whether they still had both breasts. Surgeons claimed the two-for-one approach spared women the ordeal of separate operations involving general anesthesia. "I wouldn't have it that way," Black later wrote. "I find . . . distasteful the prospects of waking up and finding that someone else had made a decision and taken an action in which I, lying quite inert on the operating table, had had no voice . . . . I signed papers that agreed only to an excisional biopsy . . . . The doctor can make the incision; I'll make the decision."[4]

Black's decision first to have a biopsy and later, if necessary, breast cancer surgery, was based on the groundbreaking research of Bernard Fisher. A native of Pittsburgh, Fisher received an undergraduate degree at the University of Pittsburgh in 1940 and a medical degree in 1943. He interned at Mercy Hospital in Pittsburgh and then did surgical residency there. Fisher finally broke away from western Pennsylvania to complete a three-year residency in experimental endocrinology at Columbia-Presbyterian in New York City, followed up by a fellowship in surgery and pathology at the University of Pennsylvania. After a two-year exchange appointment at the London Postgraduate Medical School, he returned as an associate professor of surgery at the University of Pittsburgh. He was destined to become the most influential surgical oncologist in the world.[5]

Fisher had the look, and the personality, of a defensive lineman on a football team. He was big and burly, with a head large enough to match his ego. His square face, large nose, and combed-back dark hair left the impression of someone in charge—all the time. Samuel Hellman, an oncologist at the University of Chicago, described him as "outspoken, very clear, strong in his views and clearly not to be pushed around by the vicissitudes of smaller issues, a guy with a great deal of character and forcefulness." James Holland of the Mount Sinai Medical Center in New York City, was even more direct: "Fisher is a self-disciplined man who knows how to discipline others . . . he had his own agenda," and because "he knew more about [breast cancer] than others, he might not have accepted every piece of advice that was offered to him."

Fisher entered the world of breast cancer in 1958. A colleague invited him to a seminar on chemotherapy protocols, where the merits of surgery and the possibilities of systemic implications were discussed. "At the time," Fisher recalled, "I had no interest in chemotherapy, clinical trials, or breast cancer." That soon changed. Never blindly loyal to tradition, he found intriguing the shrill opposition of so many colleagues to conservative breast cancer surgery. He could understand such reactions to quacks and the alternative therapists, but not to respectable clinical evidence. Hyperbolic opposition smacked of dogma, not science. Bernard Fisher was a surgeon and a pathologist, but above all else he was a scientist who demanded data—data hard enough to withstand the scrutiny of the most sophisticated statisticians.[6]

Ten years later, after a series of experiments and clinical trials, he turned upside down the prevailing logic of malignancy and metastasis. The consensus that had blossomed in the fertile minds of Rudolf Virchow, William Stewart Halsted, and William S. Handley insisted that breast cancer cells did not spread through the bloodstream but along major tissue lines and in the lymphatic system. Lymph nodes, the founding fathers of modern oncology argued, served as barriers to tumor spread, trapping errant cancer cells in their fluid pools. Only after a long period of time, in which the tumors took root and spread from node to node, could the cancer break out of nature's trap and spread to distant sites.

Thus the urgency of the surgeon. Anxious to get the cells before they fled the original site or the lymph nodes, surgeons hurried patients, insisting on operating immediately, and doing so in a single procedure—putting a woman under an anesthetic, excising the tumor for biopsy, and waiting in the operating room for the pathology report. If the tumor was benign, a few sutures closed the wound and ended the operation. But if the pathologist reported cancer, the surgeon performed the mastectomy. Subsequent reports on the excised lymph nodes, according to the conventional wisdom, revealed whether the cancer had spread. If the lymph nodes were negative, physicians believed that they had "got the cancer in time." If the nodes were positive, the dissemination process had already started, but since the nodes trapped cancer cells and held them hostage for a long period of time, removal of the cancer-filled nodes might save the patient.

Fisher would have none of it. The wisdom of the masters did not hold up to laboratory scrutiny. In 1966 he published a series of articles in medical journals, all presenting a new logic of metastasis. He argued that the lymph nodes, if traps at all, were not very effective, and that cancer cells from the breast do not remain long in a lymph node, often traversing the closest nodes and lodging in distant ones. "The majority of tumor cells entering the node," he wrote, "fail to maintain permanent residence." For Fisher, breast cancer could spread through both the lymphatic system and the bloodstream, since "the two vascular systems are so unified . . . it is no longer realistic to consider them independently as routes of neoplastic dissemination." In fact, Fisher argued, breast cancer cells from the beginning of a tumor's life sloughed off into the lymphatic system and into the bloodstream. Cells without a future succumbed to the immune system, but the others, the embryonic tumors, waited to take root somewhere else in the body. Breast cancer was, without question, a systemic disease from the very beginning.[7]

The argument had enormous ramifications. The frenetic, almost obsessive insistence on immediately putting a woman under the knife lost its urgency. Since there probably was no single moment when the tumor broke out of its cage to race through the rest of the body, women had more time to ponder their situation, explore options, and prepare themselves emotionally for the ordeal. Unnecessary delays should be avoided, but emergency breast cancer surgery for early stage disease was not necessary either, except in the most unusual circumstances. Nor was there any compelling reason for combining the biopsy and mastectomy in a single procedure. Except for the inconvenience of two operations, and the small risks inherent in twice putting a patient under general anesthesia, a woman could feel safe having a surgical biopsy and then waiting several weeks before undergoing more surgery.

Fisher's research broke new ground, and in 1967 the National Cancer Institute selected him to head its National Surgical Adjuvant Breast Project, a cooperative, long-term study of breast cancer treatment involving thirty-five medical schools and cancer centers in the United States and Canada. He was the natural choice. He had long ago rejected the superradical mastectomy, arguing that "there is no definite evidence to substantiate the worth of the extended operation." At the same time, he was a prudent scientist, not ready to endorse the promoters of simple mastectomies, quadrantectomies, and lumpectomies. In November 1970, Fisher wrote, "Right now, nobody really knows what the best treatment for breast cancer is. But no clinical therapy should be determined by emotion or conviction—the determinant must be the scientific method." He then set out to solve the breast cancer riddle.[8]

While Fisher tried to solve the riddle, Shirley Temple Black had decisions to make. She understood the implications of his research, choosing the two-stage procedure. The biopsy—performed at the Stanford University Medical Center—revealed a two-centimeter malignant tumor. During the next several weeks, she explored her options, reviewing the merits of a lumpectomy, a simple, or total, mastectomy, a modified radical mastectomy, a Halsted radical mastectomy, and a superradical mastectomy. She knew that "in European countries surgeons had all but given up such drastic procedures when removing a breast." Stanford surgeons recommended a modified radical—removal of the breast, axilla lymph nodes, and some chest muscle tissue. Black balked, and they cautioned her about making a life-threatening choice. She called their bluff, agreeing to a simple mastectomy which involved only removal of the breast. She stipulated in the consent form, however, that surgeons could remove a few lower nodes if they decided it was absolutely necessary. Not surprisingly,

Bathsheba's Breast

they did so. The twelve removed lymph nodes proved negative. Pathologists could not find any other cancer cells in the removed breast.

For all the adoration and special treatment she had received as a child star, Black had grown up to be a remarkably well-adjusted woman. When she took her first look at the mastectomy, she felt "unattractive" but refused to let the feeling linger. She adjusted to the changes in her body, exercising her arm and shoulder regularly and resuming normal activities. "Leave the questions of beauty and vanity aside," she wrote a month after the operation. "In a well-balanced existence, these are unhealthy virtues. Consider instead, as I do, the more fundamental virtues of enthusiasm, intellectual vigor, and the unquenchable desire to serve others until the final bell rings. With or without a breast, I plan to keep doing. Only better." She did just that. In 1974 President Gerald Ford named her U.S. ambassador to Ghana, and she later became ambassador and chief of protocol, the first woman to hold the post. She completed the first volume of her autobiography, *Child Star*, in 1988.[9]

Black's announcement reverberated throughout the country. More than fifty thousand letters poured into Stanford University and Redwood City, California, praising Temple for her courage in going public. In the 1970s cancer was the dread disease; most people held it in awe and terror, not unlike the way their ancestors reacted to leprosy and mental illness. Although breast cancer victims were not exiled to leper colonies or insane asylums, the disease was banished from the public consciousness, swept under the cultural rug, and talked about only in hushed whispers. Black's announcement late in 1972 was a frontal attack on the taboo, boldly proclaiming her "right to do with my body exactly what I wish to do"—and insisting that her womanhood was intact.[10]

Shirley Temple Black's experience coincided with a change in medical thinking. By 1977, only 22 percent of American breast cancer patients received radical mastectomies. Black's insistence on less radical surgery would not have happened without the women's movement, the breast obsession of American popular culture, the clinical trials of courageous physicians willing to test alternatives to the radical mastectomy, and the development of mammography, which permitted earlier diagnosis. Eighty years earlier, Wilhelm Roentgen had discovered x-rays, but it was Adolf Saloman, a German surgeon practicing in Berlin, who first applied diagnostic radiology to breast cancer. By then it was clear that a woman's chances of surviving the disease were directly related to its stage. The earlier she reported to a surgeon, the longer her probable life span. Intent on correlating the gross, radiographic, and microscopic appearance of normal and malignant tissues, Saloman began collecting amputated breasts in 1898. By 1912, his collection filled more than three thousand glass jars. He carefully examined each with x-rays and a microscope, and in 1913 he announced the ability to recognize occult breast tumors—tumors too small to be detected by touch—on the film.

It was not until 1960, however, with the work of Thomas Egan at M. D. Anderson Hospital, that mammography developed into a reliable diagnostic tool. Egan developed an easily reproducible, low-kilovoltage technique using inexpensive film. In 1965 the American College of Radiology (ACR) established a Committee on Mammography, and with funding from the U.S. Public Health Service the ACR began training radiologists and technicians around the country. Within five years, mammography had become a potent diagnostic tool in detecting clinically occult tumors. The Health Insurance Plan of Greater New York reported five-year results in 1973. In a control group of women with no visible or palpable symptoms, who received mammography and physical examinations, mortality rates from breast cancer were down by nearly one-third. With increasing numbers of women reporting to physicians earlier in the disease process, surgeons became more willing to consider less radical forms of surgery.[11]

The availability of less mutilating surgeries encouraged women to seek early treatment. But so did the media focus on prominent Americans suffering from breast cancer, especially in 1974 when Betty Ford and Happy Rockefeller contracted the disease. Betty Ford moved into the White House in August 1974, when Richard Nixon's resignation over Watergate made Gerald Ford the thirty-eighth president of the United States. Several days after taking the oath of office, Ford extended a general pardon to Nixon for any crimes he had committed while serving as president. Controversy engulfed the White House. At the time, Betty Ford was trying to move from their home so that family life could settle into at least a semblance of routine.

Six weeks later, on September 26, 1974, when her aide Nancy Howe had an appointment for a physical at the National Naval Medical Center in Bethesda, Maryland, the First Lady decided to go along and have a physical of her own. Howe's was routine. Ford's was not. The gynecologist suddenly stopped, midway through the breast examination, and excused himself from the room. "I thought that was kind of strange," she wrote later, "leaving right in the middle of the check-up." He was not gone for long, returning in a few minutes with William Fouty, the hospital's chief of surgery, who completed the examination. Somewhat ominously, the physicians said nothing to the First Lady. When she got back to the White House, a message awaited her. At seven o'clock that evening, she was to meet with William Lukash, the White House physician. "During that afternoon," the First Lady recalled, "I began to have my first suspicion that something might be seriously wrong." That night, Lukash and Richard Thistlethwaite, a surgeon at George Washington University, examined her again and confirmed the presence of a lump in the right breast. They scheduled a biopsy for the next Saturday, reassuring her that nine out of ten biopsies end up negative. She felt a little better, knowing that "the odds are in your favor and you don't really believe that you'll be that one woman."

Fouty, who headed the surgical team, opposed a lumpectomy. As far as he was concerned, surgeons who recommended more limited procedures placed their patients at risk by leaving behind invisible tumors. He wanted to put the First Lady under a general anesthetic, remove the lump, wait for the frozen section, and, if the tumor was malignant, remove the breast then and there. He wanted to perform a more aggressive operation. "There is a much greater risk," he told the Fords, "with anything less because lymph nodes can't, in many cases, be clinically tested for cancer." Betty Ford listened quietly and accepted the recommendation. "I'd rather have them take the whole breast area and not leave any residue which could cause complications in the future."

She checked into Bethesda on the night before the surgery, staying in the presidential suite. A small party of family and friends joined the Fords for dinner at the hospital. As they dined, the White House press secretary announced to assembled reporters that the First Lady had entered the hospital for a breast biopsy. The story was on the front pages of newspapers across the country the next morning when the operation took place. As the orderlies wheeled her into the operating room, Betty Ford already suspected that the tumor was malignant. "I know that wasn't really logical, but somehow I think I went into that operating room with a pretty clear belief that the biopsy would show a malignancy." Fouty and the surgical team waited for the frozen sections of the excised tumor tissue, and when pathologists confirmed the malignancy, they performed a modified radical mastectomy. On Saturday afternoon, another press conference broke the news. Naval hospital pathologists completed their examination of the lymph nodes four days later. Several contained tumor cells, but most were clear. Betty Ford later wrote, "When they found that the cancer had already spread to a couple of lymph nodes, it made me even more certain that they did the right thing [modified radical mastectomy]. What it really amounts to is that it should be [removing] the cancer—not the vanity of losing a breast."[12]

Three weeks after Betty Ford's surgery, Nelson Rockefeller scheduled a press conference. It came as no surprise to reporters covering the ex-governor of New York, whose battle to win Senate confirmation as the next vice-president of the United States was reaching a climax. With Spiro Agnew gone after federal felony charges had led to his resignation, Gerald Ford needed a vice-president, and he had given the nod to Rockefeller. The nomination generated controversy. Conservative Republicans had never forgiven Rockefeller for not supporting Barry Goldwater in the election of 1964, and rumors of trouble with the Internal Revenue Service also dogged him. Supporters scoffed at the rumors that he had underpaid his income taxes. With a net worth in the hundreds of millions of dollars, Nelson Rockefeller was not about to risk presidential ambitions for a measly million dollars in taxes. Reporters and cameramen jostling for position in the office expected him to respond to the rumors.

The sharks in the press corps smelled blood as the grim-faced Rockefeller settled in behind the microphones. "Ladies and gentlemen," he announced, "you're not going to believe what I'm going to tell you. Happy has just had a radical mastectomy of the left breast, or at least she's under operation right now." Caught off-guard, the reporters quietly absorbed the news. Rockefeller went on to explain that the surgery was very similar to what Betty Ford had experienced three weeks earlier. When the reporters then tried to shift the focus of the press conference back to politics, he shot back, "I think at this time perhaps all of us should think about Happy's future, which is the one concern I have."

When Betty Ford announced her mastectomy early in October, Happy's stomach had twisted a bit, as did those of millions of other women. Although she had undergone a physical examination back in June, complete with a careful breast examination by a skilled surgeon, she found Ford's announcement unsettling. Later that evening, before going to bed, she examined both breasts and panicked. A hard lump the size of the tip of her finger was lodged in the outer, upper quadrant of her left breast. The next day, a radiologist diagnosed the presence of a solid mass. A subsequent needle biopsy confirmed her worst fears: the tumor was malignant.

The wife of one of the world's richest and most powerful men can afford the best treatment money can buy, and the best place on earth to be treated for breast cancer in 1974 was Memorial Sloan-Kettering Hospital, at 68th Street and First Avenue on the east side of Manhattan. Entering through a side door, Happy checked into the hospital on October 16 and settled into a sunny, corner suite. Secret Service agents detailed the hallway and special-duty nurses kept a constant vigil. Happy and Nelson enjoyed a quiet dinner—filet mignon with mushroom sauce—catered by a favorite restaurant, and a glass of sherry on mastectomy's eve. Just before she retired for the evening, Jerome Urban, her surgeon and the father of the superradical mastectomy, visited for the third time that day, making sure Happy was comfortable and ready.

Urban had already spent considerably more time with Happy Rockefeller than he had with any other preoperative patient in his career. In the previous ten years, the Rockefeller family had bestowed more than $20 million on Sloan-Kettering, and Rockefeller's brother, Lawrence, sat on the hospital's board of directors. Sloan-Kettering administrators were determined to give Happy the full benefit of state-of-the-art technology and to handle her case with patience, sensitivity, and skill. Urban no longer performed superradical mastectomies; he was now an advocate of the radical mastectomy. Happy opted for more conservative surgery. Urban acceded to her wishes, making sure to explain carefully all of her options and their ramifications. The next morning, he removed the breast, pulled thirty-two lymph nodes out of the axilla, and dissected a small portion of Happy's chest muscles—a modified radical mastectomy. He took more time than usual—a total of three and a half hours.

The anesthesiologists carefully put Happy to sleep, planning to drug her enough to achieve pain-free unconsciousness but not enough to prolong her postoperative recovery. In fact, they were too stingy with the drugs. Happy awoke while Urban was still dressing the wound. She opened her eyes and whispered, "Where am I?" The startled surgical team took quick breaths, and Urban calmly replied, "Everything is finished." Slipping back into a languid semiconsciousness, she sighed, "Thank goodness."

Only good news greeted Happy Rockefeller during her week-long stay at Memorial. Free of nausea, she ate real food nine hours after the operation, walked down the halls with a portable tube draining the surgical wound, and was able to visit with close friends. The pathology reports could not have been better; none of the nodes contained cancer cells. She was relieved but not completely surprised. Urban had reassured her that if someone has to get breast cancer, one of the best places to get it is the upper, outer quadrant of the breast.[13]

But cancer still lurked in her body. Ever cautious, Urban had biopsied Happy's right breast during the mastectomy. Biostatisticians have known for years that women with cancer in one breast have a small but nevertheless very real chance of developing a malignant tumor in the other breast. Beginning early in the 1960s, during mastectomies, Urban routinely cut out a wedge of tissue from the corresponding position of the patient's other breast, on the chance of discovering early cancers. He removed a wedge of Happy's right breast just above the nipple. Most surgeons refused to perform prophylactic biopsies, arguing that they were "eyeball procedures" with little chance of success. Many surgeons also believed such an operation was dangerous, since it left a scar which would make future mammograms less effective. Still, Urban went ahead. He was an exceedingly meticulous doctor; if there was a loose cancer cell anywhere, he wanted to cut it out.[14]

His hunch and "eyeball" examination played out well this time. Frozen sections from that excised tissue returned from the lab before he finished the mastectomy on Rockefeller's left breast. The results were inconclusive. But a day later, the permanent slides revealed several tiny, pin-head-size tumors. Urban told Nelson Rockefeller the news, but they decided not to break it to Happy until she had recovered from surgery. The doctor then left for a two-week medical conference in Rome. When Edward Beattie, who had assisted with the first mastectomy, learned of the new tumors, he wanted to tell her and announce it publicly, hoping to promote public health campaigns about breast cancer. But Nelson Rockefeller

Bathsheba's Breast

demurred, gently at first but adamantly at last, testily insisting to Beattie, "You are responsible not only for her physical condition but for her psychological and emotional condition. You will not say anything to her or to anyone else."[15]

Three weeks later, during a follow-up visit with Urban, Happy casually inquired about the results of the right breast biopsy. He told her the bad news and she accepted it stoically. Urban reassured her that the tumors were too small to be felt by hand and too little to show up on a mammogram. They were microscopic in size and confined within the walls of the milk ducts. When she asked about treatment, he played his aggressive hand, promoting a simple mastectomy to remove the right breast but not any lymph nodes. The Rockefellers spent a few days exploring the alternatives, consulting with more conservative surgeons as well as radiotherapists and chemotherapists, all of whom argued that even a simple mastectomy was too much. But Urban prevailed. In a press conference, Nelson explained his wife's decision: "Her doctor [Urban] is of the school that thinks to operate and remove the source is the best way to protect her future . . . . She has total confidence in him." The editors of the *British Medical Journal* did not share her faith. "Few surgeons," they argued, "have been tempted to follow Dr. Urban's lead."[16]

On November 24, five weeks after the removal of her left breast, Happy Rockefeller returned to Memorial Sloan-Kettering. Early that evening, Nelson Rockefeller held another press conference, telling America that his wife was going under the scalpel again. The surgery was uneventful. Urban removed the breast and then had pathologists examine some of the small lymph nodes within the excised tissue. They found no cancer cells. He confidently told the Rockefellers that Happy's chance of living out her normal life span was better than 90 percent. There would be no need for radiotherapy or chemotherapy. When Nelson left Memorial after spending the evening with Happy on the day of the surgery, reporters inquired about her condition. He assured them, "She's sitting up and is very grateful for all the messages of good will." They quickly turned to politics, asking about the vice-presidential confirmation and recent stories that he owed more than a million dollars in back taxes. Shaking his head in exasperation, Rockefeller cut them short: "I want to tell you how well Happy is. On some other occasion, I'll discuss politics with you." Happy Rockefeller survived her breast cancers.[17]

So did Betty Rollin, an NBC news correspondent who reported the Ford and Rockefeller stories, not even knowing that she "had it herself." At the time, she knew of a hard lump on the outer side of her left breast, but mammograms had missed it and several physicians told her not to worry. Raised in a health-conscious Jewish household, Rollin knew that the disease was unusually common among "first-generation Jewish women of East European extraction," but her mother's obsessive dietary regimen had always seemed to offer some protection. Rollin was a thirty-seven-year-old woman at the pinnacle of her profession. "I was confident and lucky," she later wrote. "My confidence, moreover, was not limited to myself but encompassed my world. I knew in my head that life was capricious and worse; I had read about the Nazi holocaust, I had a sense of what was going on in remote places like Vietnam and around the corner in Harlem. But—I couldn't help it—none of the bad stuff had ever touched me directly. In my life, deprivation, injustice, disease were as remote as Bangladesh . . . as unlikely as cancer."

But safety was an illusion. The lump did not go away, and in the spring of 1975, a year after being told it was nothing, Rollin learned it was everything. Several whirlwind days of examinations, mammograms, and tests led to a biopsy and a modified radical mastectomy. When she awoke to a heavily bandaged chest and the realization that her left breast was gone, frustration at the physicians who had told her a year before not to worry exploded into rage. "I wanted to kill them both," Rollin thought, and she wanted to tell them, "What if I were your wife? Would you have let your wife sit around for a year with a lump, a hard, cancerous lump? Would you? Would you?" Waiting for the lymph nodes reports was excruciatingly difficult; she wondered if the delay in treatment had allowed the disease to spread. Mercifully, her excised nodes were negative.

She never rehearsed any "why me" dialogues, perhaps because "it had something to do with the Vietnamese war, which happened to be ending while I was in the hospital, and like everyone else I watched it on television . . . . I marveled at the pure unluckiness of being born a Vietnamese in the twentieth century . . . . I felt that losing a breast was lousy, but I never felt that losing a breast was unfair. Not really." That did not make coming to terms with the mastectomy any easier. She felt mutilated, her chest a "flat, lumpy surface like the ground, covered with, instead of dirt, skin. Across the surface, a long, horizontal, red, puffy welt meandered crazily from the center of my chest, where a cleavage once was, to the other side, under the arm, and around toward the back. And alongside this little Hiroshima of the torso, on the unbombed half, grotesque by contrast, lay a right breast, pretty and whole as a healthy baby."

Time helped Betty Rollin heal. So did writing. The revelations of Shirley Temple Black, Marvella Bayh, Betty Ford, and Happy Rockefeller had illuminated breast cancer, making it the most talked-about disease in the country. One afternoon after Rollin went back to work, she encountered another NBC woman reporter in the hallway. "I hear you've got this year's chick disease," the colleague remarked. The woman may have been grossly insensitive or just nervous, trying awkwardly to make conversation, but she had hit on a reality. With the disease out of the closet, a market existed for a good book, a personal narrative detailing an encounter with breast cancer. Rollin decided to write it. A year later, in 1976, *First, You Cry* was on the best-seller list. Two years after that, Mary Tyler Moore played Betty Rollin in *First, You Cry,* a highly acclaimed made-for-television movie.[18]

Betty Rollin did not have chemotherapy. In the 1970s oncologists reserved chemo for women with positive lymph nodes. Betty Ford's decision to undergo chemotherapy was directly linked to Bernard Fisher's research. The ferocious arguments over the relative merits of the super-radical, radical, modified radical, and simple mastectomies, he claimed, had been debated in the flawed context of outmoded theories of metastasis. If malignant cells had already broken away from the original tumor, and if the patient's immunological system could not handle them, no surgical procedure—radical or conservative—was going to save the patient. It was certainly no coincidence, he claimed, that the trend had been toward less radical, less damaging surgery. The new, modern challenge for surgeons was to develop less destructive operations without compromising survival rates. Significant improvements in survival rates would come in the pharmacy, not the operating theater. Many women already had metastases before they even felt the tumor, before a mammogram ever picked up the tumor, before the surgeon ever excised it. Surgery could never remove every malignant cell, nor could radiotherapy ionize all of them; they were already floating in the circulatory system.

Scientists would have to continue their search for effective anticancer drugs which could reach every cell in the body. Although most surgeons disliked the news, Fisher argued that the only hope of ever curing breast cancer would be for surgeons "to reduce the tumor burden to a number of viable cells [which can be] entirely destroyed" by anticancer drugs and the patient's immune system. He even predicted, "It is likely that at some time in the not too distant future, when diagnostic methodology has improved so that earlier cancers are detected, and when there is a better understanding regarding the proper use of anti-cancer agents in concert so as to maximize effectiveness, surgery will play a subsidiary role in the management of solid tumors and may be entirely supplanted by other modalities."[19]

By the mid-1970s, most of the anticancer drugs in use today had already been synthesized. The anticancer pharmacopia was diverse, with a number of bizarrely-labeled drugs showing some promise in treating malignancies: methotrexate, 5-fluorouracil, 6-thioguanine, actinomycin D, busulfan, cisplatin, 6-mercaptopurine, cyclophosphamide, melphalan, triethylene thiophosphoramide, bleomycin, vincristine, vinblastine, nitrosoureas, streptozocin, daunorubicin, procarbazine, cytosine, Adriamycin, L-asparaginase, cycloytidine, rubidozone, maytansine, hexamethylmelmine, prednisone, vindesine, and pyrazofurin, to name a few. Of these drugs, only five had positive effects on breast cancer: cyclophosphamide, methotrexate, 5-fluorouracil, Adriamycin, and vincristine.

Cyclophosphamide, or Cytoxan, is an alkylating agent which attacks malignant cells by binding to their DNA as they divide, preventing the cell from replicating successfully. Methotrexate and 5-flourouracil are antimetabolites, which resemble cellular nutrients. The cancer cell mistakes the drug for food and ingests it, after which the drug interrupts the cell's ability to reproduce because the cell, thinking it is well-nourished, starves to death. Adriamycin is an antibiotic cancer drug with extremely powerful properties. Antibiotics fight infectious diseases, but adriamycin is too toxic for such uses. In cancer patients, the drug kills malignant cells by inserting itself into strands of DNA and disturbing normal cellular processes. Vincristine, a derivative from the periwinkle plant, is also toxic to malignant cells.[20]

As clinical trials evolved in the 1970s, physicians learned the limits of single agent chemotherapy. Only 20 to 33 percent of women experienced at least some regression in their tumors. Most did not respond. Scientists today know that all cells carry a protein, called P-glycoprotein, that acts like a pump, controlling the passage of drugs into and out of a cell.

Tumor cells with large amounts of P-glycoprotein block the admission of anticancer drugs and remain unscathed. Tumor cells with insufficent P-glycoprotein are vulnerable. Clinical trials also revealed that women who did respond did so only for a while. Over time the drug lost its effectiveness, perhaps because some tumor cells possessed greater amounts of P-glycoprotein than others. Tumor cells with insufficient amounts of the protein died out, bringing about a regression of the tumor, but those with sufficient amounts survived. When they reproduced, the new cells were biochemical clones, loaded with P-glycoprotein and resistant to chemotherapy. At that point, the tumors reasserted themselves.[21]

Richard Cooper, a Harvard-trained oncologist at the University of Rochester, came up with the idea of combination chemotherapy—different drugs affect cancer cells at different stages of cell division. By administering several drugs simultaneously, or in carefully measured sequences, more cells would die, reducing the number of resistant cells and delaying their evolution into new tumors. The goal of combination chemotherapy was to reduce the number of malignant cells—the "malignant burden"—to zero, or at least to levels manageable by the immune system. In the original combinations he used, Cooper increased response rates to 50 percent—half the women taking the drugs enjoyed reductions in the size and activity of their tumors. The best results—a response rate of two-thirds—came from the combination of Cytoxan, Adriamycin, and 5-fluorouracil.[22]

In 1979 Bernard Fisher delivered an obituary on the Halsted radical mastectomy. Most American surgeons had already abandoned it. Since 1967, as director of the National Surgical Adjuvant Breast Project, Fisher had carefully accumulated data and was ready with the first of many conclusions. From thirty-five cooperating medical centers in the United States and Canada, he had tracked 1,680 women for at least six years. Each had undergone a radical mastectomy or a simple mastectomy followed up by radiotherapy. For women whose diseases had not spread to the lymph nodes, the results were virtually identical, regardless of the treatment protocol they had received. Just over 73.1 percent had survived cancer-free for at least six years. The results were similar for patients whose lymph nodes were involved. Of those receiving the radical mastectomy, 57.9 percent survived. Simple mastectomy recipients who had also undergone radiotherapy survived at a rate of 55.4 percent. The National Cancer Institute, after reviewing the report early in June 1979, formally recommended the modified radical mastectomy—removal of the breast and axilla lymph nodes—as the treatment of choice for women suffering from single-site breast cancer. Bernard Fisher had closed the lid on Halsted's coffin once and for all.[23]

On the surface, at least, an illusion of real progress dominated public discussion in the 1970s. The frankness and courage of Shirley Temple Black, Betty Ford, Happy Rockefeller, and Betty Rollin forced breast cancer out of its cultural closet, demystified its sexual implications, and allowed millions of women to discuss the disease openly and overcome any reluctance to seek early treatment. Breast cancer's stigma began to disappear. Science offered new technologies for treating the disease. Mammography provided a cost-effective means of detecting small tumors long before they were palpable to touch. Women received treatment at earlier, more curable stages of the disease, and surgeons employed less mutilating operations. Fisher's research into the nature of metastasis had confirmed the theory that breast cancer was a systemic disease from the very beginning and needed systemic treatment, and new chemotherapy regimens were available for women. More informed and empowered than ever before, American women played direct roles in determining their own treatment.

But for all the encouraging developments, breast cancer remained a killer. At the end of the 1970s, the disease was claiming forty thousand women a year. One of them was Minnie Riperton. The popular African-American vocalist caught Flip Wilson off-guard one October evening in 1976. The comedian, substituting for Johnny Carson on *The Tonight Show*, had just completed a "devil made me do it" monologue, and Riperton was the first guest. At the time, Wilson was serving as honorary chairman of the 1976 American Cancer Society's National Cancer Fund. After a few moments of small talk, Riperton dropped the bombshell: "You know, Flip, I found out I had breast cancer last month and had a mastectomy." For once in his life, Wilson was speechless. He let her continue: "Just because a woman has had a mastectomy and now has one breast, there's no reason to think her life has been ruined—sexually or physically. I have three scars—one on my leg, where I was hit by a car when I was a kid, one from having my babies, and now this one." Wilson kissed her cheek. The studio audience applauded spontaneously. "There's nothing different about me except I've had the operation. I'm young and strong and I have a full life ahead of me."

Minnie Riperton was twenty-eight at the time. The lump in her right breast had been a small one. A health food enthusiast who felt "in tune" with her body, Riperton experienced an unsettling, if imprecise, sense of misgiving in the summer of 1976, suspecting something was wrong but not knowing exactly what. She kept up a steady examination of her breasts, focusing on them as the source of her inexplicable sense of unease, and late in September she felt the lump. She visited her physician immediately. "But I knew from the beginning that everything would turn out well," she recalled. "For instance, it so happened that one of the best surgeons in the country was in his office right down the hall. My doctor took me in to meet him." Minnie Riperton was the most positive of positive thinkers.

Even positive thinking cannot help many African-American women suffering from breast cancer. Their death rates from the disease are substantially higher than those of white women. Epidemiologists have tried to explain the phenomenon. Poor women—black and white—often postpone treatment until it is too late because they cannot afford the cost of American medicine. They are also less likely to receive regular mammograms and perform breast self-examination. But socioeconomic factors alone cannot explain the discrepancy. The tumors black women get are often more aggressive and virulent than those of white women. A different biology is at work. Breast cancers in black women are less likely to be hormone dependent and, therefore, are harder to treat. Their tumor cells often divide more rapidly and metastasize more quickly. Minnie Riperton had one of those nasty, dangerous lesions.

A few days later, she had a modified radical mastectomy. The tumor was small, but her lymph nodes were already heavily involved. Chemotherapy was essential. Tomeo Hirahira, her Los Angeles chemotherapist, prescribed a standard regimen of combined drug therapy. Meanwhile, Riperton got on with her life. She continued to speak openly about breast cancer, reassuring tens of millions of American women that "this is not something you have to hide from. It doesn't change your sex life." She worked actively with the American Cancer Society, serving as its education chairman in 1978—the first black woman to occupy the post—and planned her fourth album, to be called *Minnie*.

She barely had enough time to finish it. In November 1978, a sizable lump popped up in her upper right arm, the result of an explosive tumor in the regional lymph nodes. Hirahira resumed the chemotherapy, which she had just finished a few months before, but it was already too late, and had been from the moment Riperton discovered the first lump two years earlier. She finished the album in February 1979 and tried to go on the road to promote it, but she did not have the energy to complete the tour. She entered Cedars-Sinai Medical Center in Los Angeles on July 10 and died two days later. Her death caught her friends off-guard, since she had not talked openly about her recurrence. One woman was shocked and remarked, "But I thought she was cured. I thought she was well after the mastectomy. She talked about it!" No amount of talk and positive thinking could save Minnie Riperton.[24]

CHAPTER EIGHT

Patient Heal Thyself

QUACKS AND CURES IN THE AGE OF NARCISSISM

*S*he hated the cure as much as she hated the disease. In 1959, before it all started, Cecile Pollack Hoffman reveled in the good life. A schoolteacher in San Diego, she basked in the ambience of southern California and the solid, upper-middle-class lifestyle two incomes provided. Her husband was a successful businessman. The Hoffmans felt in control, at least until Cecile found the lump. She sought medical assistance immediately, and her surgeon operated the next day, performing a biopsy and then a radical mastectomy, all in the same procedure. She recovered slowly. Constant pain afflicted her left side, and severe swelling limited her arm's mobility. Nor could she wear the dresses she liked so much. The cancer recurred three years later, even though the surgeons had supposedly "gotten it all." The new tumor in the skin of her chest required another operation which in her mind only magnified the original mutilation. Cecile Hoffman was angry and depressed.

A few months after the second surgery, her husband missed a flight on a business trip and spent several hours in the airport. Anxious for something to read, he picked up a copy of Glenn Kittler's *Laetrile: Control of Cancer*. The book was an answer to his prayers. Laetrile could cure Cecile's cancer without any more operations and restore the quality of their lives. Cecile devoured the book in one sitting and embarked on an

Ivy, a leading physiologist at the University of Illinois and former chairman of the National Advisory Council on Cancer, an arm of the National Cancer Institute. At Ivy's urging, the ordinarily astute Senator Paul Douglas of Illinois sponsored legislation to allow the Durovics to become permanent residents of the United States. Throughout the 1950s and early 1960s, they marketed "Krebiozen." The FDA would not allow the drug to be sold in interstate commerce because Durovic refused to explain how he made it. When scientists from the American Medical Association learned that it consisted of nothing more than mineral water and horse blood, it labeled Krebiozen "one of the greatest frauds of the 20th century." The FDA started judicial proceedings against Durovic in the 1960s; he fled the country in 1966 to avoid prosecution for tax evasion.[4]

The Koches, Hoxeys, and Durovics disappeared, but cultural change and scientific controversy in the 1960s created fertile ground for a new generation of medical charlatans. Patriotism and love of country were not the only casualties of Vietnam and Watergate. Americans rebelled against many of their institutions, including the medical establishment. They revered Dr. Kildare, Ben Casey, and Marcus Welby—television physicians who supposedly really cared about their patients—but such concerned healers were relics of the past, gone the way of Model-T Fords, soda fountains, and band concerts in the park. Americans found themselves dealing with skyrocketing health care costs, overpaid physicians masquerading as demigods, and huge insurance companies systematically excluding the sickest people from coverage. Doctors and hospitals appeared stricken with a case of terminal greed.

The fact that technology offered so little to cancer patients reinforced public resentment. In 1967, oncologist Michael Shimkin wrote, "So far as the therapeutic effect on this entity is concerned, we have been on a plateau for approximately the last thirty years . . . with all our medical advances, the best figures we can gather indicate that we have not improved markedly the prognosis of, and salvage from, cancer of the breast." More than a decade later, John S. Stehlin of M. D. Anderson Hospital, echoed that frustration: "Whether the physician advocates standard radical mastectomy, modified radical mastectomy, simple mastectomy with or without radiation therapy, or local excision plus radiation therapy, the survival rates are so similar as to produce discouragement about which procedure is best." A 1972 editorial in the *British Medical Journal* summed up the chaos: "There is more controversy about the management of breast cancer than almost any other topic in tumor therapy, and more so than ever before."[5]

Controversy infected every element of breast cancer treatment. The debate over surgery was as intense as ever. The National Cancer Institute's vote in 1979 to endorse modified radical mastectomies over radical mastectomies for early stage disease did little to subdue the dissension. European surgeons were still muddying the medical waters. Since 1973, Umberto Veronesi, head of Italy's National Cancer Institute, had tracked 150 women treated for small breast tumors that had not spread to neighboring lymph nodes. He biopsied patients before adding them to the clinical trials. Women whose lymph nodes showed any sign of cancer were eliminated from the study. Women who became part of the trial could choose a simple mastectomy—removal of the breast—or a lumpectomy. Five-year cancer-free survival rates exceeded 90 percent for both groups. Guy's Hospital in London reported similar results. Their study involved women over the age of fifty with tumors less than five centimeters in size and whose axillary nodes were not involved or, if involved, were movable to the touch. One group received a local excision of the tumor and the other a radical mastectomy. Both groups received radiotherapy. Ten-year survival rates were the same. Almost as soon as the radical mastectomy had been defeated, an attack on the modified radical mastectomy was under way.[6]

A few mavericks questioned the wisdom of any surgery for breast cancer. George Crile speculated in the late 1960s that major surgery might, in some cases, encourage metastasis. He was not sure how, but he wondered if the shock of major surgery might somehow compromise the immune system. Major surgery always takes a toll, temporarily at least, on patients. He also questioned the practice of routinely removing axillary lymph nodes. Between 1957 and 1964, Crile conducted a study in which 116 women received total mastectomies—removal of only the breast, not the lymph nodes—and sixty received traditional radical or modified radical surgery. Five-year survival rates astonished him. Almost 85 percent of the women whose lymph nodes had been preserved survived, while only 70 percent of those undergoing radical surgery made it. He concluded that the lymph nodes actually had a furtive immunological function, and that women without them were at risk because their own bodies were less capable of fighting back. Few oncologists shared his convictions, but the discussion made its way into the popular press and magnified the prevailing confusion.[7]

Controversy was not just confined to surgeons. Early in the 1970s, several European and American oncologists raised doubts about the usefulness of radiotherapy. Jan Stjerneswärd, an oncologist with the Swiss Institute for Experimental Research, reported bad news to radiotherapists in November 1974. In six separate clinical trials involving women with early stage breast cancer, half the patients received a radical mastectomy, while the others received radical surgery and follow-up radiotherapy. "Survival rates," he concluded, "were significantly lower among those women who were irradiated than among those who were treated by mastectomy alone." Stjerneswärd went on to argue that the routine use of what he called "prophylactic local radio-therapy after radical mastectomy" should be stopped. Dr. Thomas Dao of the Roswell Park Cancer Institute in New York had already reached the same conclusion. His own studies revealed that postoperative radiotherapy actually increased the chances of distant metastasis.[8]

Radiotherapy, in some instances, produced dangerous, long-term side effects. Within a few years of the atomic bombings of Japan, leukemia and lymphoma rates in Hiroshima and Nagasaki spiked, proving the connection between cancer and exposure to radiation. Oncologists wondered about the relationship between radiotherapy for cancer and the chance of developing subsequent, radiation-induced tumors. Data confirmed their fears. Patients with Hodgkin's disease risked developing thyroid cancer and breast cancer later in life if they were treated with radiotherapy. Retinoblastoma patients sometimes end up with osteosarcomas and soft tissue sarcomas after radiation. Breast cancer radiotherapy led to a slightly increased risk of several different tumors within the radiation field. While most cancer survivors who received radiation therapy did not fall victim to so-called "second cancers," their chances of contracting another malignancy appeared to be about three times higher than those of the rest of the population.[9]

Several celebrity deaths deepened the fear. In 1954 RKO made the film *The Conqueror*, starring John Wayne, Dick Powell, Pedro Armendariz, Susan Hayward, and Agnes Moorehead, in St. George, Utah. Of the 220 members of the cast and crew, ninety-one came down with cancer later in their lives, a number three times higher than actuarial tables would suggest. Forty-six people had died of the disease by 1980. Wayne survived lung cancer in 1964 but later succumbed to stomach cancer. Pedro Armendariz contracted kidney cancer in 1959 and then committed suicide in 1963 when diagnosed with cancer of the larynx. Dick Powell fell victim to lung cancer. Agnes Moorehead died of uterine cancer, and Susan Hayward ended up with cancers of the skin, breast, uterus, and brain. Dr. Robert Pendleton, a radiologist at the University of Utah, claimed that with "these numbers, this case could qualify as an epidemic."[10]

Epidemiologists searching for an explanation noted that most of the dead had been smokers, but they also knew that *The Conqueror* was filmed in the Escalante Valley of southern Utah. The Atomic Energy Commission detonated eleven atomic bombs in the dry lake bed of Yucca Flats, Nevada, in 1953. Two of them were especially "dirty" with strontium 90 and cesium 137 isotopes. "Dirty Simon" exploded on April 25, and "Dirty Harry" went off on May 19. Both fireballs covered the surrounding desert with a fine gray ash. An aberrant wind carried Dirty Harry's fallout 150 miles to the east, blanketing St. George, Utah, and the Escalante Valley. The "hot" ash soon disappeared into southern Utah's red sands, but winds blew radioactive dust into the dunes of Snow Canyon, which served as a natural reservoir. Most of *The Conqueror*'s battle scenes were filmed there. Levels of strontium 90 and cesium 137 were high enough to set off wild ticks in Geiger counters. Crew members were covered in dust by the end of each day, and cast members had to be frequently blown clean of dust with compressed air and given time to rinse the dirt out of their mouths and eyes. Powell then trucked more than sixty tons of Snow Canyon dirt back to Culver City, California, to make sure the interior scenes had the same color texture, and for another two months the cast and crew wallowed in the radioactive mix.[11]

Chemotherapy also had long-term risks. Several antibiotic chemotherapy drugs—such as daunorubicin and Adriamycin—can lead to congestive heart failure in some patients. Bleomycin can poison lung tissues and stimulate lung fibrosis. Cisplatin damages kidneys and can cause hearing loss in others. Vincristine often produces numbness in the fingers and toes, as well as a permanent, painful jaw ache. Some chemotherapy agents induce sterility. Alkylating agents like Cytoxan are capable of causing genetic damage. A few anticancer drugs are carcinogenic. Chlorambusil is used to treat certain leukemias and lymphomas, but it is also known to cause leukemia in some recipients. Cytoxan, a treatment for a variety of malignancies, including breast cancer, can trigger outbreaks of leukemia and bladder cancer. Women who take diethylstilbesterol and naturally occurring estrogens for cancer may have increased risk of getting endometrial, ovarian, and breast cancer. Melphalan, a drug for breast cancer, multiple myeloma, and ovarian cancer, triggers leukemia in some patients.[12]

In the age of the credibility gap, the Pentagon Papers, the Nixon and Agnew resignations, and the assassinations of John Kennedy, Martin Luther King, Jr., and Robert Kennedy, when millions of Americans questioned traditional institutions, the controversies surrounding cancer treatment proved to be a politically combustible combination. Extremists detected a sinister cabal to keep cancer cures off the market, and medical entrepreneurs profited from the misery.

The medicine cabinet of the counterculture contained a host of dubious remedies. Some masqueraded as anticancer chemotherapies. In Denver, Philip Schuch promoted an anticancer magic potion called Radio-Sulfo Brew. It was actually a Limburger cheese poultice, which patients applied—assuming they survived the smell—to tumors every twelve hours. Virginia Livingston, a Pennsylvania physician, said cancer was caused by a bacterium which invaded nutritionally weakened tissues. Her medicine—a concoction of the patient's own urine supplemented with various vitamins and minerals—supposedly strengthened normal cells and blocked the invasion of cancer-causing agents. In 1979 CBS-TV's *60 Minutes* praised the virtues of Lawrence Burton, a zoologist whose so-called "Immuno-Augmentative Therapy" (IAT) allegedly energized the immune system. Subsequent investigations by the Congressional Office of Technology Assessment found no anticancer properties in IAT. In 1988 talk-show hostess Sally Jesse Raphael promoted Stanislaw R. Burzynski's "antineoplastons," which, he claimed, can "normalize" cancer cells. Another wonder drug of the cancer counterculture was "Iscador," a mistletoe extract marketed by Swiss physician Rudolph Steiner, who claimed that for the drug to be truly effective, the mistletoe had to be picked at the proper time, "since plants not only react to the influences of the sun and moon, but also to those of the planets."[13]

The modern successor to the legacy of the Glover Serum, the Koch Antitoxin, Harry Hoxey's Herbal Tonic, and Krebiozen was the laetrile in which Cecile Hoffman invested her hopes. While Harry Hoxey tried to fend off the federal government, Ernest Krebs, Sr., a California physician, developed laetrile. He first announced the discovery in 1951, claiming to have extracted a cancer cure from apricot pits. Unlike most cancer quacks, he supplied a biochemical explanation. When laetrile reached a cancer cell, he claimed, the enzyme beta-glucosidase hydrolized it, releasing tumorcidal hydrogen into the malignant cell. Normal cells did not die because rhodanase, another enzyme, detoxified the cyanides. The FDA conducted clinical trials of laetrile in the early 1960s and announced that the drug had no effect and warned that its cyanide derivatives might actually be toxic.

But just when the FDA banned laetrile, Canadian entrepreneur Andrew Robert McNaughton took up the cause, establishing laetrile clinics in Canada and Mexico and conducting a public relations blitz in the United States. Extreme right-wing groups like the John Birch Society climbed on the laetrile bandwagon. An ultraconservative, anticommunist organization, the John Birch Society demanded complete freedom of choice in treatment selection. They claimed that big government had joined hands with big medicine in a great conspiracy to keep cancer cures off the market. "Orthodox physicians," the society claimed in 1975, "are futilely cutting, burning, and poisoning their victims, and rejecting hopeful treatments like laetrile for fears of doing themselves out of a job."[14]

Over the years, laetrile promoters changed their story many times, eventually hedging all bets. For years, they promised that laetrile could prevent and cure cancer. In 1953 the California Medical Society concluded that the drug had no impact on the disease. In the 1960s, laetrile advocates changed their testimonials, declaring that the drug "controlled" cancer and enhanced the patient's sense of well-being. After more clinical trials at the National Cancer Institute and the Mayo Clinic in the late 1970s and early 1980s, and reports that respected epidemiologists could find no positive results, the promotional rhetoric changed again. Advocates no longer claimed that laetrile cured cancer or controlled it, but that when used as part of a comprehensive program of "metabolic therapy"—which included frequent coffee enemas, a nonfat diet, and megadoses of proteins—laetrile could "help" cancer sufferers.

The apricot pit extract did not help Cecile Hoffman. Buying into the rhetoric, she became a laetrile user and founded the International Association of Cancer Victors and Friends to "restore the cancer victim's life and free choice of treatment and doctor." Along with the John Birch Society and a host of other far right political action and alternative medicine organizations, she lambasted the FDA for cutting off access to laetrile. She believed that a secret conspiracy was at work; research universities, the federal government, and the medical establishment kept cancer cures like laetrile off the market to perpetuate their own power.

Hoffman cited her own case to illustrate the evil. Because the FDA banned laetrile, she had not known of its curative powers at the time of her radical mastectomy in 1959, nor when she had surgery for a recurrence in 1962. Rather than provide a "proven cure," the medical establishment had mutilated her. She even claimed that the FDA and establishment physicians would have let her die rather than prescribe laetrile. In the mid-1960s, she delivered testimonials all over southern California, claiming that had she not lived in San Diego and enjoyed access to laetrile in Tijuana, Mexico, she would already be dead. The testimonials stopped in 1967. The cancer was back. She died in 1969.[15]

Laetrile was the most prominent of the alternative therapies, but nutrition cultists also thrived in the cancer counterculture, attributing the disease to toxins, poisons, and impurities in body tissues. Johanna Brand, a naturopath, wrote a best-selling book recommending a diet of water and three to four pounds of mixed grapes a day for two weeks, followed by a more liberal regimen of grapes, acidophilus culture milk, raw vegetables, dried fruits, nuts, honey, and olive oil. The diet would detoxify the body. Another cultist, the German-born physician Max Gerson, claimed that fresh fruits, fresh vegetables, and frequent enemas cured cancer. His daughter, who ran a Gerson Clinic in Tijuana long after her father's death in 1959, claimed that "by healing the body, you can heal cancer and almost any other chronic disease and it doesn't matter what the cause. All chronic diseases are deficiency diseases." Romanian immigrant Emanuel Revici recommended a more complicated diet of "anabolic" lipid alcohols, zinc, iron, and caffeine, and "catabolic" fatty acids, sulfur, selenium, and magnesium. He claimed to be able to trace a patient's progress in fighting cancer through a urine test. And there was a host of other diets, including the Beverly Hills diet, macrobiotic diets, and the Edgar Cayce Diet. Clinical studies by the National Cancer Institute and the FDA discredited all of them.[16]

Adelle Davis was the godmother of nutrition. Except for lengthening crow's feet around her blue eyes, the guru of supernutrition hardly looked her age. She was sixty-nine years old in 1973, but she moved like a much younger woman, with coordination and confidence. During an interview that year, she insisted that her eyes had been gray-green before several years of psychoanalysis. "The shrinks changed my eye color," she laughed. Davis was the reigning prophetess of the health food movement. She played tennis five times a week and swam nude every morning. When asked about her swimming attire, she retorted, "Nobody takes a bath with their clothes on, do they?"

During the mid–twentieth century, Davis conducted a war against the "multi-billion dollar food processing establishment." All processed food, she advised, should be avoided because industrial food manufacturers had replaced nature's healthy ingredients with chemical poisons. "A woman who wants to murder her husband can do it thoroughly in the kitchen," she once said. "There won't even be an inquest."

Adelle Davis was born in Indiana in 1904 and raised on a farm. She studied nutrition at Purdue and the University of California at Berkeley and worked several years as a dietician before moving to Los Angeles in 1934, where she earned a graduate degree in biochemistry at the University of Southern California. As a young woman, she was a devotee of Frederick Hoffman, a Prudential Insurance Company actuary whose books *Mortality from Cancer throughout the World* (1915) and *Diet and Cancer* (1937) held that cancer was a byproduct of modern society's taste for fatty, sugary, highly processed foods. Hoffman promised that a return to a low-fat, unprocessed diet would reduce the incidence of cancer, and Adelle Davis became a convert.

After a painful divorce, Davis spent several years in psychoanalysis, moving from Freudian to Jungian to Reichian therapy and then back to Freud. What she needed was something monumental, a crusade to save the world, and she found it in nutrition and health therapy. In best-selling books—*Let's Cook It Right, Let's Get Well, Let's Eat Right to Keep Fit*, and *Let's Have Healthy Children*—Davis preached a simple, clear message: "Nutritional research, like a modern star of Bethlehem, brings hope that sickness need not be a part of life." She did not offer immortality, but her promise was close: a long, fulfilling life free of illness. Many Americans bought her message. Davis sold ten million copies of her books in the 1950s and 1960s.[17]

Her faith in nutrition knew no bounds. It was a panacea of cosmic dimensions, the key to all contemporary problems and a way of unlocking the mysteries of the past. "Where the diet is good," she proclaimed, "there is no crime." When a family eats right, there is no drug abuse, no rebellious teenagers, and no divorce. In World War II, Germany defeated France, she postulated, because of its stockpile of dietic weapons: German beer and black bread, loaded with whole grains and yeasts, were much healthier than the white bread and wine consumed by the French. Even the outcome of the Cold War was in doubt, since the Russians consumed more whole grains and less processed food than Americans. "This nutrition consciousness had better grow," she warned, "or we're going under. We're watching the fall of Rome right now, very definitely, because Americans are getting more than half their calories from food with no nutrients. People are exhausted."

Critics accused Davis of sloppy research, reckless diagnoses, and gross hyperbole. A professor at the University of Southern California argued that she was "scientifically uncritical, accepting any research from any source that fit her preconceived notions about health. If some veterinary journal argued that a daily gram of rat brain will cure cat leukemia, Davis would tell her readers to start eating some rat brain." Roslyn Alfin-Slaver, a UCLA nutritionist, was familiar with the mentality of Davis's followers: "People want miracles. Some people think if you follow supernutrition, you can be cured for the rest of your life of all ailments and live to a very old age. Unfortunately, life just isn't that simple." Edward Rynearson of the Mayo Clinic was more abrupt: "Any physician or dietician will find *Let's Get Well* loaded with inaccuracies, misquotations, and unsubstantiated statements." Davis frequently faced personal injury lawsuits. Susan Pitzer sued her after the death of her infant son, Ryan. To cure colic in infants, Davis recommended potassium chloride. Pitzer followed the instructions, but since Ryan was already dehydrated, the potassium chloride sent his heart into a fatal arrhythmia.[18]

Adelle Davis was undaunted. Breast cancer, she claimed, was a disease of malnutrition, "which invariably precedes all malignancies." Too many processed foods, too many chemical additives, and too little protein were the culprits. "I have yet to know of a single adult to develop cancer who has habitually drunk a quart of milk a day," she claimed. If breast cancer victims had any hope of survival, they had to change their diet. Since

Bathsheba's Breast

the incidence of breast cancer in mice was lowest among control groups consuming prodigious quantities of vitamin E, women with breast cancer should do the same. Victims of breast cancer had only themselves to blame, Davis argued, and if they were going to get better, they needed to consume organically grown fruits and vegetables, raw milk, breads made from fresh whole grains, fertilized eggs, wheat germ, unsweetened yogurt, brewer's yeast, small portions of meats from range-fed, hormone-free chickens, sheep, and cattle, and megadoses of vitamins and trace elements. Instead of soft drinks, patients should drink several glasses a day of her famous "Pep-Up," a tasty brew of egg yolks, lecithin, vegetable oil, calcium lactate, yogurt, acidophilous culture, calcium- and magnesium-enriched yeast, soy flour, seaweed, vanilla, cinnamon, nutmeg, frozen orange juice, and magnesium oxide, all whipped into a frothy drink.[19]

But during the 1973 interview for *The New York Times Magazine*, while she preached a sermonette on the virtues of supernutrition, Davis kept fidgeting in her chair, shifting back and forth, trying to dispel a persistent ache in her hips. Perhaps she had strained a muscle playing tennis or swimming. Over the next several weeks, she increased the volume of daily "Pep-Up" cocktails, doubled up on vitamins C and E, and consumed more brewer's yeast and wheat germ. But the pain did not go away; in fact, it spread to her legs. Finally, late in 1973, she visited a UCLA oncologist. After a battery of tests, she received what was, in her mind, an incredible diagnosis: she had a terminal case of multiple myeloma—cancer of the bone marrow.

Davis reacted with disbelief. "I thought this was for people who drink soft drinks, who eat white bread, who eat refined sugar." Disbelief surrendered to depression. Thirty years earlier, the crusade for supernutrition had lifted her out of an emotional crisis. Now, with her reason for being gone, she sank again. "My whole life is a failure," she told an interviewer. In what can only be described as a terrible irony, she turned to her old nemesis—the chemical industry—in a desperate attempt to live. Davis agreed to a rigorous regimen of chemotherapy, which she was taking when she died on May 31, 1974. Before the end, however, she experienced a revelation that made her believe she had been right, after all: "I ate too much junk food in college."[20]

Nutrition fads and bogus medicines had always existed, but in the 1970s, anticancer psychotherapy added a new wrinkle, supplying an anti-establishment, self-help emotional regimen consistent with the cultural atmosphere of the times. A veritable legion of barely trained psychotherapists crowded their way into oncology, offering cancer patients treatment options that were, to say the least, extraordinarily controversial. As early as 1885, New York physician William Parker had detected, he thought, a connection between emotional depression and cancer. "Great mental depression," he noted, "particularly grief, induces a predisposition to such a disease as cancer, or becomes an exciting cause under circumstances where the predisposition had already been acquired."[21]

In the 1940s, Austrian psychotherapist Wilhelm Reich reinforced such notions. Reich had earned a medical degree at the University of Vienna, becoming a disciple of Sigmund Freud. Blessed with intense, dark eyes and a shock of black, unruly hair, Reich possessed a powerful presence, which he used to great benefit as a psychotherapist. From 1924 to 1930, he directed the seminar for psychoanalytic therapy at Freud's clinic, but as his views of personality disorders wandered outside the mainstream, the two men grew apart. During the 1920s, Reich came to see a direct correlation between what he called "orgastic potency" and personality disorders. Men and women who had experienced difficulty moving through the "genital stage" of childhood were more likely to find themselves deficient sexually, unable to achieve "orgastic potency." Freud rejected his theories, and subsequent critics labeled Reich the "prophet of the better orgasm" and the "founder of the genital utopia." Later in his career, after coming to the United States, Reich claimed to have discovered "orgone energy," a hitherto unknown physical force in the universe. "There is a deadly orgone energy," he wrote. "It is in the atmosphere. It's a swampy quality. Stagnant, deadly water which does not flow." Chemists and physicists rejected "orgone" as the silly-minded excesses of a poorly trained scientist, but Reich's followers in the psychoanalytic community became true believers.

Orgone energy, he explained, was not just confined to the subatomic world of protons, neutrons, electrons, and alpha, beta, gamma, and x-rays; it also manifested itself within human beings by controlling sexual drives and governing "orgastic potency." Such sexual forces, if lost, could trigger a variety of illnesses; healing could only come through Reichian therapy, which restored orgone energy. By the 1940s, he had come up with "orgone accumulators," which he sold to practitioners to use in psychoanalyzing patients. The accumulator was a contraption of sheet metal and cardboard, shaped like a telephone booth. Patients were to sit inside the accumulator, absorb sexually refreshing volumes of orgone, and restore balance to their "distorted sexconomies."

Cancer patients occupied a special place in Reichian theory. He insisted that disease was a function of their personalities, an idea that was hardly new. Early in the 1700s, Pierre Dionis, a surgeon in Paris, wondered if such psychic forces as sorrow and anger might cause a coagulation of lymphatic fluids in a woman's breast and produce a tumor. James Paget, the brilliant nineteenth-century British surgeon, wrote in his text *Surgical Pathology* that "mental depression is a weighty additive to the other influences favoring the development of the cancerous constitution." Cancer often appeared, he claimed, in the lives of people experiencing "deep anxiety, deferred hope, and disappointment." But Reich thought he was on to something new, that he had discovered what he called a "cancer biopathy." Typical cancer patients possessed a "bio-emotional disposition to cancer" because of their "orgone depletions." "Cancer," he claimed, "is due to the stagnation of the flow of the life energy of the organism." Cancer patients have mild emotions and live in a state of perpetual resignation and "painful acquiescence." They have no hope about life. At the core of their being, they suffer from "chronic emotional calm," which depletes orgone from their cells and triggers malignancies. They are sexually repressed and dysfunctional, unable to achieve normal orgasm. Aversion to sex, he argued, is definitely carcinogenic. Reichian psychotherapy, to lift patients from the bondage of sexual repression, and orgone-replacing stints in the accumulators, could help cure cancer patients.[22]

In 1954 the Food and Drug Administration went after Reich and his orgone accumulators. When FDA scientists asked him to explain the biology and physics of orgone energy, he responded that they were not sophisticated enough to understand his work. He refused to defend his theories or provide data proving their effectiveness. The FDA secured a court order prohibiting Reich from selling accumulators, but he ignored the injunction. Federal courts found him in contempt and sentenced him to two years in the federal penitentiary in Lewisburg, Pennsylvania. He died there in 1957. Although the American College of Orgonomy still exists, and practitioners can acquire accumulators, blankets, vests, mitts, and magic orgone wands, few self-respecting psychiatrists or psychologists give any credence to orgone therapy.[23]

The notion of a "cancer personality," however, survived Reich, floating around in the scientifically thin theoretical air of modern psychotherapy, where logic, culture, and the personal dilemmas of therapists collide. In the 1950s, when scientists established a link between emotional stress and the onset of illness, some psychotherapists took the logic a giant step forward, speculating that psyches affected immunological systems. Some described cancer as the disease of a compromised immunological system. No longer able to use the rationale of orgone energy, they bought into an equally theoretical notion, arguing that "cancer personalities" damaged their own immune systems, giving tumors a chance to take root. Sexually repressed, emotionally contained cancer victims were responsible for their own illnesses.

The idea of the cancer personality escaped the jargon-cluttered world of psychotherapy for the larger popular culture in the 1970s. A new rhetoric of self-help through psychoanalysis—what historian Christopher Lasch described as the "therapeutic culture"—became the defining characteristic of middle- and upper-class society. Throughout United States history, Americans had worshiped rugged individualism and its emphasis on competition, responsibility, and self-reliance. Popular culture—dime novels, films, radio, and television—made heroes out of cowboys, Indian fighters, explorers, hunters, and trappers, those who had carved a new life out of the wilderness. But American individualism had always expressed itself within the larger context of powerful, compelling institutions demanding loyalty for the benefit of the group. Rugged individuals always found themselves confronting the demands of family, community, church, and country, which offered support and sustenance in return for sacrifice. Worship of self was not a traditional part of American individualism.[24]

In the 1960s and early 1970s, however, Americans lost faith in their institutions. The civil rights movement, economic malaise, rising divorce rates, the youth rebellion, and the Vietnam War all combined to force a loss of innocence and to weaken traditional faith in family, community, church, and country. Without the checks and balances of traditional institutions, the American belief in rugged individualism evolved into a love of self, setting millions of middle- and upper-class Americans on a desperate search for the meaning of life. Jerry Rubin, a leader of the yippies in the 1960s, left New York for San Francisco in 1971. "In five years," he later wrote, "from 1971 to 1975, I directly experienced est, gestalt therapy,

bioenergetics, rolfing, massage, jogging, health foods, tai chi, Esalen, hypnotism, modern dance, meditation, Silva Mind Control, Arica, acupuncture, sex therapy, Reichian therapy, and More House—a smorgasbord course in New Consciousness."[25]

In the narcissistic culture of the 1960s and 1970s, such psychological seeds spread like weeds. Glib psychotherapists fashioned stark stereotypes, accusing cancer patients of emotional dysfunction. Caroline Thomas of the Johns Hopkins University claimed that cancer patients "are low-gear persons, seldom prey to outbursts of emotion. They have feelings of isolation from their parents dating back to childhood." Claus and Marjorie Benson of the Eastern Pennsylvania Psychiatric Institute believed that cancer patients "charted a personality pattern of denial of hostility, depression and of memory of emotional deprivation in childhood." Lawrence LeShan, a UCLA psychologist, helped popularize the theory of cancer personalities. Convinced that he had his finger on the emotional pulse of cancer victims, he wrote that they are people who have "a childhood or adolescence marked by feelings of isolation . . . and the conviction that life holds no hope." Making another giant leap, he claimed, "The cancer patient almost invariably is contemptuous of himself, and of his abilities and possibilities. He is empty of feelings and devoid of self."[26]

The cure was psychotherapy. If people contracted cancer because they refuse to share their innermost feelings, then the cure can be found in the confessional, preferably on a therapist's couch at $100 an hour. Since hundreds of thousands of Americans annually developed malignant tumors, cancer patients constituted a potentially huge new market for psychotherapists. The leading cancer psychotherapists were O. Carl Simonton and Stephanie Matthews-Simonton. A radiotherapist, Carl Simonton trained at the University of Oregon in the late 1960s. Oncology proved to be a challenge. Mortality rates were high enough to discourage even the most callous physicians. He began looking for some way of giving his patients an edge. His wife Stephanie, a psychologist, came up with a possible solution. She specialized in goal setting, relaxation therapy, and imaging for corporate executives. When they learned of the cancer personality theories of Wilhelm Reich and Lawrence LeShan, the Simontons decided to treat cancer patients with Stephanie's relaxation and imaging therapies.

In the early 1970s, the Simontons established the Cancer Counseling and Research Center in Fort Worth, Texas. Their 1978 book *Getting*

Well Again became a best-seller, and with free publicity from such television programs as *60 Minutes* and articles in such magazines as *Smithsonian,* they attracted thousands of psychologists, naturopaths, faith healers, counselors, and homeopaths to Fort Worth, where they taught their anticancer psychotherapy techniques. By the early 1980s, they had trained nearly ten thousand therapists—at $250 to $500 each. They became household words in the oncology business. Wendy Schain, a counselor at the National Cancer Institute who worked with breast cancer patients, claimed in 1980 that two of every five of her patients at the NCI knew of the Simonton technique, having heard of it from the media or by word of mouth.

During medical school and his oncology residency, Simonton worried that he might have a "cancer personality." Treating cancer patients was depressing business, and depression caused cancer. Physicians and psychologists who identified too closely with their patients could become depressed and end up with the disease themselves. One solution, which academic medicine had long employed, was to erect barriers between physician and patient, to create a protective emotional distance. But that entailed its own risks, since another dimension of the "cancer personality" was the "isolation of self." Believing his own rhetoric, Simonton faced a terrible dilemma: to risk getting cancer by getting too close to patients, to risk it by becoming emotionally distant, or to risk it by agonizing over the other risks. "I have been so devastated," he later recalled, "that I thought I would die when patients died. I have nearly destroyed myself because I was too invested in patient outcome."

Continuous psychotherapy was the answer, and the Cancer Counseling and Research Center was a hotbed of intense psychoanalysis for the Simontons' disciples. The primary clientele was other therapists, not cancer patients. On any given day, the Simontons presided over a virtual lovefest at their heavily wooded retreat. At the time, they were halfway between being hippies and being yuppies, between their peace-and-love undergraduate days in the 1960s and their status as multimillionaires in the 1980s. A touchy-feely-hugging atmosphere prevailed, as did the grabbag lexicon of pop psychology: participants were to "get in touch with their feelings," "empower themselves," "find the inner self," obliterate the "cancer personality," "confess their secrets," "abandon their guilts," "raise their consciousness," and "take control of their lives."

There was nothing profound about the Simontons, who acknowledged the carcinogenic role of tobacco, chemicals, diet, radiation, and genetic predisposition. What intrigued them was why some individuals exposed to carcinogens developed cancer and others did not, why the immunological system of some people handled miscreant cells and why others did not. Carl Simonton tried to make the case for the "immune surveillance" theory—that cancer cells are produced on a steady basis in all human beings, but they are destroyed by the body's white blood cells, which also handle bacterial and viral infections. Cancer occurs, according to this logic, when some of malignant cells "get away," escaping the body's surveillance system. Among people with a "cancer personality," such escapes are more likely to occur.

From that logic, they claimed that psychotherapy could restore balance to the immune system, enabling it to round up and destroy wayward cells. Regular psychotherapy would allow patients to become more sexually liberated, emotionally mature, psychologically expressive, and personally empowered. The Simontons encouraged patients to enhance their immunological systems through meditation. Convinced that the brain can stimulate the endocrine glands to strengthen the immunological system, they taught patients stress-reducing relaxation techniques and coached them to "image" their personal battle against cancer, to meditate several times daily and command their white blood cells to destroy the cancer cells. The specific images would vary from patient to patient. A billiards player might imagine his immune system as the cue ball knocking all the cancer "balls" into the pockets. A teenager might see the disease in terms of a video game, with "Pac-Man" white blood cells devouring the cancer dots. Successful patients stayed in therapy, religiously "imaged" their cancers, and lived.[27]

The Simontons also had an easy explanation for recurrences. They did not consider the grade, stage, tissue type, genetic markers, or cell differentiation of the tumors—tested tools to explain recurrence and metastasis. Just as the etiology of cancer was psychological, so was the etiology of recurrence. People with recurring tumors, they claimed, "may have unconsciously surrendered to the emotional conflicts they face," or their bodies were screaming out "for the help of a therapist." Cancer victims confronting a return of their disease have "not yet found ways of giving themselves permission to meet their emotional needs except through illness." They had "slacked off and grown complacent" about changing their personalities. The Simontons believed that some patients loved and needed their disease. Such flawed personalities must stop using cancer "to meet their needs." If they were going to put away their cancers and live, they had to terminate "self-destructive behavior" and start "taking care of themselves emotionally."[28]

Others jumped on the bandwagon, hawking psychological cures. Cancer therapists framed devastating portraits of patients, diagnosing them as victims of emotional pathologies, arguing that the source of their tumors could be found in psychic handicaps. Norman Cousins attributed his spontaneous recovery from ankylosing spondylitis—the degeneration of connective tissues in the spine—to a regimen of good nutrition and laughter. Spontaneous remissions from the disorder are not at all unusual, but Cousins parlayed his experience into a faculty position at the UCLA medical school and a best-selling book, *The Anatomy of an Illness* (1979). A proponent of holistic medicine—high-quality medical care, good nutrition, and psychological stability—he believed that cancer is "connected to intensive states of grief or anger or fear."[29]

Bernie Siegel was another best-selling believer in cancer psychotherapy. A trained surgeon burdened with a heavy caseload of patients, he went into a depression early in the 1970s. On January 1, 1974, he wrote plaintively in his personal journal, "At times it seems the world is dying of cancer. Every abdomen you open is filled with it." Four years later, he discovered the Simonton technique, entered therapy himself, and emerged from his depression convinced that sick people have the power to assist the healing process. Cancer victims, he claimed, were the most psychologically unhealthy people in the world. They grow up "believing there is some terrible flaw at the center of their being, a defect they must hide if they are to have a chance for love. Feeling unlovable and condemned to loneliness if their true selves become known, [they] set up defenses against sharing their innermost feelings with anyone. They feel their love shriveling up, which leads to further despair." He wrote a best-seller—*Love, Medicine, and Miracles*. He marketed it, along with tapes and seminars, in bookstores and hotel meeting rooms throughout the country.[30]

The Reichs and Simontons and LeShans and Siegels could never provide anything more than anecdotal testimonials to prove a correlation between personality type and vulnerability to cancer. Reliable clinical evidence was paltry at best. Critics of cancer psychotherapy cited severe weaknesses in their logic. Zoologists pointed out that cancer is not just a disease of human beings. It occurs in most vertebrate species and in a variety of plants. Tumors in redwood trees or feline leukemia cannot be attributed to emotional depression in the giant sequoias or the neighborhood cat. Neuroblastomas in two-week-old infants can hardly be explained as consequences of personality portraits, unless the babies developed personality flaws while still in the womb. Do all of the preadolescent children in a pediatric cancer ward possess sexually repressed, emotionally retarded, self-loathing personalities? If depression causes cancer, why does history not record cancer epidemics in the wake of wars, economic depressions, and holocausts? Why is there no evidence of increased cancer rates among depressed patients receiving long-term care in psychiatric facilities?[31]

In response to the claims of the cancer psychotherapists, oncologists launched a number of clinical studies in the 1970s. Only one reported any correlation, claiming that middle-aged men with the highest depression levels had a 2.3 times greater risk of developing cancer over a seventeen-year period than men who were not depressed. But a follow-up study three years later showed a rapidly declining correlation. A study of the cancer risk among 95,647 widows and widowers showed no statistically significant elevations because of bereavement-based depression. A look at nine thousand women at the Kaiser Permanente Medical Center in Walnut Creek, California, showed no statistical increase of breast cancer because of depression. In 1989, the American Medical Association concluded that there is "much doubt about the correctness of the view held by many that those with depressive symptoms are at excess risk of cancer. It is clearly not consistent with a strong relationship between depressive symptoms and cancer among major segments of the population."[32]

Most oncologists also rejected the notion of a "cancer personality." The work of people like Wilhelm Reich and Lawrence LeShan, they argued, occupied ground between bad science and no science—poorly designed research whose conclusions rested heavily on preconceived notions. Performing personality tests on cancer patients was foolhardy at best, especially if correlations were going to be drawn between a personality type and vulnerability to cancer. Faced with a life-threatening illness, cancer patients naturally exhibited various degrees of depression, anxiety, concern, doubt, and hopelessness, feelings that psychiatrist Elisabeth Kübler-Ross said all seriously and terminally ill people experience. David K. Wellisch and Joel Yeager of UCLA concluded that "the cancer-prone personality has been elusive and perhaps non-existent." Taking a psychological profile of an individual with cancer revealed little about that patient's precancer personality, and certainly not enough to draw elaborate conclusions about the relationship between personality and disease. In a 1978 study, B. H. Fox claimed "that because it is so difficult for science to determine whether there is such a personality, it is doubtful that we will ever know."[33]

Other critics of the cancer psychotherapy worried about the guilt that psychotherapeutic treatments often imposed on patients. A logic of individual responsibility was built into the therapy. If patients were indeed emotionally accountable for their disease, they were also at fault if they failed to recover from it. Karen Ritchie, a psychiatrist at M. D. Anderson Hospital, worried that the "problem may be most severe when the patient is dying. Now, in addition to all the real losses that must be grieved and loose ends that must be tied up, the patient feels the burden of guilt and failure at not being strong enough to cure the cancer." In 1985 Carl Simonton had told one patient, "You are living a very unhealthy lifestyle. If you don't change it and start honoring yourself and taking care of your needs, you will die." A Simonton-trained therapist later asked her, "Are you ready to give up your cancer by changing your lifestyle?" Apparently, according to the Simontons, she was not ready. She was the culprit. Three hundred years ago, Anne of Austria felt responsible for her breast cancer. A life of vanity and excess, she was convinced, had angered God, who had then punished her with a horrible illness. But God was more forgiving than the Simontons. God promised Anne a place in heaven after she had completed her penance. The Simontons offered nothing. Richard Evans, a social psychologist at the University of Houston, placed the Simontons in the larger context of American culture. "This is one aspect of the social psychology of hope and despair," he commented. "But if you're dealing with bogus hope, that's really sad."[34]

Continous psychotherapy could not save the Simonton marriage. They parted company in the mid-1980s. She moved to Little Rock, Arkansas, and launched the Health Training and Research Center, a private psychotherapy treatment and training facility. Carl moved west to southern California, where he established the Simonton Cancer Center in Pacific Palisades. The American Medical Association launched a careful investigation of the Simonton method in the 1980s. The association discovered that although Carl and Stephanie had urged patients to combine psychotherapy with standard care, their professional converts in the psychoanalytic community were not as careful. Many were poorly trained and nurtured hostile feelings for the medical establishment. Some promised cures using psychotherapy alone and steered patients away from medical oncologists. Alarmed about the emotional consequences of the technique, and unable to find any clinical evidence that it worked, the AMA added the Simontons to its official list of unproven cancer therapies.[35]

Susan Sontag was convinced they were quacks long before the AMA said so. A novelist and cultural critic, she had wielded a sharp pen over the years that dripped sarcasm as she pilloried the values and institutions of modern society. Sontag was born in New York City in 1933, raised in Tucson and Los Angeles, and educated at Berkeley and Harvard. Brilliant and intellectually fashionable, she wrote *Benefactor* (1963), *Against Interpretation* (1966), *Death Kit* (1967), *Trip to Hanoi* (1968), *Styles of Radical Will* (1969), and *Art of Revolution* (1970). "Most people in this society," she wrote, "who aren't utterly mad are . . . reformed or potential lunatics." After visiting North Vietnam, she decided the country epitomized patriotism, neighborliness, and faith in the human condition. She reserved the sharpest barbs for her own culture. There is no hope for the West, no redemption for "what this particular civilization has wrought upon the world. The white race is the cancer of human history." Sontag was especially eloquent describing American degradation, a decline inherent in a lack of genuine guilt over rampant consumerism, social alienation, bourgeois expectations, moral bankruptcy, psychological impotency, and the inability to communicate or sustain relationships.

Nor did intellectuals escape her wrath. In what many critics considered an anti-intellectual diatribe, she raged against the flight from feeling in modern literary criticism, the futile attempt to interpret literature, to reduce its contents to convenient intellectual categories. All it created, she argued, was the "perennial, never consummated project of interpretation," which is inherently "reactionary, impertinent, cowardly, and stifling." She went on to argue that "the world, our world, is depleted, impoverished enough. Away with all duplicates of it, until we again experience more immediately what we have." Interpretation buries the aesthetic experience, preventing people from coming to terms emotionally with art. "The effusion of interpretation of art today poisons our sensibilities." The plague of the modern mind, Sontag reasoned, is too much thinking, not enough feeling.[36]

In 1975 Sontag had to come to terms with some of her own rhetoric. She found a tumor in her breast. Instead of wallowing in an emotional crisis, she embarked on a personal crusade. When her surgeon put "tremendous pressure" on her to have a single procedure biopsy, then if necessary, a mastectomy, she rebelled, insisting, as Shirley Temple Black had, on a biopsy and then a few weeks' treatment delay to consider her options. When the pathologist told her that the tumor was "virulently malignant," Sontag secured a second, though similar, opinion. Conversant with the debate over breast cancer surgery, she visited the Cleveland Clinic to discuss her options with George Crile, where she learned that because breast cancer was a systemic disease from the very beginning, conservative surgery was just as effective as radical surgery. She weighed the options and ultimately agreed to a radical mastectomy. "So little was known," she told *Family Health* magazine, "that if there was only a tiny advantage to the radical, I would do it. I certainly didn't want any additional mutilation, but I wanted to live." She then opted for aggressive chemotherapy, over the protests of several New York surgeons who warned her about potentially lethal side effects. Eventually, she had a French chemotherapist design a radical, multiple-drug therapy that she received at Memorial Sloan-Kettering. After more than two and a half years of chemotherapy, she volunteered for an experimental program of immunotherapy. "It was unpleasant, but I certainly wouldn't call it agony. And it sure beats dying."

Within a month of finding the lump, Sontag wanted to write a book. As she considered the "How could this happen?" "Why me?" and "What am I going to do?" questions, she confronted the theoretical world of Wilhelm Reich, Lawrence LeShan, and O. Carl Simonton, and the possibility that she possessed a cancer personality, a sexually inhibited, emotionally resigned, anger-suppressing makeup that had brought on cancer. Of course, nobody who knew Susan Sontag considered her a cancer personality. In fact, she appeared to be a boldly expressive woman, in person and on the printed page, hardly the guilt-ridden, self-loathing, emotionally crippled individual the cancer psychotherapists portrayed.[37]

Sontag proved her point in 1977 when the book came out. *Illness as*

Metaphor rests on the premise that cultures mythologize what they do not understand, producing an endless series of very potent, and potentially misleading, metaphors. "Nothing is more punitive," Sontag claims,

> than to give a disease a meaning—that meaning being invariably a moralistic one. Any important disease whose causality is murky, and for which treatment is ineffectual, tends to be awash in significance. First, the subjects of deepest dread (corruption, decay, pollution, anomie, weakness) are identified with the disease. The disease itself becomes a metaphor. Then, in the name of the disease (that is, using it as a metaphor) that horror is imposed on other things. The disease becomes adjectival. Something is said to be disease-like, meaning it is disgusting or ugly.

Since cancer defies understanding, it has produced a large and intoxicating lexicon of metaphors. Cancer is "malignant" disease and "invades" its "victims" and "devours" them. In the literary symbolism of Western civilization, the term "cancer" became a synonym for the fatalistic, the catastrophic, the disastrous, and the evil. Sontag herself had joined the throng when she described white people as the "cancer" of civilization. Such metaphors have created fear and resignation among cancer patients, leaving them with the impression that the disease takes an inexorable course to death. Too many patients, she claimed, react to a cancer diagnosis in one of two ways: "'I have cancer and I'm going to die' or 'I have cancer and I don't want to think about it.'" The images frustrated her: "I am so angry at the way the cultural clichés operate to disarm people and make them helpless instead of active on their own behalf."[38]

For Susan Sontag, psychotherapists like Wilhelm Reich, Lawrence LeShan, and O. Carl Simonton, with their cancer personality theories, made life and death worse, not better, for cancer sufferers. Their arguments were moralistic, punitive, and condescending. Such theories will survive only as long as the cause of cancer remains a mystery. "Theories that diseases are caused by mental states," she wrote, "and can be cured by will power are always an index of how much is not understood about the physical terrain of a disease." In the Middle Ages, priests and physicians—who knew nothing about the relationship between rats, fleas, and the bubonic bacterium—argued that the best defense against the plague was a positive attitude. "The happy man would not get the plague," one of them claimed. William H. Welch's medical textbook, *The Principles and Practices of Medicine* (1881), attributed tuberculosis to hereditary disposition, a sedentary lifestyle, poor ventilation, and "depressing emotions." Others saw the roots of the disease in emotional excess—too much sex, too much rich food, and too much alcohol. But once the real etiology of the disease was understood, the psychological portrait vanished. Robert Koch discovered the tubercle bacillus in 1882; the next edition of Welch's medical textbook said nothing about a connection between emotions and the disease.

Cancer psychotherapists were the inevitable products of modern American culture. In a secularized society searching for transcendent meaning and a democratic culture of individual rights, they provided a seductive illusion of power. "Psychologizing seems to provide," Sontag claimed, "control over the experiences and events (like grave illnesses) over which people have in fact little or no control." And for her, the cancer psychotherapists were a temporary phenomenon. Once the true sources of cancer are identified—viral, environmental, bacterial, or genetic—the Reichs and LeShans and Simontons will disappear. "The language about cancer will evolve in the coming years. It must change, decisively, when the disease is finally understood and the rate of cure becomes much higher . . . the cancer metaphor will be made obsolete."[39]

Sontag battled the metaphors as well as her own cancer, even though, in the beginning, "I discovered that I believed all of them." In a 1978 interview with *Family Health* magazine, a reporter asked her if she felt good about her chances for survival. She responded honestly, "It's funny, I have a kind of double consciousness. I know the odds are against me, and yet I feel I should proceed as if I am going to live and have a normal life." She did.[40]

CHAPTER NINE

Choices

MEDICAL TREATMENT IN THE
AGE OF LIBERATION

Rose Kushner saw wrongs and tried to right them. Even when she was a small child, her moral sense was finely tuned. Coming of age in the late 1950s, she committed herself to all the right causes—civil rights, the women's movement, the environment, and peace in Vietnam. With her husband Harvey and their children Gantt, Todd, and Lesley, Kushner lived in Kensington, Maryland, raising her family and dabbling in Beltway politics. Her legacy to modern America, however, would come in a new political arena.[1]

It started on Saturday night, June 15, 1974. Kushner was luxuriating in a hot bath, anticipating a quiet evening watching Archie Bunker and *M*A*S*H**. While shaving under her arm, her finger brushed across a tiny, dense mass of tissue near the surface of her left breast. "It was so small," she later wrote, "that I was not sure there was really anything different about the spot. But if my head pretended for a moment that nothing was there, my stomach knew immediately something was wrong. It coiled into a tight ball and stayed that way for weeks." On Monday morning, her physician confirmed the presence of a solid mass and ordered a mammogram. In the three days she had before seeing the radiologist, Kushner staked out a carrel in the National Library of Medicine and read everything she could find on breast cancer.

The radiologist's good news late in the week—"Everything is fine . . . . It's just benign fibrocystic disease—nothing to worry about"—brought little comfort. Kushner had read about the unlikely but real possibility of false negatives. The only way to be sure was to have a surgical biopsy. She then made the first of many independent decisions, disregarding the optimistic mammogram and deciding to see a surgeon.

A second choice soon faced her. Like Shirley Temple Black, she did not want a single-procedure biopsy-mastectomy. "My lump was small," she remembered, "and I was no surgical risk. I made up my mind to have a biopsy first and then wait." If the tumor was malignant, she wanted time to adjust psychologically and sort out options. The decision put her on a collision course with the surgical establishment. She started shopping around for a surgeon willing to perform the biopsy and encountered nothing but hostility. "No patient is going to tell me how to do my surgery," one shouted. "I've never heard of such a thing." Another was even more vitriolic. "You're absolutely ridiculous! If the diagnosis is positive on frozen section, the breast must come off immediately." Kushner went through nineteen surgeons before she found one willing to do it her way. He removed a tiny tumor, and pathologists quickly diagnosed its malignancy.

Then a third choice. Determined to keep control of her life, Kushner evaluated the options and decided on a modified radical mastectomy. Her initial confrontations with so many surgeons left her wary of their arrogance and reluctant to dictate to a surgeon what type of operation he was going to perform. A few days at Memorial Sloan-Kettering overcame her last shreds of deference. The surgeons there would not listen to her, insisting on a radical mastectomy, even though her tumor was only one centimeter. When she returned to Kensington, Kushner told her husband, "Forget it! I'm not having a Halsted. We've got to find out where I can get a modified." An internist told Kushner to call the Roswell Park Memorial Institute in Buffalo, New York. When Kushner asked why he suggested Roswell Park, the doctor told her, "Because they haven't done Halsteds there for years." She flew to Buffalo that evening.

Only when she met Thomas Dao, chief of surgery at Roswell Park, did Kushner get any satisfaction. He repeated several tests, asked hospital pathologists to examine biopsy samples, listened to Kushner argue the merits of modified versus radical surgery, and then agreed with her. He neither blustered, argued, postured, nor demeaned. In his opinion, Kushner had assessed her own situation and decided on a reasonable course of treatment. Dao performed a modified radical mastectomy.

As soon as she awoke in the recovery room, Kushner started worrying about the next decision. By the 1970s follow-up radiotherapy was commonplace, whether the operation had been radical, modified radical, or simple. A number of oncologists, including Bernard Fisher of the National Surgical Adjuvant Breast Project, doubted the wisdom of radiation after a radical mastectomy, since no proof existed that recipients lived any longer than those who had only surgery. But Dao was even more opinionated. From his own studies, he had concluded that radiotherapy, for reasons he could not explain, actually increased the likelihood of metastases and reduced long-term survival odds. Most oncologists, especially radiation specialists, heatedly rejected his point of view, but in 1962 he had stopped employing radiation except for bone metastases and palliation. Kushner decided to stay with Dao on the issue.

She had one more decision to make—whether to have breast reconstruction surgery. Scientific and cultural issues were at stake. Like everything else in the breast cancer arena, reconstructive surgery stirred up intense debate. Although most studies supported the safety of breast reconstruction, some surgeons worried that a silicone implant in the chest wall might camouflage recurring tumors, making them more difficult to detect. Reconstructive surgery was a relatively new phenomenon, and reliable data on its long-term effects were not yet available. Restoring the breast required major surgery and a general anesthetic, with all of their inherent risks. Why should a woman put herself through such an ordeal for purely cosmetic reasons?

Kushner weighed the problem, reading dozens of articles in surgical journals and consulting several physicians. "Over the years," she remarked in 1983, "I researched the question . . . and soon there were fewer and fewer reasons not to do it." Physicians assured her that silicone was not carcinogenic, and that mammograms, properly administered, could detect any recurrences. "What convinced me most, though, was that I couldn't find a single woman who was sorry she had decided to have reconstructive surgery." She had the operation in 1978.

For a while, Rose Kushner did not have to face urgent decisions.

Questions surrounding the lump, the biopsy, the mammogram, the mastectomy, radiotherapy, and reconstruction were gone. But peace of mind did not return. She was angry, not so much about the disease, or about the toll it had taken on her, but about the cavalier masculine certainty characterizing so many surgeons. It was all terribly ironic. Although breast cancer was modern medicine's most controversial disease, she had come across only a handful of men who possessed even the slightest humility about it. With confusion and controversy endemic, the right of a woman to choose her treatment, Kushner concluded, assumed even more importance. If the medical community was incapable of arriving at a consensus, why bully women into a treatment? "We women," Kushner wrote in her best-selling *Breast Cancer* (1975), "should be free, knowledgeable, and completely conscious when the time comes for decision, so that we can make it for ourselves. *Our* lives are at stake, not a surgeon's."[2]

Rose Kushner searched for culprits. In her mind, cancer was not simply a matter of tissues and cells, of genetic codes gone awry. She wanted reasons why cancer had selected her, and why the medical establishment had behaved so badly. Never one to acquiesce, in 1975 she launched a public health, consumer rights campaign to educate women about breast cancer. Determined to provide the information women needed to make choices, Kushner established the Breast Cancer Advisory Center in Kensington, Maryland, and pushed a broad agenda—making Americans aware of the evils of the single-step biopsy-then-mastectomy, alternatives to the Halsted radical mastectomy, and the dangers of estrogen.

Setting her sights high, Kushner approached the White House as the first order of business. She had a friend in the press corps who told her that Betty Ford would soon undergo a radical mastectomy. Worried that the First Lady was not getting good advice from physicians at Bethesda Naval Hospital, Kushner managed to get presidential press secretary Ronald Nessen on the phone and told him that the single-stage biopsy-mastectomy was unnecessary, as was the Halsted radical mastectomy. She asked Nessen to pass the message on to the president and get him to postpone the surgery. Nessen talked with the president and then told Kushner, "I am sorry, Mrs. Kushner. The president has made his decision." Enraged, Kushner blurted back, "The president has made *his* decision. It's not his decision to make. Mrs. Ford should make that decision, don't you think?" It was to no avail. Betty Ford underwent a modified radical mastectomy the next day.

Bathsheba's Breast

Undaunted, Kushner launched the breast cancer movement, targeting the single-stage biopsy-mastectomy first. American loyalty to the one-stage procedure baffled European physicians, who had long since abandoned it. There were just too many compelling reasons for separating biopsies and mastectomies into two procedures. The most obvious was the possibility of false positives from a frozen section. The risks were rare but real that a pathologist could incorrectly diagnose benign tissue as malignant. The surgeon, waiting in the operating room, would proceed on the basis of a misdiagnosis and unnecessarily remove a breast. Kushner argued that separating the biopsy from the mastectomy by several days or several weeks would provide time for permanent tissue slides and a more reliable analysis. The number of unnecessary mastectomies would fall.

Unnecessary mastectomies occurred for other reasons. Most American surgeons in the 1970s scheduled women with lumps for a biopsy-then-mastectomy without determining if the cancer had already metastasized. Typically, a woman would have a biopsy and then a radical mastectomy. Her physician would then conduct a series of brain, lung, liver, and bone scans. If other tumors appeared, subsequent radiotherapy and chemotherapy might be planned. But in some cases, physicians discovered that the disease had spread widely and that the woman's case was terminal. Had they done such scans before the biopsy, they might have decided that since the patient was going to die anyway, putting her through radical surgery was unnecessary.

Kushner also attacked the single-stage procedure because it prevented physicians from staging tumors before treating the disease. In Europe, surgeons performed an initial biopsy and then, if indicated, a battery of scans and tests to identify metastases. Pathologists carefully graded the tumor to determine its aggressiveness and hormone dependency. Once the tests were completed, a team of oncologists decided on treatment—a radical mastectomy, modified radical mastectomy, total mastectomy, lumpectomy, or quadrantectomy, and whether to follow up with radiotherapy and chemotherapy. American surgeons, Kushner claimed, "are so hell-bent on radical mastectomies that the grade or stage of a tumor is irrelevant to surgical treatment." More sophisticated approaches, individualized to a woman and her disease, required separation of biopsies and mastectomies. Helen Westerberg, a breast cancer specialist at the Karolinska Institute in Stockholm, told Kushner, "You can't plan rational treatment unless you know the extent of the surgery without first doing the staging. Any kind of mastectomy is pointless if a patient's cancer is already far advanced."

Kushner also argued that mental health reasons alone dictated an end to the single-stage procedure. Usually done within hours or a few days of the discovery of the lump, the one-stage biopsy and mastectomy posed an acute emotional trauma. Going into the operation, a woman had no idea about the outcome. By using two-stage approaches, physicians gave patients time to adjust psychologically to the reality of having cancer and a future without a breast. Post-surgical recovery—emotionally and physically—would be enhanced.

Kushner also conducted a public relations blitz against the Halsted radical mastectomy; it was, she argued, an outmoded procedure from another era which European surgeons no longer routinely performed. She traveled widely in Europe during the late 1970s, visiting major cancer centers and taking note of the startling number of women who were members of surgical oncology teams. It did not take her long to conclude that "breast cancer surgery is not as extensive in countries where there are more women practicing medicine than in the United States." One of her missions in life was to let as many women as possible know about surgical alternatives to Halsted.

Finally, Kushner warned America about possible links between breast cancer and estrogen. "I had never taken birth control pills," she wrote in 1975, "but now I was thinking of the pill as a female hormone, an estrogen, rather than as a contraceptive. I realized how many times I had been given prescriptions for one estrogen or another: to regulate menstrual periods, or prevent miscarriage, or to 'dry up' after weaning my children from the breast. And who knew how much diethylstilbesterol (DES)—the hormone used to fatten livestock—I have eaten in chopped liver and chicken soup?"

Warning flags waved everywhere. After World War II, gynecologists prescribed DES to patients with histories of multiple miscarriages. The drug stabilized the uterus and helped bring fetuses to full term. For women plagued with miscarriages, DES was a godsend. According to the FDA, it did not have any dangerous side effects for patients or their babies. But in this case, FDA clinical trials had not been sufficiently long-term. A generation later, epidemiologists made a gruesome discovery. In 1969 physicians began reporting a startlingly high incidence of vaginal carcinomas in adolescent girls. Epidemiologists searched for a clue, and by

1971 they had learned that all of the young women with vaginal adeno-carcinoma shared one trait: their mothers had taken DES during pregnancy. The drug moved through the placentas into the circulatory systems of their babies, inflicting genetic damage to embryonic vaginal tissues. Twelve to fifteen years later, with the onset of puberty, the adenocarcinomas appeared in their daughters.[3]

Vaginal cancer was not the only long-term side effect of taking DES. Epidemiologists determined in 1984, after a ten-year study, that women who had taken DES during pregnancy had a 47 percent increased risk of breast cancer. Since more than four million women had used the drug during the 1940s and 1950s, several thousand cases of breast cancer each year could be attributed to synthetic estrogen. What epidemiologists could not reliably determine, but what they suspected, were the indirect effects of DES use among animals. While obstetricians routinely prescribed DES for patients threatening to miscarry, farmers had long added DES to cattle, sheep, and chicken feed. DES acted as a growth hormone, accelerating muscle development and shortening the time it took to get livestock ready for slaughter. When Americans ate hamburgers and chicken soup, they also consumed diethylstilbesterol. The FDA banned the use of DES in chicken feed in 1959 and cattle and sheep feed in 1972. But the long-term capacity of previously absorbed DES to trigger breast cancer could not be stopped.[4]

Birth control pills were another culprit. In May 1960, the Food and Drug Administration stamped its approval on the birth control pill, a combination of estrogen and progesterone. G. D. Searle and Company of Chicago named the drug Enovid-10. It proved successful, with only minimal short-term side effects, in preventing pregnancy. Searle marketed the drug in twenty-pill dispensers, enough to last a month, at about ten dollars each. As news of the product made its way into the popular press, millions of women "went on the pill." Few consumer products, let alone a drug, have enjoyed such an immediate reception from an entire society. It seemed a safe, inexpensive way of giving women reproductive freedom.

Epidemiologists, however, soon became alarmed about long-term effects. The pill "tricked the body." During the first weeks of a woman's hormonal cycle, elevated estrogen levels create a state of artificial pregnancy, and ovulation does not occur. At the end of the cycle, the progesterone induces menstruation. Ever since the 1930s, scientists had known that excess estrogen triggered breast tumors in mice, but they had no evidence of similar responses in humans. When the incidence of breast cancer accelerated in the United States in the 1960s and 1970s, epidemiologists speculated about a correlation.

By 1970 more than ten million American women used birth control pills, but complaints about side effects—nausea, headaches, weight gain, blood clots, and strokes—became more frequent. So did lawsuits against G. D. Searle and Company. In January 1970, Senator Gaylord Nelson, a Wisconsin Democrat, opened an official congressional inquiry into the safety of oral contraceptives. During the next two months, dozens of scientists and pharmaceutical company executives appeared before the committee, some of them warning about the pill's dangers, others reassuring America of its safety.

One of the witnesses, however, offered testimony that electrified the hearings. Roy Hertz, a physician and scientist with the National Institutes of Health, had spent his career exploring the biochemical and pharmacological properties of estrogen. Hertz argued that even though ten million American women used the pill, it was still an experimental drug. "All we really know about the pill," he testified, "is that it prevents conception and causes blood clots." He then dropped a bombshell—the long-term effects of the pill might be carcinogenic, because "estrogen is to cancer what fertilizer is to the wheat crop." Fifteen hundred pages of testimony later, the hearings were over, and their impact had been enormous. More than a million women switched to other birth control techniques; the American College of Obstetricians and Gynecologists drafted an insert to be placed in birth control dispensers warning that use of the pill increased a woman's risk of blood clots and strokes; and the American Medical Association warned of possible links between pill use and breast and endometrial cancers. "Patients should be carefully examined periodically," the AMA advised, "and those who have or have had a known or suspected hormone-dependent tumor should not use this method of contraception."[5]

Many epidemiologists wanted another look, especially Ralph Paffenbarger. Trained as a pediatrician, Paffenbarger moved into epidemiology during the 1950s, specializing in polio research for the National Institutes of Health. Once the polio vaccine had been developed, he left the NIH and moved to the state public health department in California, where he spent the next decade working on chronic diseases. Looking for a new re-

Bathsheba's Breast

search focus, his attention fell on breast cancer. "We had done studies on heart disease and cancer," Paffenbarger recalled, "and breast cancer was clearly one of the more important cancers. We were looking for new things that might explain the rising incidence. Was the pill involved? It was an obvious question."

Teaming up with Elfriede Fasal, a gynecologist and epidemiologist, Paffenbarger designed a study involving thousands of women admitted to nineteen San Francisco hospitals between 1970 and 1972. Each woman answered detailed questions about her menstrual history, use of estrogen, birth control techniques, general health, and history of breast disease. Fasal and Paffenbarger spent three years sifting through the data, and in 1975, when Rose Kushner started hunting down breast cancer bogeymen, they published their results. Women who took birth control pills from two to four years nearly doubled the chance of getting breast cancer. Also, women with a history of benign breast disease before they started taking birth control pills, and who then used the pill for more than six years, had anywhere from a 600 to 1,000 percent higher risk of getting breast cancer than women who did not use it.[6]

For Kushner, the study was all the proof needed to demand warning labels on birth control pills. In 1979 Paffenbarger and Fasal could say with complete confidence that women who used birth control pills for more than a year had an elevated risk for breast cancer. Malcolm Pike, a biostatistician at the University of Southern California, reported in 1981 that women who began using birth control pills during their teenage years, before a full-term pregnancy, doubled their risk for "early onset breast cancer"—cancer before they were forty-five years old. If they used the pill for eight years before a full-term pregnancy, they tripled the risk. In a 1983 article, Pike upped the risk. After one year on the pill, the chances of being diagnosed with early breast cancer increased by 30 percent; after eight years, the risk was 400 percent.[7]

Government agencies reacted to Paffenbarger like a besieged army. They criticized his methodology and questioned Pike's sampling techniques. The FDA, the Centers for Disease Control, and the National Institute of Child Health and Development launched the Cancer and Steroid Hormones Study (CASH) to study the problem, and between 1980 and 1987, CASH conducted several studies of its own. Not surprisingly, each repudiated the notion that there was any correlation between birth control pills and breast cancer. Throughout the 1980s, federal agencies maintained that stand. Louise Tryer, vice-president of Planned Parenthood of America, decided that the CASH reports were "reassuring, particularly for women in the United States," and that there should be no changes in current uses of the birth control pill.[8]

In 1987 CASH lowered its level of certainty. Between 1986 and 1989, five studies provided disturbing evidence. In 1986 Swedish and Danish epidemiologists reported an increase in breast cancer among women who took birth control pills for more than seven years. A New Zealand study in 1987 noted higher odds among women who took the pill for more than ten years. A 1988 CASH study revealed a nearly 600 percent increased risk of breast cancer for childless women who had had their first period before age thirteen, took the pill before their twentieth birthday, and remained on the pill for at least eight years. In 1989 British researchers with the Imperial Cancer Research Fund concluded that women who had used birth control pills for more than four years had a 43 percent higher risk for breast cancer than women who had never used the pill, and that the risk increased to 74 percent after eight years. Finally, oncologists at the University Hospital in Lund, Sweden, claimed that women who used birth control pills from three to five years before the age of twenty-five doubled the odds of getting breast cancer; after five years of use the risk jumped to more than 500 percent.[9]

Other estrogen products came under scrutiny too. Kushner called estrogen replacement therapy (ERT) into question. The guru of ERT in the United States was Robert Wilson, a New York obstetrician-gynecologist. For Wilson, menopause was a deficiency disease caused by lack of estrogen, just as insulin shortages caused diabetes. In the 1950s he began treating women with estrogen replacement therapy, calibrating doses according to a "Femininity Index"—enough mature cells in the lining of the vagina to keep it moist and supple. If Wilson found that 80 percent of a woman's cells were mature, she was "still feminine" because her estrogen levels were sufficient. Anything less indicated that her "femininity was waning." Early in the 1960s, he trumpeted his crusade to keep women from "being condemned to witness the death of their own womanhood." What the women needed, he pronounced, was "hormone replacement therapy, preferably beginning as early as age thirty." The key to everlasting femininity, Wilson claimed, was estrogen replacement therapy.

In 1966 Wilson wrote *Feminine Forever,* which rocketed to the top of the nonfiction best-seller list when more than 100,000 copies sold in the first seven months after publication. ERT answered a host of female problems, or at least problems a male physician perceived in women he knew. Only a man could have described the therapy with such gender-loaded excesses:

> Women rich in estrogen tend to have a certain mental vigor that gives them self-confidence, a sense of mastery over their destiny, the ability to think out problems effectively, resistance to mental and physical fatigue, and emotional self-control. Their emotional reactions are proportional to the occasion. They neither over-react hysterically, nor do they tend toward apathy. They are, as a rule, capable of facing the world with a healthful relaxed attitude and thereby to enjoy their daily life. They are seldom depressed. Irrational crying spells are virtually unknown among them. In a family situation, estrogen makes women adorable, even-tempered, and generally easy to live with. Consequently a woman's estrogen carries significance beyond her own well-being. It also contributes toward the happiness of her family and all those with whom she is in daily contact.

He also rhapsodized about ERT's ability to keep a woman's hair shiny, hips thin, breasts firm, and skin tight.

Ayerst Laboratories, the manufacturers of Premarin, a post-menopausal estrogen treatment, celebrated geometric increases in sales that accompanied publication of *Feminine Forever.* ERT boomed. But disturbing news soon appeared. In October 1975, Donald Austin of the California Tumor Registry announced that uterine cancer in the San Francisco Bay area was 50 percent higher in 1973 than it had been in 1969. Affluent white women over the age of fifty, the prime users of ERT, were the most vulnerable. Two months later, epidemiologists at the Kaiser-Permanente Medical Center in Los Angeles confirmed Austin's suspicions. Endometrial cancer was on the rise, especially among middle-aged women receiving ERT.[10]

Not much time passed before speculation about the relationship between ERT and breast cancer ceased to be rumor and acquired scientific credibility. Such relationships in laboratory animals had been documented for decades. A 1976 issue of *The New England Journal of Medicine* reported the histories of 1,891 menopausal women who had received long-term ERT. Their rate of breast cancer was 30 percent higher than normal. Throughout the 1970s and 1980s, evidence mounted, and in 1991 the Centers for Disease Control completed a meta-analysis of sixteen other studies completed between 1976 and 1989. They reminded readers of the health benefits of ERT—stronger bones and healthier hearts—but minced no words about the relationship between ERT and breast cancer. There was no doubt, and they even quantified their conclusions. "On the basis of our estimate," they claimed, "approximately 4,708 new cases and 1,468 breast cancer deaths would occur each year because of estrogen use."[11]

While fighting other women's battles, Rose Kushner discovered in 1982 that her own struggle was not over. Breast cancer has a long lead time. Oncologists are not comfortable calling a woman "cured" until ten cancer-free years have passed after initial treatments. Kushner did not make the benchmark. In June 1982, eight years after the mastectomy, physicians at Roswell Park found a tiny, four-millimeter malignant tumor in the chest wall near her implant. "After eight years, it was a shock to have the cancer come back, but my experience shows the importance of having regular checkups," she told reporters. Surgeons removed the lesion and pathologists determined the malignant cells possessed estrogen receptors. In earlier days, she would have faced oophorectomy, adrenalectomy, and hypophysectomy to stop the flow of estrogen to the tumor, but times had changed. A new antiestrogen drug had appeared, and Kushner took advantage of it.[12]

Hormonal therapy bounded forward in the 1980s. Physicians had known for almost a century that some breast cancers respond to endocrine therapy. In the cruder days of surgery, before estrogen-blocking drugs were available, surgeons cut off the supply of estrogen to breast cancer cells by removing ovaries, adrenal glands, and the pituitary. Because they had no way of determining which breast tumors were estrogen dependent, surgeons performed oophorectomies, adrenalectomies, and hypophysectomies on advanced cancer patients, knowing that most would not respond. During the 1940s and 1950s, scientists gathered data and came to a modest conclusion. Older women were more likely to benefit from hormonal therapy than younger ones. Patients with long disease-free intervals between their mastectomy and the recurrence of tumors, like Kushner, benefitted more than women whose recurrences appeared soon after the operation. Hormonal therapy was more likely to shrink skin and lymph node metastases but was less successful with bone and brain metastases. Still, oncologists could not predict with any precision which women were candidates for hormonal therapy.

Research in the late 1960s and early 1970s provided tools for predicting which patients might benefit from hormonal treatments. British scientists traced the amounts of gonadal and adrenal steroids excreted in the urine of breast cancer patients and found a measurable, if modest, correlation. Patients who excreted the steroids had a somewhat better chance of responding to hormonal therapy. More successful, however, were the studies of estrogen receptors in laboratory animals. At the end of the 1960s, American, Dutch, British, and French biochemists discovered that the reproductive tissues of mice and rats demonstrated a striking capacity to absorb hexestrol and estradiol, two steroid estrogens. Eventually, they learned that steroid estrogens bind with cytoplasmic proteins in the tumor cells of some breast cancer patients, and that these women will benefit from hormonal therapy. Physicians no longer had to use a shotgun approach; they could now predict which patients would benefit from endocrine treatments and which would not.[13]

The treatment, however, was almost worse than the disease. Removal of ovaries, adrenal glands, and pituitaries left women wounded and debilitated. Without those organs, they experienced long-term problems from low blood sugar, obesity, depression, and dizziness. In the late 1950s, physicians tried to compensate for the body's inability to produce the necessary hormones by prescribing daily injections of cortisone, but adjusting dosages to different individuals proved daunting. Too little cortisone left patients with all the side effects of hormone starvation, but too much cortisone caused liver damage, fluid retention, and the telltale, moon-faced, humpbacked appearance. A nonsurgical option for women whose breast tumors were hormone dependent became available in the 1960s. Patients kept their ovaries, adrenal glands, and pituitary, but to block the flow of estrogen to hormone-dependent tumors, physicians loaded them with such male hormones as androgen and testosterone. Those too had serious side effects. What breast cancer patients really needed was a drug that would block estrogen but do so without the side effects of steroids and male hormones.

That drug, a nonsteroidal antiestrogen, first emerged in the British laboratories of Imperial Chemical Industries (ICI). Arthur Walpole worked at ICI in the 1940s and 1950s, where he developed several anti-cancer drugs. He also discovered tamoxifen in 1962, when he was testing it as a contraceptive in rats. Walpole learned that tamoxifen was effective as a "morning after" drug, preventing a fertilized egg from taking root in uterine tissues. His high hopes for using tamoxifen as a "morning after" drug in human beings were never realized. Tamoxifen reduced fertility in rats, but it actually stimulated ovulation in women. At Walpole's suggestion, Mary Cole of the Christie Hospital in Manchester, England, began clinical trials on advanced breast cancer patients whose tumor cells possessed estrogen receptor cells. They found that tamoxifen had a strong affinity for estrogen receptors on cancer cells and prevented estrogen from binding to them, depriving the cell of an essential ingredient. Oophorectomies, adrenalectomies, and hypophysectomies became unnecessary. Because it was not a steroid, tamoxifen had none of the damaging side effects of cortisone replacement therapy.[14]

Putting her hopes in tamoxifen, Kushner shifted her crusade into high gear. She established a breast cancer information hotline that fielded hundreds of calls each week from frightened, angry women and evolved into a strong combination umbrella group of breast cancer groups—the National Alliance for Breast Cancer Organizations. Her two books—*Breast Cancer* (1975) and *Why Me?* (1982)—were best-sellers. Kushner's articles on breast cancer appeared in major newspapers and magazines around the country. She filed lawsuits against the federal government and the cancer establishment demanding treatment reforms. She made a nuisance of herself at medical meetings, asked pointed questions during scientific presentations, and collared officials from the American Cancer Society (ACS), the American Medical Association, and various physicians organizations. She walked the halls of Congress, lobbying for changes in policy at the National Institutes of Health (NIH) and the Food and Drug Administration.

In the late 1970s, her lobbying yielded results. Convinced that widespread adoption of birth control pills by American women at least in part explained the increased incidence of breast cancer, Kushner filed suit against the U.S. Department of Health, Education and Welfare and the Food and Drug Administration, demanding the placement of warning labels on birth control pills so that women would know the risks. In 1978, federal courts ruled in Kushner's favor and required all manufacturers of birth control pills to provide the warnings to consumers.

She had similar success battling the single-stage biopsy-mastectomy procedure. Kushner had not been alone, of course, in her assault on the one-stage operation. George Rosemond, former president of the ACS, called for the end of the one-stage procedure in 1973, as did Gordon F. Schwartz of the Jefferson Medical College in 1975. Both had been around long enough to remember the old days, when the two-stage approach had been the norm. Most women went to a family physician or local surgeon who biopsied the lump in an office or clinic. Pathologists at major urban medical centers then diagnosed the tissue, and if it was malignant, the patient went there for surgery. But in 1946, Congress passed the Hill-Burton Act providing tens of millions of dollars each year for the construction of hospitals in smaller cities and towns throughout the United States. In the 1950s large numbers of the new, smaller hospitals began treating cancer, and the one-stage procedure was proving to be more efficient. It tied up the operating room only once, not twice. Within a few years, the one-stage procedure had become the norm.[15]

By the late 1970s, an increasing number of surgeons, especially those at major cancer centers, agreed with Kushner that there was no compelling medical reason for doing a biopsy and mastectomy at the same time. Of course, many women wanted the one-stage procedure to avoid the inconvenience and risk of two surgical procedures. Others just wanted to get it all "over with." But science was heading in the other direction. Shirley Temple Black rejected the one-stage approach in 1972 with her catchy statement, "The doctor can make the incision; I'll make the decision." Women, demanding control over their own bodies, insisted on a voice in their medical treatment. The one-stage procedure had become a medical and cultural anachronism; the days of omnipotent physicians were drawing to a close. In 1979 the NIH formally recommended that biopsies and mastectomies be performed as separate procedures. Kushner shared victory champagne with her husband the night of the decision. "A mastectomy is bad enough," she later recalled, "but not to have time to adjust to the idea in advance is barbaric."[16]

Kushner hailed the 1979 decisions by the ACS and the NIH to formally endorse Bernard Fisher's work. The ACS, long a bastion of radical surgery, began helping to fund his research, and Arthur I. Holleb, its chief medical officer, acknowledged that for early-stage breast cancer, lumpectomy (which Fisher preferred to call segmental mastectomy) and radiotherapy were perfectly acceptable treatment options. In June 1979, the NIH convened a conference entitled "The Treatment of Primary Breast Cancer: Management of Local Disease." The NIH had established a ten-person panel that included Bernard Fisher, Jerome Urban, and Rose Kushner, and they announced at the conference, with Urban dissenting, that the standard treatment for Stage 1 and Stage 2 breast cancer was no longer the radical mastectomy or even the modified radical mastectomy but the simple (total) mastectomy with lymph node dissection. Fisher and Kushner had made common cause in what some called the "Rose and Bernie" show, and the conjunction of his science and her passion had finally managed to bulldoze the surgical establishment. In 1974, surgeons performed nearly 46,000 radical mastectomies for breast cancer. That number fell to 17,000 in 1979 and 2,500 in 1987.

Fisher's argument that breast cancer was a systemic disease from the very beginning was tragically supported on April 24, 1979, with the death of Marvella Bayh. Ever since her decision in October 1971 to go public with her disease, Bayh had been the American Cancer Society's poster child for early detection and breast self-examination. In 1974, she had cochaired the ACS National Cancer Crusade and had toured the country speaking to a variety of public health groups. Women's magazines had regularly featured her as a "breast cancer survivor." But in February 1978, Bayh learned that her cancer had metastasized and was incurable. She kept up the crusade, traveling and speaking up to the very end, but her death dampened much of the prevailing optimism about the efficacy of breast cancer treatment.

Kushner also celebrated Bernard Fisher's landmark studies of the 1980s, which resolved several breast cancer controversies. Between 1985 and 1989, Fisher reported the results of his long-term study of breast cancer treatment protocols. In 1985, he reported in *The New England Journal of Medicine* research results in 1,843 women. After recommending the end of the Halsted radical mastectomy in 1979, he had set out to evaluate the modified radical mastectomy for women with early-stage breast cancer. The patients selected for the study all had tumors four centimeters or less in size. Fisher randomly divided the women into three groups. One group received a "total" mastectomy with an axillary lymph node dissection; a second group received a lumpectomy and an axillary node dissection; and a third group received a lumpectomy, axillary dissection, and follow-up radiotherapy. The tumors removed in lumpectomies all had margins free of malignant cells. The five-year survival rates for recipients of the total mastectomy were not as good as those for women who had undergone only lumpectomies. Women receiving lumpectomies and radiation were much better off than those receiving only mastectomies.

Four years later, Fisher updated his research on the same 1,843 women. Of those who had received lumpectomies and radiotherapy, 85 percent were still alive five years after treatment, compared to 76 percent for those receiving total mastectomies. As a result, Fisher concluded that for women with early-stage breast cancer—tumors four centimeters in size or less—lumpectomy combined with radiotherapy could replace the modified radical and total mastectomies as treatments of choice. Still, there was a higher incidence of local recurrence in the affected breast after lumpectomy, requiring careful vigilance and a willingness on the part of the patient to assume that increased risk.

In that same 1989 issue of *The New England Journal of Medicine,* Fisher reported on his tamoxifen studies. A total of 2,644 women participated in the study. All had been treated for breast cancer, and none had tumor cells in the lymph nodes. Each possessed tumors with estrogen receptors. Half the women received a placebo, and half received tamoxifen. Although long-term survival rates were the same for both groups, tamoxifen reduced the rate of local recurrence and new tumors in the opposite breast. Women taking tamoxifen enjoyed a longer period of disease-free survival than those getting the placebo. Fisher recommended the use of tamoxifen for women whose tumors were estrogen positive.

Finally, Fisher reported his clinical trials of chemotherapy in 1989. He had studied 679 women with breast cancers that had no axillary node involvement and no estrogen receptors. Half the women received a chemotherapy regimen of methotrexate and fluorouracil. The others had no chemotherapy follow-up. Four years later, Fisher could report that the women receiving chemotherapy enjoyed a longer disease-free period than the women without the treatments, but survival rates for both groups were identical. The methotrexate-fluorouracil combination was not a cure but did extend life.[17]

Warnings were now on birth control pills, the safety of the lumpectomy was confirmed, and the single-stage biopsy-mastectomy had been formally rejected by the National Institutes of Health. Rose Kushner felt some satisfaction, at least until she heard about Nancy Reagan.

October 1987 posed difficult challenges for the First Family. On October 19, the stock market crashed, losing more value in one day than it had on Black Tuesday in 1929. President Ronald Reagan was in the midst of a bitter, and ultimately unsuccessful, battle to convince the Senate to confirm the nomination of Robert Bork to the Supreme Court. Negotiations with Mikhail Gorbachev and the Soviet Union to reduce stockpiles of strategic nuclear weapons had reached a critical stage. The Reagans faced a personal crisis as well. Early in the month, physicians at the National Institutes of Health gave Nancy Reagan her annual physical. John Hutton, the White House physician, accompanied her. When the mammogram films were developed, a nurse came and told the First Lady that they needed a couple of extra exposures. "I felt my stomach tighten," Nancy Reagan later wrote. Hutton came back about thirty minutes later to report, "We think we've seen something. We think it's a tumor in the left breast. We'll need a biopsy." A tiny lump of no more than seven millimeters—the smallest tumor detectable by mammography—showed up because its denser tissues blocked out x-ray beams.

Because of a busy schedule and, no doubt, her emotional need to sort out the frightening information, the First Lady postponed the operation, filling ten days and nights with banquets, speeches, and meetings in her campaign against drug abuse. If the tumor proved to be malignant, she had to choose among four alternatives. The most aggressive approach was a modified radical mastectomy, an operation to remove the breast, the axilla nodes, and a small portion of chest muscle. A less physically damaging option was a total mastectomy—that is, removing the breast and the axilla nodes. The third was a lumpectomy—cutting out the lump and a small portion of adjacent tissue—followed up by radiotherapy. The final option was to remove only the tumor itself.

Medical technology offered Nancy Reagan an opportunity few women had ever enjoyed in the past, a choice between several scientifically rational options, each of which had its supporters and detractors whose arguments regularly appeared in medical journals and popular magazines. But the opportunity itself was daunting, for it forced her to weigh the options and evaluate the alternatives, to accept the counsel of one set of experts but to reject that of other, equally qualified physicians and scientists.

For Nancy Reagan the decision was a relatively easy one. There was only one expert she really trusted, Dr. Loyal Davis, her stepfather. While growing up, she had enjoyed a close relationship with Davis, a distinguished neurosurgeon at the Mayo Clinic. Many times over the course of his career they had talked about breast cancer. In their discussions, she had listened to him criticize the Halsted radical and the Urban superradical as unnecessarily aggressive for Stage 1 disease, but she had also listened to his warnings about lumpectomies. In his opinion, women receiving lumpectomies left themselves with a higher risk of recurrence. Davis's *Textbook of Surgery: The Biological Basis of Modern Surgical Practice* was in its twelfth edition when he died in 1982. He was blunt about breast cancer options: "Modified radical mastectomy has become the procedure of choice for most surgeons in the United States." That was all Nancy Reagan needed to know. She did not want to spend the next six weeks making daily pilgrimages to the radiotherapy machines at Bethesda. Most of all, she wanted to get rid of the cancer and to get on with her life. She decided to have a modified radical mastectomy. "A lumpectomy seemed too inconclusive," she wrote in her diary on October 6, 1987. "I know, given my nature, that I'd be worried to death. It will be hard enough to go through the ten days of waiting, and I know I can't spend months, or years, wondering."

Nancy Reagan opted for a single-stage biopsy-mastectomy rather than the recently recommended two-step procedure. She insisted that Ollie Beahrs, one of her father's colleagues at Mayo, assist the Bethesda surgeons. Just before orderlies wheeled her into the operating room, Beahrs and Hutton again reviewed the options with her. She was insistent: "Look, if you get in there and find out that's what it is, please don't wake me to have a conversation about it. Just do it. It shouldn't take you long, because there isn't much there to take off. Dolly Parton I'm not." Her modest statement was all too correct. The lump was so small that the surgeons had a difficult time locating it, but when they did, pathologists composed a frozen section and decided it was malignant. With the First Lady still under anesthesia, surgeons performed the mastectomy. Several days after the operation, pathologists sent good news to the White House. All the axillary nodes were cancer-free.

It should have been a happy ending, but breast cancer politics dictated differently. In the mid-1980s, the debate over the mastectomy was at its most intense. Progressive surgeons and critics in the women's movement held radical surgeons in low esteem, often describing them as insensitive, egotistical men who butchered women for no good reason. The campaign against the mastectomy was at its peak in 1987 when Nancy Reagan made her decision. She was a perfect candidate for lumpectomy and radiation—a woman with a tiny, Stage 1 tumor and negative nodes. The fact that she was also one of the most prominent women in the world, a role model with the power to set the record straight and make a persuasive statement in behalf of lumpectomies, was not lost on advocates of the procedure. Her decision for aggressive treatment angered many people, who showered her with criticism. That breast cancer is an intensely personal disease requiring intensely personal decisions mattered little to those who wanted the First Lady to do what they considered the right thing. Rose Kushner, after admitting that such decisions were very personal, lambasted the First Lady, angrily proclaiming that her decision has "set us back ten years. I'm not recommending that anyone do it her way." But C. Norman Coleman of the Harvard Medical School supported the First Lady: "I really can't overstate the emotion that goes into decision making," he told a *New York Times* reporter. "If you are worried about a recurrence of cancer in the breast at any time—ever—if you take the breast off, you obviously won't have a recurrence."

The criticisms stung. Nancy Reagan not only had to mourn the loss of her breast; she had to defend her decision. "I resented these statements," she wrote in her memoirs, "and I still do. This is a very personal decision, one that each woman must make for herself. This was my choice, and I don't believe I should have been criticized for it. For some women, it would have been wrong, but for me it was right. Perhaps, if I had been twenty years old and unmarried, I would have made a different decision . . . . For me, a mastectomy seemed the sensible thing to do, and the best way to get it all over with."[18]

Kushner interpreted Nancy Reagan's decision as a setback for her cause, but it was only a minor one. For a few months in late 1987, an abnormally large number of breast cancer patients opted for mastectomies, but the numbers soon returned to normal. People in the women's movement acknowledged Kushner as a major figure in the crusade to change breast cancer treatment; finally, late in the 1980s, the medical establishment afforded her similar recognition. Commenting on the demise of the single-stage biopsy-mastectomy, Bruce Chabner, director of the division of cancer treatment for the National Cancer Institute, praised Kushner as the "single most important person in leading to this major change in breast surgery." From 1980 to 1986 she served as a member of the National Breast Cancer Advisory Force, and in 1989 she became a member of the American Cancer Society's Breast Cancer Task Force.[19]

Late in 1989, Kushner learned that the Society of Surgical Oncology had selected her as the 1990 recipient of the James Ewing Award for outstanding contributions in the fight against cancer. When news of the award reached her, she smirked through a deep cough. The tamoxifen treatments to deal with the small recurrent lesion on her chest had not done the job. The cancer had spread, and by December 1989 Kushner was barely hanging on to life. She thoroughly enjoyed the irony of the Ewing prize. It's "poetic justice," her husband said. "They booed her off their stage in 1975." The Society of Surgical Oncology made the award posthumously. Rose Kushner died of breast cancer on January 9, 1990.[20]

CHAPTER TEN

The Breast Cancer Wars

The data was political dynamite—a laser-printed, computer-paper explosive—and Janet Daling knew it as soon as her software began sorting out the oncological categories. An epidemiologist at the Fred Hutchinson Cancer Research Center in Seattle, Daling had uncovered a statistical correlation between abortion and breast cancer. During the 1980s, European scientists had speculated about the risk, but critics noted flaws in the experimental design and discounted the warnings. Daling had been one of the skeptics. In her own research, she had failed more than once to find a correlation, and she knew, given the political climate, that abortion opponents would grasp at any alleged connection and hype it shamelessly.

Personally committed to reproductive freedom, Daling decided to answer the question definitively, to put the controversy to rest in a flawlessly designed, critic-proof study. She tracked 1,800 women—half of whom had already been diagnosed with breast cancer—over a seven-year period, starting with detailed health histories from each and then monitoring them in regular follow-ups. The results were unexpected. Women aged forty-five or younger who had undergone an induced abortion ran a 50 percent higher risk of contracting breast cancer than women who had never had an abortion. Women under the age of eighteen who underwent an abortion after the eighth week of pregnancy increased by 800 percent their risks of premenopausal breast cancer. During pregnancy, Daling speculated, new breast cells proliferate rapidly and do not stabilize until the last trimester when hormones help them mature. Interrupting a pregnancy may fill the breast with large numbers of primitive—and potentially dangerous—cells. Women who had experienced natural miscarriages did not have an elevated risk of breast cancer, perhaps because the pregnancies were hormonally flawed from the very beginning and had not induced changes in breast tissues.

Daling's conclusions were certain to inspire controversy and give abortion opponents a new political weapon. Right-to-life groups hounded her for information, naively hoping to enlist her as a pro-life volunteer. But they did not know her. She did not suffer ideologues lightly. In the summer of 1993, a particularly obnoxious pro-life attorney from Virginia finally got under her skin, forcing Daling to remove her placid scientific mask. "I told him," she mentioned to a reporter for *Time,* "I don't think you care one bit about breast cancer and women's health. You just want to help your cause." She did not want to supply pro-lifers with scientific ammunition, but she was not about to bury her research either, even though some pro-choice advocates would have preferred to see the data remain unpublished. "Scientists have to put their political and personal views aside and report the data," she told a reporter. *The Journal of the National Cancer Institute* published her article in its November 2, 1994, issue.

Anticipating the debate, Daling hedged her scientific bet just a bit. The 800 percent increased risk for younger women was particularly alarming, certain to be misunderstood and taken out of context, so she tucked the number away, giving the 50 percent general risk full play but burying the rest into a table. "We didn't say that in our report," she told *Time,* "because we didn't want to alarm anyone before more research is done." That was a naive pipe dream. Her research was picked up by every wire service and network news station in the country, precipitating the most predictable of reactions. "I'm absolutely appalled that politics is entering into the science of this study," Daling protested. "No one is getting any of the correct information out to the public."

Pro-choice public relations groups shifted into high gear, trying to cast doubt on her findings. Dozens of animal studies, they argued, had failed to establish any correlation. Some abortion rights advocates made light of the 50 percent increased risk, calling it infinitesimal compared to the 3,000 percent higher risk for lung cancer that smokers possess. In its own attempt at damage control, *The Journal of the National Cancer Institute* published a contrary editorial in the same issue. Lynn Rosenberg, a

Boston University epidemiologist, wrote the piece, insisting that a 50 percent risk "is small in epidemiologic terms and severely challenges our ability to distinguish if it reflects cause and effect or if it simply reflects bias . . . the overall results as well as the particulars are far from conclusive, and it is difficult to see how they will be informative to the public."

Pro-lifers reacted just as predictably. Paige Cunningham, president of Americans United for Life, argued that even "if you want to say the study is inconclusive, I think women have a right to know. Physicians routinely tell patients about much smaller risks than this." Anti-abortionists called for congressional hearings, and the Republican triumph in the elections of 1994 whetted their appetites. They realized that the issue would have to wait one hundred days in 1995 until after Speaker of the House Newt Gingrich had disposed of his "Contract with America," but "on Day 101," promised John Wilke of the Life Issues Institute in Cincinnati, "it's our turn." Congressman Christopher Smith, a pro-life Republican from New Jersey, could hardly wait. "I have absolutely no doubt that these issues will be aired," he told *Newsweek*. By March 1995, the pro-life group Abortion Industry Monitor had distributed tens of thousands of copies of its pamphlet *Before You Choose: The Link between Abortion & Breast Cancer*.[1]

In the 1990s, everything about breast cancer seemed controversial. The disease revealed its biological secrets grudgingly, and each new discovery or teasing epidemiological clue produced as many questions as answers, generated complex philosophical and political dilemmas, and triggered new controversies. Almost weekly, some laboratory issued a press release announcing the latest findings, warning women of some new risk. In 1994, the *New York Times* reported that women who do not breast-feed their babies have an elevated risk for premenopausal breast cancer, as do women who do not exercise regularly. It was not at all unusual for the news to be poorly handled by reporters anxious to sell copy. Wire services could not print quickly enough the news that lesbians had a higher than average risk for getting breast cancer than the population at large, as if sexual orientation caused the disease. Talk shows buzzed with the news that well-educated career women were similarly at risk, as if college degrees and good jobs were carcinogenic. The facts that lesbians and career women were more likely than the population at large to postpone childbirth or not have children at all—both risk factors—were barely mentioned.[2]

Breast cancer was the hottest of topics—in molecular laboratories, legal conference rooms, legislative corridors, White House offices, and surgical suites. The disease had negotiated its way to the forefront of the women's health movement. For twenty years, feminists had focused increasing attention on gender issues in medicine. Cindy Pearson, executive director of the National Women's Health Network, compared breast cancer with heart disease. "In the late fifties to the mid-sixties," she remarked in 1993, "[we] became incredibly conscious of the fact that men were dying or becoming disabled at a very early age by heart disease and stroke. Heart disease became a big issue, got a lot of funding, the American Heart Association got really active on it, and it's a big success. Heart disease rates have been dropping for thirty years." Breast cancer, however, was a different story. "Today it is just barely being seen as the same kind of premature killer and disabler of women. It took an extra twenty years to see breast cancer in the light that we so easily and quickly saw heart disease. I don't think we've responded with equivalent emphasis to the high proportion of breast cancer in women as we did to the high incidence of heart disease in men thirty years ago. The reason? Sexism."[3]

Medical sexism was never more evident than in the National Cancer Institute's decision to cancel the "Women's Health Trial." In 1984 the NCI and the American Cancer Society launched a long-term, $25 million "Women's Health Trial" involving six thousand women to determine if dietary reductions of fat would change the incidence of breast cancer. But when NCI statisticians reevaluated the study's design and decided that 32,000 women would need to be involved for the results to be reliable, projected costs skyrocketed from $25 million to more than $100 million. The NCI summarily canceled the project. David Korn, head of the Stanford University Medical School, defended the decision, claiming that "there is no way to measure fat intake. The only thing you can do is rely on memory. By the time you've reached the latter part of the study, you would have a rather elderly population—how accurate would their dietary memories be? Where would they be? Would half of them be in nursing homes with various kinds of senility and forgetfulness?" Congresswoman Patricia Schroeder of Colorado was livid. "We were sickened," she claimed, "by the reasons they gave us—that you couldn't teach women to keep records or change their diets."[4]

Sexism had always straitjacketed breast cancer treatment. Women got the disease; men tried to fix it. Women suffered; men talked, decided, operated, and radiated. Women asked what to do and men told them. Breast cancer was a disease of women, but men controlled its social, political, and scientific agenda. Until the 1990s, at least, when a cultural earthquake shifted breast cancer's fault lines. In the pantheon of cancer stars, women like Rose Kushner were about to eclipse the likes of William Stewart Halsted and Jerome Urban. As they asserted themselves, they shook the foundations of American oncology.

No place better symbolized the new era than the UCLA Breast Center. Tastefully appointed furnishings, thoughtful decor, and soft, pastel colors blanketed the waiting and examining rooms in a warm glow. The interior designers who fashioned the suites had comfort in mind, for patients destined to spend time there would be preoccupied and nervous. If decor could heal, the center had the look of good medicine. Late in June 1994, a young woman with breast cancer watched her doctor enter the room. With a commanding physical presence, a bold, outspoken confidence, and strong, powerful arms, the physician looked every bit a surgeon. When the patient asked if the cancer was lethal, the doctor chuckled, wheeled a chair up to the examining table, patted her on the legs, and cheerfully, but intimately and reassuringly, reminded her that "driving in L.A. is lethal. Your mammogram doesn't say anything about death. We're not talking doom." The surgeon began a careful discussion of the breast, its functions, and cancer. Then, when the young patient appeared somewhat bewildered, Dr. Susan Love, director of the UCLA Breast Center, did what few breast surgeons ever do: she unbuttoned her own blouse, exposed her own left breast, and used it to describe mammary anatomy and malignant disease. Forty minutes later, she told the young woman, "There are options. And you have time to think about it." "Will you take care of me?" the patient inquired. "I'll take good care of you," Love answered, embracing the young woman in a sincere, heartfelt hug.

Thousands of women around the country credited Susan Love with saving their lives. She was born in 1948 in Long Branch, New Jersey, to Irish Catholic parents. Educated at parochial schools, Love spent two years taking premed courses at the College of Notre Dame. Throughout her sophomore year, she pondered a career as a nun and then joined a convent. But the cloistered life proved too esoteric, too abstract, more given to contemplation than action. "They wanted to save their souls," Love recalled, "and I wanted to save the world." She left the convent after four months, enrolled at Fordham University, and finished a bachelor's degree. After a stellar career at the State University of New York's Downtown Medical Center in Brooklyn, she completed a surgical residency at Beth Israel Hospital in Boston. Love put up with all the abuse male surgeons dished out to female residents. "It's so pragmatic, so tactile," she told a *New York Times* reporter. "You can fix things."

After finishing her residency, she moved to Boston and went on to become chief breast surgeon at the Dana Farber Cancer Institute. She also came out of the closet, acknowledging a lesbian identity and falling in love with Helen Cooksey, a surgical colleague. In 1989 Love became pregnant through artificial insemination and gave birth to a daughter, Katie Love Cooksey. The two women formally adopted Katie, though only after an extended legal battle. Adoption was a political and social statement, a declaration of lesbian independence. "Helen and I have money and privilege," she argued, "so it's our obligation to pave the way." Her *Susan Love's Breast Book* became a best-seller in 1990, and two years later UCLA enticed her into taking over the Breast Center. Cooksey postponed her surgical career to raise Katie.

In the world of breast cancer surgery, Susan Love was an iconoclast, an outspoken, strong-willed woman bent on transforming medicine and politics. She was convinced that the traditional protocol of surgery, radiotherapy, and chemotherapy—"slash, burn, and poison" as she called them—would never effect a real cure. Still, she commented in 1993, "[T]he research establishment continues to spend enormous sums of money on them, asking tired, old questions like 'Should we give chemotherapy for three months or four months?' and 'Should we give patients four drugs or five drugs?' What we need to do instead is put more of our funds into figuring how the disease progresses at the molecular level, because that's where the real answers are going to be."

Nor did she put undue faith in breast self-examination or mammography. Love did not dispute the effectiveness of early detection as a means of reducing breast cancer mortality rates, and she regularly had mammograms of her own, but mammography and self-examination, she was certain, would soon reach their limits as diagnostic tools. Breast self-examination, she claimed, "is an overrated activity. The medical establishment would like you to believe that breast cancer starts as a grain of sand, grows to be the size of a pea and on and on until it becomes a grape-fruit. Breast cancer doesn't work like that. It grows slow and it's sneaky. You could examine yourself every day and suddenly find a walnut." By the time lumps are discovered, even tiny ones, they have existed for years. "You know," she explained to a reporter for *Technology Review,* "women are al-ways being told about the importance of early detection, but in the cur-rent state of the art, we can detect breast cancer only at a relatively late stage. The cancer has typically been there for 6 years if it shows up on a mammogram and 8 to 10 years if you can feel the lump."

Love also expressed strong opinions about the role of gender in sci-ence and medicine. Surgical oncology, especially breast cancer surgery, was far from an exact science. "Often," she preached, "the result is that the val-ues of a white, middle-aged man are imposed on a patient who is female and maybe older or younger, maybe white and maybe not." To an older widow, Love recalled, a young male surgeon recommended removal of the breast: "Well, you're elderly and you're widowed—you don't need your breast anymore. Why don't you just have a mastectomy? It'll be easier." He could not fathom an elderly woman who might want to keep her breast. In a 1994 interview with NBC's *Dateline,* Love recounted another example. When a young patient asked her male surgeon what a recon-structed, postmastectomy breast would feel like, he reassured her, "It will feel perfectly normal, no different from your other breast." Actually, mas-tectomies sever nerves in the chest and axilla. The new breast and the area surrounding it feel odd and different, numb and insensitive, attached to the body but not really part of it. The doctor had misconstrued her ques-tion. What he was telling the young woman was that it would feel nor-mal to the touch of any man. It would feel normal to *him.*

After Rose Kushner died in 1990, Love emerged as the leading gen-eral in the breast cancer wars. She exhibited all of Kushner's emotional commitment, but the cold logic of science leavened her passion. While Kushner lambasted Nancy Reagan's decision to have a mastectomy, Love paid more than lip service to the merits of individual choice. The decision to have a lumpectomy or a mastectomy, she argued, "is not the momen-tous sort of choice people often imagine it is . . . either of those treatments will work as well as the others, so really you're deciding between two routes to the same goal. A woman determined to keep her breast is usually will-ing to put up with the six-week . . . radiation treatments, while a woman who isn't so determined and who has an especially demanding schedule, like former First Lady Nancy Reagan, might well choose mastectomy." She was not as convinced as Kushner that birth control pills, fertility drugs, and estrogen replacement therapy explained the rising incidence of breast cancer, but she was cautious. "Doctors are just passing them out like M&Ms," Love warned.

She was not the least bit cautious, however, about preaching that breast cancer had been largely ignored in the United States because it was a disease of women. Marginalized groups do not receive adequate health care, and women were no exception. In a call to arms, Love asked women to marshal their political resources and go on the offensive. "Women, whether they're doctors or not," she said in 1993, "also need to take to the streets and yell and scream. That's something we've learned from the AIDS movement: nothing gets done unless you make a loud noise. Women are angry that the breast cancer epidemic continues without much change, and it's crucial to focus that anger and put it to good use. Our lives depend on it. We can't let this disease pass on to another generation of women."[5]

Epidemiologists provided women like Susan Love with all the evidence they needed to justify a new political movement. By the mid-1980s, dramatic changes in the incidence of breast cancer precipitated talk of an epidemic. The numbers had the look of a national disaster. In 1940 the annual incidence of breast cancer was fifty-nine cases for every 100,000 women in the country. Ten years later, the rate had jumped to sixty-five cases per 100,000. It ticked up to seventy-two cases in 1960, seventy-four in 1970, and ninety in 1980. In 1990 there were 105 new cases of breast cancer for every 100,000 women in the United States. In 1940 more than 37,000 women discovered malignant lumps in their breasts. The number increased to roughly 49,000 in 1950, 65,000 in 1960, 75,000 in 1970, 105,000 in 1980, and 138,000 in 1990. By the mid-1990s, more than 180,000 new cases appeared annually. Of the women living in the United States in 1940, one in twenty was destined to develop breast cancer. By 1950 the ratio had dropped to one in fifteen, and it continued to fall, to one in fourteen in 1960, one in thirteen in 1970, one in eleven in 1980, and one in nine in 1990. In June 1993 National Cancer Institute (NCI) statisticians recrunched the numbers, and one in nine gave way to one in eight. Actually, one in eight was a deceptive figure. The NCI report said that one in eight American women who live to age ninety-five will get breast cancer. Since few women live that long, the one in eight risk was not widely applicable, but in the hands of sound-bite news broadcasters, the numbers crunched alarmingly. Establishment medicine appeared to be losing the war.[6]

Talk of defeat worked into the headlines, especially when the optimistic predictions by leading oncologists in the 1980s went unfulfilled. Scientists are often their own worst enemies, purveyors of optimism too quick to pronounce cancer's demise. After the oncogenes responsible for "turning on" some cancer cells were discovered, Lewis Thomas, head of Memorial Sloan-Kettering, naively predicted the disappearance of cancer "before this century is over." He should have known better. Vincent T. DeVita, director of the NCI and equally given to hyperbole, speculated that "by the year 2000 we may not have cancer . . . . The speed of advance has been enormous." In the early 1970s, when he had launched the "War on Cancer," President Richard Nixon resonated with similar confidence, but at least his rosy predictions had been widely recognized as a naive concoction of sincere hope and political hype.

Empty promises gave birth to new skepticism. Cancer was not going to go away by the year 2000 because it consisted of more than two hundred extremely complicated diseases about which science still knew comparatively little. Although the government had poured $25 billion into cancer research during the 1970s and 1980s, long-term survival rates for breast, lung, and colon cancer had changed very little. President Donald Kennedy of Stanford University likened the "war on cancer" to a "medical Vietnam," and James Watson, the molecular biologist and codiscoverer of the DNA molecule, dismissed the so-called "war" as a "bunch of shit."[7]

Epidemiologist John Bailar was the most outspoken critic, regularly tweaking the cancer establishment. A biostatistician with a medical degree from Yale and a Ph.D. from American University, Bailar had the look, and the tact, of a labor union recruiter. His round, ruddy face was topped with a full head of grayish streaked dark hair, and he spoke his mind—all the time. He had left the editorship of *The Journal of the National Cancer Institute* for Harvard in 1980 after earning the enmity of the American Cancer Society for denigrating its heralded mammography screening program. Harvard Yard did not temper him. In a 1986 edition of *The New England Journal of Medicine,* Bailar claimed that the war against cancer was being lost. "The ugly fact," he announced, "remains that overall cancer mortality is rising . . . . This cannot be explained away as a statistical artifact obscured by the clear evidence of progress here and there, or submerged by rosy rhetoric about research results still in the pipeline." Newspapers published Bailar's remarks widely, inspiring him to escalate his attack. At the fall 1993 meetings of President Bill Clinton's Cancer Panel, after listening to a number of rosy pronouncements, Bailar stood up and announced, "I . . . again conclude, as I did seven years ago, that our decades of war against cancer have been a qualified failure. Thank you."[8]

Out of that failure emerged the breast cancer advocacy movement. Shirley Temple Black, Betty Ford, Happy Rockefeller, and Betty Rollin dramatically elevated America's breast cancer consciousness in the 1970s, but it took another decade before awareness assumed a political dimension. Local groups providing emotional support to breast cancer patients—such as Reach to Recovery—had been around for years, and Rose Kushner had brought them together in her National Alliance for Breast Cancer Organizations. Throughout the 1980s, membership continued to grow and new groups proliferated, such as One in Nine (Long Island), the Y-Me Bay Area Breast Cancer Network (San Francisco–Oakland), and the Susan G. Komen Foundation (Now Breast Cancer Foundation) (Dallas). Increasingly, women were getting the disease and needed to talk about it. Such support groups were popular among feminists, who found them useful vehicles for empowerment. Science even promoted them. Stanford epidemiologist David Spiegel demonstrated that women active in support groups lived longer than other breast cancer patients, perhaps because sharing pain, hope, and fear strengthened their immune systems.[9]

Only the shortest of steps separated emotional support from political activism. As women spoke about the disease in support groups, they became increasingly politicized. The fact that insurance companies did not routinely cover mammograms became an early rallying cry. One enraged women's health advocate insisted, "You can be damn well sure that if there was a way of diagnosing testicular or penis cancer early, those bastards in the legislatures and board rooms would fund it for every man in the country!" Women's groups lobbied state legislatures to force insurance companies to cover routine mammograms, and by 1993 forty-five states had done so.

Medicare payments for mammograms became a national issue during the Reagan years. Although routine mammograms clearly saved lives among elderly women, Medicare still would not cover the procedure unless it was used to investigate suspicious lumps. Several congresswomen, led by Pat Schroeder of Colorado, called for expanding Medicare coverage to include routine annual mammograms. The bill did not survive an all-male House subcommittee in 1988. Schroeder resurrected the proposal during the first Bush administration and, with the president's support, oversaw its passage. On January 1, 1991, Medicare began offering reimbursement for screening mammography.

Oddly enough, Bush's 1991 nomination of Clarence Thomas to the Supreme Court galvanized congressional backing for more breast cancer funding. When University of Oklahoma law professor Anita Hill accused Thomas of sexual harassment, the confirmation hearings became a three-ring circus, with an all-male Senate Judiciary Committee grilling Hill about her accusations. Tens of millions of women watched the televised proceedings and took offense at the one-sided inquisition. Thomas was confirmed, but in the wake of the hearings, hundreds of congressmen began casting about for a politically safe way to demonstrate their sensitivity to "women's concerns." Unlike abortion or gay rights, breast cancer was perfect, a "win-win" game to solicit women's votes.

Just as the political climate changed, the National Breast Cancer Coalition exercised its own political muscle. In December 1990 Susan Love met with Susan Hester, director of the Washington, D.C.–based Mary-Helen Mautner Project for Lesbians With Cancer. AIDS activists, whose militant demands had produced a tenfold increase in AIDS funding, inspired them. Acquired immune deficiency syndrome early on generated little political interest because it was a "gay disease," and few politicians wanted to be on the cutting edge of that controversy. Not until the mid-1980s, when gay activists demanded attention and wielded enough political clout to get it, did AIDS receive the dollars it deserved. "The AIDS activists were our model," remembered Francine Kritchek of One in Nine. "They showed that if the populace became very concerned, then the politicians would respond." Susan Love and Susan Hester, along with Sharon Green of Y-Me, Ann McGuire of the Women's Community Cancer Project, and Pam Onder of the Greater Washington Coalition for Cancer Survivorship, established the National Breast Cancer Coalition (NBCC), an umbrella organization of more than 180 breast cancer advocacy groups. "We have to be the voice, the obnoxious voice," Susan Love claimed. "We can't shut up now."

Fran Visco, a liberal activist and feminist, became president of the NBCC. She had not worried much about breast cancer before 1987. Until then, she had enjoyed good health, a one-year-old baby boy, and a successful career as a Philadelphia attorney. A breast cancer diagnosis caught her off-guard, upsetting a near perfect world and stirring up the juices of political passion again. "I wasn't a famous activist, but I protested the war in the 60s, and I spoke out for women's rights in the 70s." She wanted answers, a reasonable explanation for what had happened and would happen to her and to millions of other women. But there were so few answers. "I had no family history," she told the *New York Times*, "and I felt that meant that I was O.K., that I didn't have to worry about it . . . . When I started reading of the disease, I thought I was seeing misprints. If this is true, why didn't I know about it?"[10]

Breast cancer advocates made more political noise than ever, and Congress listened. Congresswoman Nita Lowey, a Democrat from New York, took up the challenge in the name of her mother and two aunts who died of the disease. So did Congresswomen Barbara Vucanovich, a Republican from Nevada, and Marilyn Lloyd, Democrat from Tennessee, both of whom were breast cancer survivors. In 1990 Congress had appropriated only $21 million for breast cancer research; in 1991 the amount more than doubled to $43 million. In 1992, the National Breast Cancer Coalition delivered a 600,000-signature petition to Congress demanding more money. Senator Tom Harkin, an Iowa Democrat who had lost two of his sisters to the disease, joined the cause and inserted a $210 million breast cancer initiative into the defense department budget. The final vote was eighty-seven to four in the Senate. The senators "didn't dare go back and tell their constituents that they had voted against this successful strategy," said Joanne Howes, an NBCC lobbyist. Including the defense budget money, funding jumped to $343 million in 1993, $449 million in 1994, and more than $500 million in 1995.

The political strength of the breast cancer lobby became abundantly clear early in 1995 when John Hamre, the Pentagon's chief budget planner, testified to the Senate Budget Committee that the Department of Defense might not spend the money earmarked for breast cancer research since the money was "unrelated to military needs." President Bill Clinton, whose mother had died of breast cancer in 1994, lost his temper when he read Hamre's testimony and sent a stinging letter to Secretary of Defense William Perry demanding that the money be allocated. Ginny Terzano, an administration spokesperson, explained the rebuke to the White House press corps: "The president feels strongly about both of these issues and thinks financial support is important and he wanted to reiterate that to Secretary Perry."[11]

On October 25, 2000, the National Breast Cancer Coalition enjoyed the fruits of another legislative victory when President Bill Clinton signed into law the Breast and Cervical Cancer Treatment Act. Beginning in 1994, low-income, uninsured women had enjoyed the right to free breast screening, but those diagnosed with malignant disease were not entitled to affordable treatment. NBCC leaders like Fran Visco made it a top priority to close that cruel gap between diagnosis and treatment, mounting a legislative crusade that stormed its way through Congress. Few members of the House of Representatives or the Senate were prepared to risk the wrath of the NBCC in opposing the measure. The Breast and Cervical Cancer Treatment Act gave poor, uninsured women access to the Medicaid program to pay the cost of treatment. Visco hailed the law. "As the bill went into effect yesterday," she said, "now is an important and appropriate time to honor those women who died before this program went into place—before diagnosis and treatment were inextricably linked."[12]

Each victory inspired new offensives. Many insurance companies refused to pay for bone marrow transplants, an increasingly common treatment for women with metastatic disease, because they were "experimental." The treatment, which had earlier proved effective in treating leukemia patients, involved massive doses of chemotherapy that wiped out surviving cancer cells but also poisoned patients' bone marrow, leaving them vulnerable to infection and death. But by harvesting bone marrow or stem cells from patients or matching donors before the killer dose of chemotherapy, physicians could then reinject them into patients after the treatment, restoring their immunological systems. Beginning in the 1980s, thousands of desperate breast cancer patients underwent the treatment before its effectiveness had even been established. Few patients could afford the $80,000 to $250,000 price tag. Lisa DeMoss, a spokesperson for Blue Cross, admitted in 1995 that it was "a serious question of who is going to pay for medical science and research. We've always excluded payment for experimental and investigation procedures." Most oncologists, on the other hand, did not consider bone marrow transplants experimental. "An experiment is a situation where you don't know the anticipated outcome, but that's not the case here," said Richard Champlin, a bone marrow specialist at M. D. Anderson Cancer Center in Houston. "There have been thousands of bone marrow transplants performed. They are done at virtually every academic center in the country. Everyone sees the same results—a very high response rate and some long-term survivors that wouldn't be expected with other forms of treatment."

Some advocacy groups tried to secure legislation forcing insurance companies to cover the procedure, but they faced stiff opposition. With health care prices escalating, employers took every opportunity to cut costs, and beginning in 1991, many state insurance boards allowed insurance companies to exclude bone marrow transplants from existing policies. Unable to provide a general solution, breast cancer advocacy groups counseled individual women to hire attorneys. Susan Stewart, a breast cancer advocate in Chicago, told a reporter in 1995, "Ninety percent of the time or better, an attorney writes a letter or makes a phone call, and it gets settled. In general, if the patient puts up a fight, the insurance companies settle." Often, litigation can cost insurance companies more than the procedure. In 1994, a California jury awarded $89 million to the family of a woman who died of breast cancer after Health Net, a health maintenance organization, denied her a bone marrow transplant.[13]

In 1999 the first good data began to appear on the efficacy of bone marrow transplants in treating breast cancer, and the results were hardly encouraging. Survival rates for women undergoing the procedure were only marginally better than those receiving standard therapies. Larry Norton of Memorial Sloan-Kettering in New York noted, "The ultimate survival was equal. There were fewer deaths in the transplant group, but more deaths in the procedure. It might turn out in the long run, another two or three years, that transplant is a little better. My guess is that the difference will be in the 5 percent range." Breast cancer advocacy groups argued about the significance of the data. The Susan G. Komen Breast Cancer Foundation in Dallas issued a press release claiming that "the results of these studies in no way suggest that this matter is settled," while Fran Visco of the National Breast Cancer Coalition countered, "We don't need to add to the confusion. We certainly don't need to encourage women to have unproven treatments like this outside of clinical trials."[14]

Always ready to make sure that women were not being exploited, women's groups took aim at various medical procedures and research protocols, often finding themselves butting heads with the cancer establishment. The mastectomy continued to be a primary target. The growing consensus in academic circles about the efficacy of lumpectomies did not always find clinical expression in private practice. By the early 1990s, most breast cancer patients came to their physicians early in the disease process, especially compared to the women who had visited William Stewart Halsted a century before. The American Cancer Society's decades-long early detection public health campaign saved lives. With tumors being detected at increasingly early stages, Sidney Salmon, head of the Arizona Cancer Center, in 1993 estimated that fewer than 10 percent of breast cancer patients really needed a mastectomy; lumpectomies and radiation were just as good in achieving cures and far less damaging.

But the number of mastectomies still being performed far exceeded 10 percent. A 1993 American Cancer Society survey revealed that in New England, 45 percent of breast cancer surgeries were mastectomies, but in the South, four out of five operations were mastectomies. Other studies confirmed the regional discrepancies. Women living in large urban areas of the Northeast and receiving treatment at teaching hospitals with radiotherapy facilities were the most likely to undergo lumpectomies, while southern women in small town hospitals were the least likely. Mastectomies continued in some regions to treat ductal carcinoma in situ, the earliest stage of the disease. European surgeons shook their heads in disbelief. Gianni Bonadonna, a renowned oncologist at the National Tumor Institute in Milan, told his American colleagues, "It's crazy to go on with mastectomies as a routine. The problem of breast cancer is not in the breast."

Poor women are far more likely to have mastectomies than middle- and upper-class women. Some avoid radiotherapy because they cannot afford to miss six weeks of work for the treatments. Many physicians are less inclined to take the time to explain the range of options to a poor Medicaid patient than to a well-to-do woman covered by insurance. Older women are also much more likely to have mastectomies than younger women, perhaps because male surgeons see little sexual utility in an elderly breast and fail to discuss the lumpectomy option.[15]

The staying power of mastectomies baffled Mark Lippman, director of the Vincent Lombardi Cancer Center in Washington, D.C. "I'm puzzled," he told a reporter in 1993, "as to what combination of educational, prejudicial, financial, and historical issues have failed to get lumpectomies going." Many surgeons did not help. Some recommended mastectomies because insurance companies paid more for the radical procedure than for the lumpectomy. Some were simply wedded to tradition and loath to change old habits. According to Lippman, "In many cases, what is happening is inappropriate encouragement to undergo a mastectomy from the first care giver a woman sees, the surgeon who does the biopsy."[16]

Some surgeons resisted the move to the modified radical mastectomy or lumpectomy for legal reasons. During the 1960s and 1970s, as changing social norms pulled physicians off the pedestal they had occupied for decades, medical malpractice lawsuits multiplied at geometric rates. For a surgeon to openly admit that he or she had been wrong in employing radical or superradical procedures, to confess that such extensive operations had been unnecessary, was to invite litigation from former patients. On the other hand, to deviate from the prevailing surgical consensus in favor of more conservative techniques was to risk litigation from patients who experienced a local recurrence. "Many surgeons felt trapped in a 'damned if you do, damned if you don't' situation," recalled Richard Martin of the University of Texas M. D. Anderson Cancer Center in Houston.

The nature of surgical practice in the United States also explains the delay in abandoning mastectomies. Unlike their European counterparts, who practice in large group and hospital settings, many American surgeons in the early 1990s still worked in small, one- or two-person fee-for-service practices. They might have read journal articles and attended annual conventions, where the latest trends were openly promoted, but they did not have the benefit of continual, daily interaction with a large number of colleagues, with its accompanying intellectual synergism and peer pressure. The surgeons most likely to perform lumpectomies worked in large academic, clinic, or hospital settings, where the latest scientific trends were most likely to be implemented. Highly independent surgeons in small practices were the least likely to abandon the mastectomy.[17]

Susan Love knew why mastectomies survive. "Lumpectomies," she insisted, "are more difficult operations. Patients expect decent cosmetic re-sults or they would not opt for the procedure in the first place, but most breast surgeons have never been trained in it, because it's a relatively new operation and they went to medical school in the days when everyone just did mastectomies." For too many women, she argued, going to a surgeon in the 1990s was not much different from showing up at Halsted's door a century before. "Women who have just learned that the lump is malignant often confront tradition-bound surgeons who say to them, 'O.K., I'll take care of you and I'll cut your breast off and everything will be fine.'" Wor-ried more about death than disfigurement, they go along. Love takes a more measured approach, urging women to be patient and thoughtful, to secure second opinions, to function from positions of emotional strength when they make such a momentous decision. "Breast cancer is not an emergency," she tells her patients. "By the time they're diagnosed, most breast cancers have been around for years, which means it's unlikely that anything too dramatic will happen right away."

But the attitudes of surgeons were not the only explanation for the slow transition to lumpectomies. Many women resist lumpectomies, pre-ferring the finality of the mastectomy to the uncertainty of more limited operations. Leaving breast tissue behind, they often fear, will increase the risk of recurrence or development of a new tumor. Nancy Brinker, head of the Susan G. Komen Breast Cancer Foundation, explained the phe-nomenon simply: "Fear of this disease has run so deep and the treatment is so harsh that women still have in their minds that the more you cut out, the more you keep it from spreading. I can't tell you how many women I talk to who say, 'I just want to get it out.'"[18]

In addition to campaigning for lumpectomies and radiation, activists opposed the use of routine, annual mammographies in younger women. In 1972 the National Cancer Institute and the American Cancer Society had established the Breast Cancer Detection Demonstration Project (BCDDP), a system of twenty-seven mammography screening centers throughout the United States to detect breast cancer at an earlier stage. Frank J. Rauscher, then director of the National Cancer Institute, told *Science* magazine, "Breast cancer is a hell of a problem. It is a major killer of women, many of them in the prime of life. And for years, the incidence of the disease and its mortality have been the same—awful." By 1976 more than 270,000 women had received one or more of the x-rays. The NCI mammographies revealed 1,100 cases of breast cancer. Of those, three hundred occurred in women under fifty. Perhaps one hundred would not have been discovered without mammography. Of the eight hundred cases of breast cancer found in women over fifty years of age, perhaps 280 were detectable by mammography alone.

The National Cancer Institute was proud of the results until 1975, when John Bailar raised doubts about the safety of mammographies. Convinced that several environmental carcinogens, including x-rays, are responsible for the rising incidence of cancer, Bailar expressed doubts about mammography. If the National Cancer Institute–American Cancer Society screening program succeeded, and millions of women underwent annual mammograms during their adult lives, the cumulative effect might be a dramatic increase in breast cancer. Bailar was Deputy Associate Director for Cancer Control at the National Cancer Institute and editor of *The Journal of the National Cancer Institute* at the time, and from that pulpit he went public with his concerns. For younger women, he argued, the annual exposure of breasts to x-rays might actually cause breast cancer later in their lives. "The risk of getting cancer from exposure to radiation," he wrote, "equals or exceeds the chance of finding a cancer early that could not be found by clinical examination." Irwin Bross, director of biostatistics at the Roswell Park Memorial Institute in Buffalo, New York, agreed. He warned that the breast cancer screening project, in which every adult woman in the country would receive a mammogram, had catastrophic potential. Mammograms are x-rays, Bross warned, and excessive x-rays over the course of decades can cause cancer. The screening program, he feared, might bring about "the worst iatrogenic [physician-induced] epidemic of breast cancer in history."

Coming from such influential epidemiologists, the warnings precipitated internecine battles at the National Cancer Institute. Walter Ross, a prominent leader of the American Cancer Society, considered the jeremiads irresponsible. "Mammography became transformed," he later wrote, "almost overnight in the public's mind from a desirable examination into an unacceptable menace." Bailar eventually left the National Cancer Institute for Harvard and then McGill University, but he remained, in Ross's mind, "a perennial critic" of the American Cancer Society. When confronted with the possibility that mammograms might actually become a new cause of breast cancer, Benjamin F. Byrd, a former president of the

American Cancer Society, dismissed the warning, smugly replying, "There's also an excellent chance that by that time science will have learned to control the disease."[19]

Publicity forced the National Cancer Institute and American Cancer Society to confront the issue. Frank Rauscher asked Lester Breslow, dean of the school of public health at UCLA, to evaluate the threat. After spending a year looking at the data, he bluntly recommended "the immediate cessation of routine mammography for screening women under 50 years of age." The only younger women getting routine mammograms, he urged, should be those in high risk groups. Unless the protocol was changed, within ten years there would be several thousand new cases of breast cancer attributed to mammograms, a far higher figure than the number of women who would have been saved by the breast x-rays.

Rauscher found himself in a tenuous position. Epidemiological evidence seemed clear enough, but political reality demanded a different response. The American Cancer Society, the NCI's greatest ally and a source of tens of millions of research dollars, remained absolutely committed to annual screenings for all women, as did the American College of Radiologists, whose members faced a loss of income if mammography screening was confined to older women. On July 29, 1976, Rauscher convened a group of four hundred women employees—secretaries, administrative assistants, technicians, nurses, and physicians—of the National Institutes of Health. He shared Breslow's conclusions and listened to them, hoping for some kind of intellectual epiphany. It did not happen. They expressed every conceivable opinion. In the end, Rauscher did what scientific bureaucrats often do; he recommended further study.

The controversy did not go away. During the 1980s and 1990s a flood of new studies reinforced the growing consensus that routine mammography screening was of little use to women under fifty. Radiologists often missed breast cancers in premenopausal women because denser breast tissues obscured small tumors. One Canadian study revealed a "false negative" rate of as high as 40 percent. A number of epidemiological studies in Canada and Sweden also indicated that women under the age of fifty who had received regular mammograms, compared to women in the same age group who had not had them, were just as likely to contract breast cancer and to die from it. And there was still the concern that mammograms might actually cause breast cancer. Although the advent of new, low-dosage x-ray technology had greatly reduced the threat of radiation-induced tumors, finite risks remained. Finally, routine screening in premenopausal women caused thousands of unnecessary biopsies each year, the scar tissue from which could obscure real breast cancers years later.

The BCDDP controversy assumed the dimensions of a national scandal, with investigative reporters burrowing into NCI records in order to find a smoking gun of some kind, prima facie evidence that the American Cancer Society and the National Cancer Institute had jumped headlong into widespread mammography screening without pondering its possible consequences and perhaps even ignoring internal warnings. Newspapers, magazines, and television news anchors broadcast the story, raising more than a little ire among women's health advocates. When the American Cancer Society admitted that nearly 250,000 women had been admitted to the BCDDP study without being warned of its potential risks, reporters had a field day.

As the evidence against routine screening of younger women mounted, the list of opposition groups grew. The American College of Physicians called for an end to routine screening, as did the American College of Family Practice. The National Women's Health Network and the Center for Medical Consumers actively advised premenopausal women to avoid mammograms except to investigate suspicious lumps. The National Cancer Institute and the American Cancer Society were the slowest to come around. In 1990 both groups shifted slightly, telling women in their forties to have a mammogram "every one or two years." Late in 1993 the NCI formally dropped even that guideline. Instead of telling younger women to avoid routine mammograms, the NCI urged them to discuss their own risk factors with a physician and then make a personal decision about screening. The proposal seemed cowardly, irritating more than a few activists. "The NCI is the repository of public trust and public dollars," complained Cindy Pearson of the National Women's Health Network. "As a consumer I want the government to say what they think the state of the science is." Only the American Cancer Society continued to support routine screening for younger women.

The Breast Cancer Detection Demonstration Project also generated a new debate about the nature of the disease and appropriate treatment. With millions of American women receiving mammograms, the number of cases of "ductal carcinoma in situ" (DCIS) skyrocketed. By the mid-

1990s, nearly 20 percent of all diagnosed cases of breast cancer would be ductal carcinoma in situ. In DCIS cases, cancerous cells are present in the milk ducts of the breast but have not broken out to invade neighboring tissues. Before the advent of mammography, they could rarely be discovered. Too small to be detected by physical examination, they produce micro calcifications, or small amounts of calcium, that show up on mammograms. Because many DCIS cases never escape the milk ducts to invade neighboring tissues, some oncologists refuse to classify them as "breast cancer," preferring the term "precancer." Just how, or if, to treat DCIS provides the controversy. Should women with DCIS undergo surgery, radiotherapy, and chemotherapy to treat a condition that may never become invasive breast cancer? Aggressive oncologists recommend prophylactically treating the disease with modified radical mastectomy so that invasive breast cancer never develops, while more conservative physicians adopt a wait-and-see attitude or recommend lumpectomy followed up with radiotherapy.[20]

Tamoxifen became another call to arms. Early in the 1990s, the long-term results of tamoxifen therapy manifested themselves. Scientists had understood for a century that depriving some breast tumors of estrogen achieved temporary remissions, and tamoxifen had made oophorectomies, adrenalectomies, and hypophysectomies obsolete. Oxford University, in a study involving 75,000 women, discovered that patients receiving two-year tamoxifen regimens improved their ten-year survival rates by 8 percent over women not receiving the treatment. Craig Henderson, an oncologist at the Dana Farber Cancer Center in Boston, found the results astonishing. "Everybody was wrong," he told the *New York Times*. "No one anticipated the benefit would be as large or persistent." He then added an obligatory disclaimer. "Although the effects are long lasting, this does not mean we are curing patients. It is a big step forward and what is likely to happen is that people with cancer will live longer and better for less cost."

Tamoxifen also yielded other unexpected benefits. The drug lowered cholesterol levels and increased bone density, reducing risks for heart disease and osteoporosis. Even more surprising, women who took the drug were less likely to develop new tumors in the other breast. In some way, tamoxifen specialists concluded, the drug not only reduced the likelihood or postponed the recurrence of cancer but also prevented the appearance of new tumors. At the University of Pittsburgh, Bernard Fisher wondered whether tamoxifen could actually kill new cancer cells before they were clinically visible and before they ever multiplied into a tumor. "Tamoxifen may have some effect on tumors that exist below the area of detection," he claimed.

Ever the scientist, Fisher wanted to test his hypothesis in clinical trials, which the National Cancer Institute approved in 1992. He launched a "prophylactic tamoxifen" study, enrolling sixteen thousand high-risk women—women who had started menstruation before the age of thirteen, or who had close relatives with the disease, or who had never had children. At the end of the trial, if the participants had reduced incidences of breast cancer, physicians would have stumbled on the first drug ever known to prevent the disease.

But while reducing recurrences, increasing bone density, and cutting cholesterol levels, tamoxifen had several harmful side effects, including hot flashes, vaginal discharges, irregular menses, skin rashes, phlebitis, lung clots, thrombocytopenia, and an increased risk of liver and endometrial cancer. Fisher's study might prevent breast cancer in an average of sixty-two women while subjecting several thousand to one or more side effects. Some feminists wondered whether he was using women as guinea pigs. Cindy Pearson questioned the wisdom of subjecting healthy women to such risks: "The tamoxifen prevention trial sets a dangerous precedent because it is the first time that a toxic drug with known health risks is to be unleashed on a healthy population."

Fisher considered the risks minor and the potential benefits considerable. "[The trial] will provide," he argued, "the vital information necessary to determine whether tamoxifen is a useful prevention drug that should be used by women in the general population who are at risk for breast cancer." He did not endear himself to women's health advocates when he failed to report a disturbing side effect of the trial. In September 1994, two years into the study, Fisher learned that twenty-three of the women with breast cancer who were taking tamoxifen had developed uterine cancer, and four had died. He waited two months before reporting the news to the NCI, and waited until January 1995 to inform the healthy women participating in the trial. A number of women accused Fisher of trying to cover up the report "because he was concerned about the bad publicity that would be generated." Adriane Fugh-Berman, a medical advisor to the National Women's Health Network, knew the answer:

"There's a certain sense of desperation in the cancer establishment, because there's been so little progress in breast cancer treatment and in reducing breast cancer mortality."[21]

Breast cancer advocates made good use of the desperation, claiming that at any given time in the 1990s, 2.6 million American women had breast cancer—1.6 million who knew about it and another million who did not. June Andlin, a Houston breast cancer survivor, in 1990 demanded justice: "These women are America's grandmothers, mothers, wives, sisters, daughters, and friends. They deserve to know what's happening to them and why. There's something broken in the cancer establishment and we intend to fix it. Too many women are suffering and dying!"[22]

The cancer establishment rejected talk of an epidemic. Both the National Cancer Institute and the American Cancer Society denied that a breast cancer "epidemic" was under way. Biostatisticians argued that the increased incidence of breast cancer was largely attributable to mammograms and the demographics of age. Because of the popularity of mammograms in the 1980s and 1990s, physicians detected many cases of breast cancer before they would have been normally discovered, creating an artificial, and temporary, bulge in the number of cases. Women were also living longer. Rapid declines in childhood illnesses, death at childbirth, and infectious diseases allowed increasing numbers of women to live into old age, when they became more susceptible to breast cancer. Even the recent increase in the number of women under fifty years of age diagnosed with breast cancer was a demographic phenomenon: the baby boom generation has simply placed more women in that age category.[23]

Establishment oncologists accused breast cancer advocates of employing shrill rhetoric and hyperbole to promote a political agenda, especially to generate more money and to change the direction of cancer research. Sarah Fox, a physician at UCLA, claimed that words like "epidemic certainly get the attention of politicians and lay people. It still seems to be that since we are a crisis-oriented society, the people who make the most noise get the most publicity. Interest groups do count as opposed to data and rationality." Larry Kessler, head of applied research at the National Cancer Institute, attributed rising breast cancer incidence rates to an aging population and increased use of mammograms. "It's inappropriate to say there's an epidemic," he told the *New York Times*. "As populations grow and women live to old age, it is just around. We don't need new hype. We don't need to make women afraid." The fact that the incidence of breast cancer increased from eighty-five cases per 100,000 women in 1980 to 112 per 100,000 in 1987 was a statistical aberration, he argued, the result of surging numbers of mammograms. He even predicted a reversal in the incidence rates late in the 1990s when the numbers of women receiving mammograms stabilized. NCI officials argued that progress could be made against the disease if Congress would just appropriate more research money and if all patients enjoyed universal access to state-of-the-art treatment.[24]

They also cited signs of recent gains in survival rates. Samuel Broder, head of the National Cancer Institute, announced early in 1995 that the death rate from breast cancer had declined 5 percent from 1989 to 1992. In 1989, there were 27.5 breast cancer deaths per 100,000 women in the United States, and that number dropped to 27.4 in 1990, 27.1 in 1991, and 26.2 in 1992. He attributed the decline to early detection and the use of "adjuvant therapy"—chemotherapy and radiation, as well as surgery. He was more cautious, however, than some of his predecessors at the NCI. "Despite the good news," Broder hedged, "we are far from satisfied. We need to make more progress against breast cancer in all women."

Breast cancer advocates were not placated. Susan Love took vigorous exception. "To me," she argued, "an epidemic is an inordinate number of women getting breast cancer. Whether we're picking them up a little early because of screening doesn't change the fact that there are huge numbers. There are too many women dying of breast cancer and we have to do something about it." Fran Visco agreed. "If you already have 1 in 8 women getting breast cancer in their lifetime," she claimed, "and you already have 2.6 million who have the disease and 50 percent of those diagnosed are dead in 10 years, those are pretty horrible statistics. I certainly believe they rise to epidemic proportions . . . . The modestly falling death rate [should not] overshadow the fact that we're still for the most part treating it with very toxic substances." She took little comfort in the fact that while hundreds more women were being cured each year, thousands more were contracting the disease.[25]

Activists were not about to acquiesce in NCI optimism, deciding instead to change the research agenda, to push the cancer establishment out of the "cure rut," to make sure that more money found its way into understanding the causes of breast cancer and its prevention, not just its treatment. Susan Love protested that "early detection is not early enough." For too many decades, she insisted, oncologists have been wedded to surgery, radiation, and chemotherapy. Real progress will not materialize until science unlocks some of breast cancer's most fundamental secrets. "Basically, all cancer is genetic," Love argued. "It's not all hereditary, but it's all genetic . . . . What are these carcinogens in breast cancer? We don't have a clue. Could they be hormones? Sure. Could they be a virus? Sure." It could be "a million" things.

The raging controversies over breast cancer diagnostic and treatment protocols, along with the glacial pace so many surgeons assumed in moving toward less radical procedures, prompted a political backlash in the women's health movement. If logic could not prevail, many activists decided, then legislation would. Beginning with Massachusetts in 1979, state after state passed informed consent laws, requiring physicians to make patients fully aware of all treatment options. The Massachusetts legislation was particularly direct, requiring doctors to tell "each patient suffering from a form of breast cancer, of all alternatives available for treatment in addition to mastectomies." Seeing more power slipping through their fingers, many surgeons squawked in protest, demanding that government stop interfering with the doctor-patient relationship, but in the end they had little choice. Most informed consent laws required physicians periodically to sign affidavits, under penalty of perjury, that they were complying with the legislation.

To the chagrin of most establishment oncologists, activists also demanded a role in deciding how government funds were used. In December 1992, Susan Love and Fran Visco met with Samuel Broder and the NCI's National Cancer Advisory Board (NCAB). They requested representation for women with breast cancer on all decision-making bodies, a seat on the NCAB, and establishment of a permanent breast cancer subcommittee of the NCAB. The National Cancer Institute responded by founding Project LEAD to assist breast cancer advocates in serving on such cooperative committees, but many NCI scientists drew the line at giving them a vote in determining research grant recipients. Richard Klausner, head of the NCI in 1995, said, "I don't think it necessarily makes sense to assign an advocate for every disease to every study section that may match his or her area of interest. Science doesn't neatly divide up that way." To many NCI officials, the demand undermined the long-held scientific tradition of competitive peer review for research funding and threatened to politicize cancer research.

When Visco heard their reactions, she exploded. "The scientific community is telling us, 'Fight for more money, but don't tell us where to spend it,' that politics doesn't belong in breast cancer. But there's politics in the scientific community, and those politics have worked in the past to the expense of breast cancer and the expense of women's lives. There has always been a limited amount of money to fund all the promising research that should be funded. People make a decision to fund X at the expense of Y. And Y too often has been breast cancer . . . . They think we're going to be there to scream. They think we're going to be there to bare our breasts. But what we want is to make sure the money we fought so hard for isn't wasted. What we want is answers."[26]

And if the cancer establishment did not have enough problems, scandal enveloped the career of its leading light, Bernard Fisher of the University of Pittsburgh. In the spring of 1994, Fisher found himself in the middle of a public relations disaster. A lifetime's work hung in the balance. When he entered the world of breast cancer in the 1950s, Fisher had confronted a surgical establishment ferociously wedded to radical treatment. More than any other American, he had been responsible for accumulating irrefutable evidence that breast cancer was a systemic disease and radical mastectomies unnecessary. William Stewart Halsted was wrong; Geoffrey Keynes was right. Surgeons could step back from the radicals. Even the most dogmatic, tradition-bound surgeons could not ignore him. Radical mastectomies gave way to modified radical and simple mastectomies, and the number of lumpectomies increased.

But Fisher's world began crumbling around him in 1990 when an NCI biostatistician noticed irregularities in data arriving from the University of Montreal's St. Luc's Hospital. Although the NCI had provided $119 million to fund breast cancer clinical trials, Fisher had channeled millions to Canadian institutions where surgeons seemed more willing than Americans to participate. One of the most enthusiastic was Roger Poisson, professor of surgery at the University of Montreal, who supplied Fisher with 16 percent of the women involved in the study. Since the NCI awarded funds on a per-patient basis, St. Luc's reaped a windfall. Fisher also listed Poisson as a contributing author to his landmark articles, giving the Canadian junior author status in the most important breast cancer research of the twentieth century.[27]

But there was less to Poisson than met the eye. A tall, thin, wide-eyed man who strategically combed his thinning hair in an unsuccessful attempt to camouflage male-pattern baldness, Poisson had manufactured a career on the tails of Fisher's lab coat, demonstrating an unfailing ability to produce women willing to participate in the trial. In fact, he was too successful. When NCI investigators audited his medical records, they discovered ninety-nine cases of data falsification, including outright fabrications serious enough to call into question Fisher's published claim that lumpectomies and radiation gave breast cancer patients survival rates equal to those of mastectomies. Anxious for more money and more coauthorships, Poisson had conjured up records, even going so far as to label some patient files as "false" so he could keep track of his real patients. In 1991, the National Cancer Institute dismissed him from the study and began legal proceedings to recover its money from St. Luc's.[28]

The scandal exploded in newspaper headlines throughout the United States and Canada when the National Cancer Institute and the *New England Journal of Medicine*, which had published the pioneer studies in the late 1980s, censured Fisher for not making the scandal public and for not publishing new conclusions based on uninfected data. He lamely defended himself, claiming that the conclusions of his original study were still valid. The editors of the *New England Journal of Medicine* would have none of it. "There is no excuse," they claimed, "for the four-year delay between the first indication of misconduct in 1990 and the publication of a re-analysis, which we hope will take place in 1994." Samuel Hellman, a University of Chicago oncologist, captured the sentiments of most American physicians who knew how important Fisher's role had been in changing breast cancer treatment. "Bernie made some mistakes and the N.C.I. made some mistakes, but I would not like to see him be the fall guy."

But the buck stopped at Fisher's desk. Late in March, two weeks after the controversy broke, the National Cancer Institute dumped him as head of its National Surgical Adjuvant Breast Project. Thomas Detre, a colleague at the University of Pittsburgh, then issued an official apology: "Women were upset and distraught, and we now understand that it was an error not to have published information about the cheating sooner and in some form that the public could understand."

Poisson remained unrepentant. When reporters confronted him, he self-righteously confessed that he had falsified data to protect his patients, to get them into a state-of-the-art clinical trial. "Those people in their ivory towers don't treat patients," he argued. "It's all very well to compare clinical experiments carried out in the laboratory. I was on the battle front with patients who were dying. There are very few people in the world who have treated as many breast-cancer patients as I have." To please anti-American patrons in the Canadian audience, he then launched into an attack on the United States, citing a sinister conspiracy to discredit him. "There is someone there [in the United States] who would like my skin. There are American senators who feel there is too much American money going outside the country . . . . I could have launched an appeal, but it would have meant fighting against American lawyers." Dwight Kaufman of the National Cancer Institute dismissed Poisson's claims as "farcical. [He] misses the point of the potential harm to women around the world that could have come from tainted and fraudulent data." Poisson likened himself to a Rudyard Kipling hero: "Man is great once he has lost everything and is capable of rising again." But Roger Poisson would not rise again.[29]

Fisher hardly endeared himself to breast cancer advocates during the controversy. He found their concern laudable but their rhetoric hyperbolic. Tremendous progress in treating breast cancer had been achieved, he believed, but the shrill accusations of advocacy groups did not really help. Angry women, whose friends and family members had died of breast cancer, or who had suffered from the disease themselves, were not always in the best position, he claimed, to make dispassionate decisions. "One of the greatest tragedies," Fisher criticized, "is to try to equate progress with your own mortality. There are many frustrated people who feel nothing has been accomplished." Science for Bernard Fisher was in the statistics, the aggregates of human beings and the extrapolations derived from them, not in the individuals.[30]

In 1990s breast cancer politics, the stars of men like Bernard Fisher and Roger Poisson were setting, while those of women like Susan Love were on the rise. More than 1.8 million readers of the *New York Times* saw graphic evidence of this on August 15, 1993. Sometime during a leisurely journey through the Sunday paper, they gawked, did a double take, and stared at the cover photo of *The New York Times Magazine*. A thin, dark-haired woman, her head wrapped in a flowing scarf, looked to her left, her right arm and torso exposed from the abdomen up. A few telltale scars indicated where a breast had once been. Mastectomy photographs are common in surgical journals and textbooks, but not on the cover of mass circulation magazines. That was exactly why Jack Rosenthal, the magazine's editor, had approved the cover photo. "You Can't Look Away Anymore," the headline blared. The photograph was a self-portrait by Matuschka, a former lingerie model who had undergone a modified radical mastectomy. "I've been accused of exploitation and going for shock value," she told a reporter, "but I tried to make it aesthetically appealing. You're looking at a beautiful model. It's a way to suck people into looking at it. Does it upset people? I don't know. I can't say. But that's me."[31]

Biology, Society, and Destiny

Cancer is a stubborn disease, revealing its secrets grudgingly, and scientific progress is measured in inches, or better yet, in extra days survived. In a country conditioned to extraordinary success—to conquering the wilderness, to winning wars, to putting men on the moon—a country where most people count on getting their own way, cancer's intransigence bears witness to human frailty. And in the early 1990s, the only certainties in the world of breast cancer revolved around gross, statistical survival rates. Oncologists were far better at classifying breast tumors into pathological categories and predicting five-year survival rates than in curing them. Infiltrating ductal carcinoma, the most common form of breast cancer with 67.9 percent of all cases, had a survival rate of 79 percent. The second largest cluster of tumors—6.3 percent—was lobular carcinoma, with a survival rate of 84 percent. Medullary carcinoma was the third most common form of the disease, with 2.8 percent of the total number of cases and a survival rate of 82 percent. Mucinous adenocarcinoma, with a survival rate of 95 percent, made up 2.2 percent of breast cancers. Only 1.4 percent of breast cancers were comedocarcinomas, and 87 percent of women with that tumor lived for at least five years. Paget's disease—1.1 percent of all cases—had a survival rate of 79 percent. More than 95 percent of women with papillary carcinoma (0.9 percent of all breast cancers) survived for five years. Even more women—96 percent—outlasted tubular adenocarcinoma, although it constituted only 0.7 percent of tumors. Inflammatory carcinoma was the worst. Only 18 percent of its victims were alive five years after diagnosis. Fortunately, it was also the least common form of the disease. Ten-year survival rates for each of these diseases, of course, were lower.[1]

Knowing the survival odds provided little comfort, especially amidst so much debate. For all the money, energy, and press poured into breast cancer research and treatment, controversy still confronted women at every turn. Although the benefits of hormonal therapy were becoming clearer, the tamoxifen debate raged on. Tamoxifen and new aromatase (an enzyme involved in the production of estrogen) inhibitor drugs—such as trioxifen, toremifene, 4-hydroxyandrostenedione, and droloxifen—produced longer periods of disease-free survival in women with estrogen receptor positive tumors, especially postmenopausal patients. More experimental hormonal treatments—such as leuprolide, buserelin, tripterelin, and goserelin—helped premenopausal women. Fewer than a third of women with metastases responded, and epidemiologists, worried about side effects, still could not say that the hormone blockers increased long-term survival. In December 1995 the National Cancer Institute, worried about tamoxifen's penchant for producing endometrial cancers, called for a five-year limit for women taking the drug. A host of scientists disagreed. Michael Baum, professor of surgery at Royal Marsden Hospital in London, termed the recommendation "a subversion of the scientific process. I suspect there is a hidden agenda—a fear of litigation if a woman gets endometrial cancer. It is wicked and cruel to frighten women about taking tamoxifen."[2]

Mammography had new critics in 1996. Because of the increased use of mammography among American women in the 1980s and 1990s, the incidence of ductal carcinoma in situ (DCIS) rose dramatically. DCIS is the earliest form of breast cancer, when malignant cells are still confined to milk ducts. Surgeons and patients naturally opted for treatment—usually lumpectomies or mastectomies and radiotherapy. Since many ductal carcinomas in situ never break out of the milk ducts to invade other breast tissues and metastasize, mammograms probably caused tens of thousands of needless operations each year. It was certainly a "catch-22." Early detection of dangerous tumors was saving lives, but it was also forcing large numbers of women to undergo painful, unnecessary medical procedures.[3]

Even the issue of when to have a mammogram erupted once again in controversy. Just when a consensus seemed to be emerging—that

women with no risk factors should wait until they are fifty to begin routine annual mammograms—Swedish oncologists confused the issue. Their own long-term study revealed higher survival rates among women who had initiated routine mammograms at forty rather than fifty. The news caught the cancer establishment and the advocacy movement off-guard. Smug "I told you so's" emanated from the American Cancer Society, while the National Cancer Institute called for a formal review of its own policies. Press releases from the National Breast Cancer Coalition advocated caution and more research.[4]

Some critics took even more radical positions on mammography. A number of studies in the 1990s cast doubt on the long-term efficacy of widespread screening. Screening ten thousand women between the ages of forty and fifty would save 1.5 lives. Adding up the direct cost of that many mammograms, as well as the cost of surgical procedures and follow-ups from false positive diagnoses, health economists estimate that it costs society approximately $2 million for each life saved. A number of experts wondered if redirecting that money to other areas of public health might save more lives. Michael Baum, director of research for the British Institute of Cancer Research, had just that concern. He had been responsible in the 1980s for establishing Great Britain's nationwide breast cancer screening program. But late in 1995, he resigned his position on the National Breast Cancer Screening Advisory Board. National screening, he told the London *Sunday Times,* "is not worth doing. There is a political correctness about screening. I took pride in setting up the service, which is as efficient as it can be, but just because you are doing something efficiently, it doesn't mean it's worth doing."[5]

Everything about cancer seemed to generate controversy and debate. Epidemiologists, for example, had long warned that obesity was a risk factor, and they suspected that women who consumed a high-fat diet were similarly vulnerable. Comparative epidemiological studies seemed to confirm that notion. Japanese women, for example, eat a low-fat diet and have low rates of breast cancer compared to American women with high levels of fat intake. Japanese women who immigrate to the United States and consume a high-fat diet, however, lose their immunity to breast cancer. Self-help and nutritional books advised women to cut down on fat consumption as a way of protecting themselves. But in the mid-1990s, a number of clinical trials investigating the issue were coming to completion, and none confirmed an association between breast cancer and dietary fat. Counting fat grams, along with calories, apparently offered little protection.[6]

Nothing better illustrated the dilemma facing women than conflicting reports concerning the tricky role estrogen played in breast cancer's origins. Epidemiologists had long suspected female hormones as a culprit in the rising incidence of the disease. Women who begin menstruation early, or who experience menopause unusually late, have higher rates of breast cancer, perhaps because of a longer exposure to estrogen. Obese women have a higher incidence, perhaps because fat cells have the capacity to produce estriol, an estrogen-like hormone. Women who exercise regularly, on the other hand, are less at risk, perhaps because physical exertion suppresses hormone production. So, apparently, are women who have children relatively early in their reproductive lives and who nurse their newborn—again, perhaps, because of the interruptions in hormonal cycles brought on by pregnancy and lactation or the more rapid maturation of breast tissues that occurs during first pregnancies.

But nothing was certain. What physicians and scientists did not know in the 1990s about women's hormones and their impact on breast cancer could fill libraries. Tantalizingly provocative and highly controversial arguments about the relationship between breast cancer surgery and menstruation appeared around the world early in the decade. Oncologists at Memorial Sloan-Kettering in New York and Guy's Hospital in London claimed that premenopausal women with breast cancer and positive lymph nodes enjoyed longer survival periods if surgery was performed during the last half of their menstrual cycle. Paul Rosen, a Sloan-Kettering pathologist, claimed, "There's something biochemical that happens when surgery is performed late in the menstrual cycle that increases the probability that tumor cells that have spread beyond the breast will die." Estrogen dominates the menstrual cycle during the first two weeks, a period described as the follicular stage, giving way to progesterone dominance for the remainder of the cycle, known as the luteal stage. The presence of estrogen, Rosen speculated, fed cancer cells distant from the original tumor and stimulated their growth. When the large tumor was removed during progesterone's dominance of the luteal stage, the distant cells might be more inclined to die.

By 1992 Guy's Hospital surgeons routinely scheduled breast cancer between twelve and sixteen days after the start of the patient's last period.

Like everything else in breast cancer treatment, the theory spawned bitter critics, some of whom claimed that women should not postpone surgery for any reason. Andrew Door of the National Cancer Institute was circumspect but skeptical. "By and large," he claimed, "scientists are not embracing this as a compelling idea, since a lot of the research has been sloppy." William Wood of Emory University, on the other hand, discounted the theory altogether, arguing that the research was ill-conceived. "To me," he claimed, "it's a superstition, like tying a rabbit's foot around your wrists."[7]

Estrogen replacement therapy posed another enigma. In the summer of 1995, within three weeks, the best medical journals in the country contradicted each other. Harvard epidemiologists tracked 121,700 breast cancer patients for fifteen years. After filtering out other risk factors, they concluded that women taking estrogen for more than five years—with or without progesterone—had a 30 to 40 percent greater risk of breast cancer than women not having hormone replacement. They also reported elevated risks of endometrial cancer in women receiving estrogen replacement without progesterone. Published in the June 15, 1995, issue of *The New England Journal of Medicine,* the article became fodder for the evening news, talk shows, news magazines, and newspaper headlines.[8]

But three weeks later, the *Journal of the American Medical Association* denied a link between hormonal replacement therapy and breast cancer, when estrogen was used alone or with progesterone. The study was conducted by the University of Washington and Fred Hutchinson Cancer Research Center. In a randomized survey of 660 women with invasive or early-stage in situ tumors, Seattle epidemiologists could not establish any increased risk among women receiving combined estrogen-progesterone therapy. They even uncovered a slight reduction in risk among women receiving combined estrogen-progesterone therapy for more than eight years. They did admit, however, that the "number of subjects who used this regimen for a long period is small, and subsequent studies will need to monitor the risk in those estrogen-progesterone HRT users who continue into their second decade of treatment." The contradictions terrified and confused HRT recipients. "My God!" remarked Joan Simons, a Houston HRT user with a family history of breast cancer. "What the hell are we supposed to do?"[9]

An even more imposing dilemma faced breast cancer patients who had been long-time users of hormone replacement therapy. If HRT triggered the disease, it seemed only logical to discontinue use. Some clinical trials among women with metastatic disease revealed temporary regressions upon cessation of estrogen use. But for many women, losing a breast as well as estrogen replacement turned out to be a double blow. Not only were they dealing with cancer, they were feeling lousy again, undergoing instantaneous menopause and being deprived of estrogen's protection against osteoporosis and heart disease. Many felt so bad without estrogen therapy that they were willing to accept a higher cancer risk, and lower survival odds, by continuing the therapy. By the mid-1990s, several large cancer centers had launched clinical trials to see if survival really was compromised by hormone replacement therapy.[10]

Nobody really understood the origins of breast cancer. Some thought they did, especially environmentalists worried about chemical pollution. Rachel Carson had been the godmother of their movement. "Can anyone believe it is possible to lay down such a barrage of poisons on the surface of the earth," she wrote in 1962, "without making it unfit for all life?" Her best-selling book *Silent Spring*, an indictment of DDT and the pesticide industry, ignited heated debate, launching the modern popular environmental movement and inspiring shrill counterattacks from the American chemical industry. *Chemical World News* termed the book "science fiction, to be read in the same way that the TV program 'The Twilight Zone' is to be watched." Some attacks were mean-spirited *and* sexist. A member of the U.S. Federal Pest Control Review Board wondered why she was so upset. "I thought she was a spinster," he argued. "What's she so worried about genetics for?" Others accused Carson of being radical, anti-American, and hysterical. She was anything but. A calm woman with a trained, scientific mind, Carson was simply convinced that the world was at risk, awash in an ocean of man-made chemicals that would eventually upset nature's delicate balance. Cancer, she thought, was nature's way of getting even. "Man alone, of all forms of life, can *create* cancer-producing substances." She knew of what she spoke. Writing *Silent Spring* was Rachel Carson's own race against death.

Born in Springdale, Pennsylvania, in 1907, Carson came by environmentalism naturally. Her mother refused to kill insects when they made their way inside the house, and her father carefully picked apples from the family orchard without breaking tree branches. "I can remember no time when I wasn't interested in the out-of-doors and the whole world of nature," she wrote. "I was rather a solitary child and spent a great deal of time in woods and beside streams, learning the birds and the insects and flowers." A brilliant child and gifted writer, she sold her first story to *St. Nicholas* magazine when she was only ten.

Although science was an inhospitable world for women in the 1920s, Carson majored in biology at the Pennsylvania College for Women and then earned a master's degree at Johns Hopkins. After a brief stint at the University of Maryland, she took a job as an aquatic biologist for the U.S. Bureau of Fisheries, making her home in Washington, D.C. Her book *Under the Sea Wind,* a lyrical description of fish and bird migratory patterns, was published two weeks before the Japanese attack on Pearl Harbor. Although *Under the Sea Wind* received rave reviews, it died on the shelves. "If I could choose what seems to me the ideal existence," Carson wrote to a friend, "it would be just to live by writing. But I have done far too little to risk it." Instead, she kept working at the Bureau of Fisheries, which had become the U.S. Fish and Wildlife Service. Her wish came true a decade later when she wrote *The Sea Around Us,* a book that popularized the vision of the ocean as the source of all life. Serialized in *The New Yorker* and recipient of the National Book Award, *The Sea Around Us* remained on best-seller lists for eighteen months, giving Carson enough money to purchase a summer home on the coast of Maine and retire. Four years later, she wrote *The Edge of the Sea,* describing the cornucopia of life in a small tide pool and cementing her reputation as a popular ecologist.

Silent Spring had its beginnings in January 1958 when Carson received a disturbing letter from Olga Huckins of Duxbury, Massachusetts. A writer for the *Boston Post,* Huckins kept a two-acre bird sanctuary behind her home. In the summer of 1957, to kill mosquitoes multiplying in the wet marshes, the state blanketed Plymouth County with an aerial mist of oil and DDT, killing flies, grasshoppers, bees, and birds in the sanctuary. Outraged at the deaths of her beloved songbirds, Huckins described the catastrophe in a letter to the *Boston Herald,* demanding a moratorium on aerial spraying. "Airspraying where it is not needed or wanted," she wrote, "is inhuman, undemocratic, and probably unconstitutional. For those who stand helpless on this tortured earth, it is intolerable." Huckins asked Carson to do something about aerial spraying.

Carson spent several years poring over thousands of scientific articles and technical reports and consulting with chemists and ecologists around the world. But in the spring of 1960, just when she was ready to begin writing, Carson discovered a lump in her breast. A year before, she had had a malignant lump excised, but her surgeon decided to withhold the news, a practice not uncommon then and one that still survives in some regions of the world. Falsely relieved, she decided to include a chapter on cancer in the *Silent Spring* manuscript. "The chemical companies won't be happy," she wrote friend Dorothy Freeman.

Several months later, Carson had a recurrence, demanded the truth, and learned that she had breast cancer. On April 4, 1960, she had a mastectomy. Along with arthritis, an ulcer, and angina, breast cancer posed another obstacle to writing *Silent Spring*, but her surgeon had reassured her that he had "gotten it all," and she felt no threat to her life.

But late in November, Carson noticed lumps under her arm and underwent more tests. "It was a difficult day," she wrote, "things seemed pretty bleak." The cancer had made its way to her lymph nodes, and writing was going to be difficult. "The time this represents now when it is all so precious is of course horribly frustrating. But naturally there is no choice." She was not, however, about to accept a verdict passively. Well aware that her survival prospects were dismal, she wanted to up the odds, to try something different. At the time, the real iconoclast in breast cancer treatment was George Crile, Jr., of the Cleveland Clinic, and Carson sought him out. A critic of the radical mastectomy, he was one of the few American surgeons in the 1960s who viewed cancer as a systemic disease and advocated conservative limited surgery combined with radiotherapy. Carson had read Crile's 1955 book *Cancer and Common Sense*. "I had admired his little book on cancer greatly when it was published," Carson wrote, "and thought then that if ever I had such a diagnosis I would want to consult him . . . . [He] is so much more than a medical man—he is also a biologist with the greatest possible breadth of understanding, with such awareness of what we don't know, and consequent unwillingness to rush in with procedures that may disrupt the little understood but all important ecology of the body cells."

Crile and Carson were kindred spirits. He became "Barnie" to her, and the fact that his wife Jane was battling cancer only endeared him more to Carson. He set up a radiotherapy regimen and sent the instructions to a technician in Silver Spring, Maryland. "I don't question whether it is the right thing," she told Dorothy Freeman. For a scientist certain that cancer lurked in the environment, submitting to megavoltage radiation was difficult: "I know that 2-million volt monster is my only ally in the major battle—but an awesome and terrible ally, for even while it is killing the cancer I know what it is doing to me. That's why it's so hard to subject myself to it each day." But she did, even though the accumulating nausea made writing difficult. *Silent Spring* finally appeared in 1962. President John F. Kennedy read the book and immediately set in motion a presidential investigation of DDT and pesticides. The modern environmental movement was under way.

Rachel Carson may have won her battle with the chemical companies, but she lost her battle with breast cancer. In April 1962 new nodules appeared under her arm, just outside the radiated field. Crile wanted to remove them surgically and then follow up with more radiation, but Carson demurred, consenting to more radiation but no more cutting. She started a new radiotherapy regimen, but as soon as one series of treatments ended, new tumors sprouted in other locations. Throughout 1963, while dealing with the acclaim and controversies surrounding *Silent Spring*, Carson endured hundreds of radiation treatments to her hips, legs, collarbones, neck, spine, torso, rib cage, and brain. The treatments and the disease made walking and swallowing painful. "These are difficult days, I must confess," she wrote. "Almost any movement now is painful, for both the large area over my ribs and my back protest when I rise from a chair, lean over to pick up something, or move in any way in bed."

By March 1963, certain that a million radiation treatments would not save her life, Carson sought out Andrew C. Ivy of the University of Illinois, hoping the drug Krebiozen might bring her some relief. She knew of the debate surrounding Krebiozen, and that her own doctors "[would] disapprove . . . . [But] instead of attacking the local manifestations of the disease, as by radiation, it really helps the whole body resist." Carson believed cancer was systemic, not local, and she turned to Krebiozen because the drug was based on at least a semblance of scientific logic. But the wonder drug did nothing for the tumors, and she turned to a liquid phosphorous concoction in October. It failed as well. As the end of her life approached, Carson expressed no regrets. "What do I most want to say?" she wrote Dorothy Freeman. "I have had a rich life, full of rewards and satisfactions that come to few, and if it must end now, I can feel that I have achieved most of what I wished to do."

Biology, Society, and Destiny

The cancer finally overwhelmed her on April 14, 1964. She was fifty-six. But in *Silent Spring*, Rachel Carson left a legacy that later empowered the breast cancer movement. "Although the search must be continued for therapeutic measures to cure those who have already become victims of cancer," she argued, "it is a disservice to humanity to hold out the hope that the solution will come suddenly, in a single master stroke. It will come slowly, one step at a time. Meanwhile as we pour our millions into research and invest all our hopes in vast programs to find cures for established cases of cancer, we are neglecting the golden opportunity to prevent, even while we seek to cure."[11]

In the 1970s Rachel Carson's environmentalism gained enormous political momentum. Congress passed the Clean Air Act and the Occupational Health and Safety Act in 1970 and created the Environmental Protection Agency in 1971. More and more epidemiologists wondered whether chemical pollution explained the geometric rise in cancer rates. Samuel Epstein was one of them. Trained as a tropical medicine specialist at London University, he immigrated to the United States in 1961 to head the toxicology and carcinogenesis laboratories at the Children's Cancer Research Foundation in Boston. His 1978 book *Politics of Cancer* argued that industrial pollutants from the steel, petrochemical, and pharmaceutical industries account for the upswing in cancer incidence, and that corporate leaders had conspired to cover up the harmful effects of their products. He accused the National Cancer Institute of succumbing to political pressures from industry lobbyists and wasting billions in a misguided search for cures. At least as much money should be invested in learning how to prevent cancer, he insisted, as in how to treat it.[12]

The conviction that chemical carcinogens explained the rising incidence of breast cancer may have been deeply held by people like Rachel Carson and Samuel Epstein, but other voices, equally passionate, took exception. Chemical company public relations offices spewed out an endless stream of self-serving, pro-industry data, but some respected scientists took on the environmentalists as well. Elizabeth Whelan, a Harvard-trained demographer and cofounder of the American Council on Science and Health, wrote *Panic in the Pantry* in 1975 and *Toxic Terror* in 1985, accusing environmentalists of exaggerating the harmful effects of pesticides, misapplying the results of animal testing to humans, and employing scare tactics to promote their agendas. She discounted industrial pollutants as a significant cause of human cancers. Bruce Ames, a prominent University of California at Berkeley biochemist, also rejected chemical pollution as a factor, arguing instead that the environment is replete with natural carcinogens that pose a greater threat than anything chemical companies produce. Nature, according to Ames, is not benign, nor is technology the reason for human misery. Edith Efron, in her 1984 book *The Apocalyptics: Cancer and the Big Lie,* accused the cancer environmentalists of sloppy research, ideological hyperbole, and scare tactics. "Carcinogens," she wrote, "are not just single entities; they are aspects of the earth, they are preconditions for birth, reproduction, and survival, they are augurs of life and death, they are an attribute of existence itself."[13]

But an influential wing of the breast cancer movement blamed pollution. Rooted in New Deal liberalism and civil rights activism, feminism and environmentalism had little faith in corporate culture, and the chemical industry public relations hype enraged them. As the political battle lines formed in the 1990s, many breast cancer activists, like labor organizers of old, targeted corporate America and its agents in the cancer establishment as purveyors of death and disease. Devra Lee Davis, founding coordinator of the Breast Cancer Prevention Collaborative Research Group, insisted that "it makes sense to say the environment may be playing a role in human breast cancer. The weight of evidence, the hundreds of articles on animals, and the growing literature on humans all point in the same direction." According to Joe Thornton, a specialist on environmental cancers, "The worldwide increase in breast cancer rates has occurred during the same period in which the global environment has become contaminated with industrial synthetic chemicals."

In May 1993, *Ms.* magazine attacked the "Cancer Establishment"— the coalition of the National Cancer Institute, the American Cancer Society, the major pharmaceutical companies, and such major hospitals as Memorial Sloan-Kettering in New York City and M. D. Anderson in Houston—accusing this "mostly male establishment of ignoring prevention and focusing on cancer 'management' and a search for a cure. What we have is a golden circle of power and money, where many of the key players are connected, either directly or indirectly, with corporations that—depending on policies and priorities the establishment sets—have much to gain or lose." Critics found conspiracies everywhere. Armand Hammer, they pointed out, chaired the National Cancer Advisory Panel during the 1980s while heading Occidental Petroleum, a leading manufacturer of chlorine and organochlorine-based chemicals, which some environmentalists identified as carcinogens. Richard Gelb, CEO of Bristol Myers Squibb, chaired the board of Memorial Sloan-Kettering in 1991. His company manufactured chemotherapeutic drugs and silicone breast implants. Ralph Moss, author of *The Cancer Industry,* made much of the fact that Leo Wade, a former corporate boss at Standard Oil of New Jersey, rose to the directorship of Memorial Sloan-Kettering in New York. And Imperial Chemical Industries, a manufacturer of explosives, plastics, paints, and pharmaceuticals, helped sponsor National Breast Cancer Awareness Month each October in the United States and Great Britain. An article in *Mother Jones* noted that General Electric and DuPont market hundreds of millions of dollars of mammography equipment and film each year. Curing cancer was politically safer than working to prevent it because fewer vested interests were threatened. Prevention programs did not get their due, critics argued, because success would cut billions in revenues from major corporations. What else could explain the fact that only three percent of the annual budget of the American Cancer Society was devoted to the study of environmental carcinogens?[14]

One in Nine, a Long Island breast cancer advocacy group, had its origins in a dispute over environmental carcinogens with the National Cancer Institute and the Centers for Disease Control. In 1992 Senator Alphonse D'Amato learned that Long Island breast cancer rates were 15 percent above the national average. When he took the issue to the Centers for Disease Control, he was told that breast cancer was common on Long Island not because of environmental factors but because of the concentration there of Jewish women—who had a higher rate of breast cancer. Such smug complacency irritated many influential Long Island women, who formed One in Nine and demanded that the government address prevention. Liz LoRusso joined the group after an encounter with an insensitive male radiotherapist, who accused her of worrying too much about modesty during the treatments. She fumed over the comment all night, and the next day told the man, "Do you remember what you said to me yesterday about modesty? Well, *you* go get your testicles cut off, lose every hair on your body from the top of your head to the tip of your toes, then lie down on this table and have someone draw all over your crotch with a Magic Marker and we'll see how *you* like it!"[15]

Prodded by powerful politicians like D'Amato, the New York State Health Department undertook a study to assess One in Nine's claims of an environmental cause of Long Island's high breast cancer rates. Its 1994 report somewhat vindicated breast cancer advocates. Focusing on Nassau County, the study determined that one in seven women who developed breast cancer after menopause lived within one kilometer of a chemical, rubber, or plastic factory. Of the women who did not develop cancer, fewer than one in ten did. Mary Lou Monahan, president of the Long Beach Breast Cancer Coalition, told a reporter, "I'm so happy that they're looking at it, that they're finally doing studies that are environmentally linked." Lorraine Pace of Breast Cancer HELP (Healthy Environment for a Living Planet) looked at it more poetically: "You used to be able to go out and fish in the bay; you could walk across the bay from clam boat to clam boat. You can't do that now. I think whatever happened to the clams is now happening to us."

Conscious of the political momentum building, the National Cancer Institute increased funding for research exploring the relationship between breast cancer and the environment. Late in 1995, the NCI launched the Long Island Breast Cancer Study Project. To test for environmental causes of the disease, NCI epidemiologists planned to visit the home of every woman with breast cancer on Long Island and to test for pollutants in tap water, house dust, and yard soil. Steven Stellman, chief epidemiologist for the American Health Foundation, took note of the NCI's decision. "Five years ago," he commented, "I don't think anybody in the scientific community took seriously the question of whether environmental exposure was related to breast cancer, with the one exception of radiation. We've seen a major sea change in the extent to which the public, the scientific communities and the public agencies that control funding regard this question. They all take it very seriously now." Geri Barish, president of One in Nine, agreed wholeheartedly. "We've waited a lifetime," she told a reporter, "for the environmental factors of this disease to be acknowledged, and for something to be done about it. I've always felt the environment was the No. 1 cause of breast cancer, and probably other diseases as well."[16]

Hard data on the relationship between pesticides and breast cancer, however, was in short supply, with good scientists lined up on both sides of the question. In 1993, for example, Mary S. Wolff of the Mount Sinai School of Medicine in New York City reported a high correlation between breast cancer and exposure to DDT. Published in *The Journal of the National Cancer Institute*, her research claimed that women with extensive DDT exposures had breast cancer rates four times higher than women with little or no exposure. One year later, the same journal reported opposite results. Nancy Krieger of the Kaiser Foundation in Oakland, California, tracked 57,000 women and found no connection. In fact, the Asian women in the study had higher rates of DDT in their blood than whites but lower rates of the disease.[17]

Tens of thousands of women who had undergone mastectomies and reconstructive surgery and had survived the disease also confronted new concerns about the chemical industry. The silicone implants now tucked away in their breasts might be as dangerous as the tumors had been. The implants were not simply restorers of form and beauty. Early in the 1990s, a huge controversy erupted over whether the implants were a source of several malignant and autoimmune diseases.

Ruth Handler was right in the middle of the controversy. She had always noticed lumps, small routine masses that physicians called "fibrocystic disease." In 1958 she discovered the first of these and became concerned. Her family doctor told her not to worry but scheduled a biopsy just to be sure. Mercifully, the microscope revealed a benign lesion. She underwent several more biopsies in the 1960s with similar results. The lump she found in her left breast early in June 1970 did not alarm her, Handler remembered, although it "felt different from all the others, and it was in a different place, too." After a cursory examination, her surgeon felt the same way. "Ruth," he told her, "this one worries me." Several days later, at a Beverly Hills hospital, she underwent a biopsy and then a modified radical mastectomy.

The irony was not lost on her. Ruth Handler, the inventor of Barbie, the woman who had put breasts on dolls—firm, uplifted, pointed, undeniable breasts—had lost one of her own. Along with her husband Elliott, she had founded the Mattel Toy Company and had watched it boom. Barbie was responsible for Mattel's phenomenal success. In the late 1940s and early 1950s, research and development at Mattel were quite simple: the Handlers watched children play. Ruth became fascinated with her daughter Barbie's affection for paper dolls. Although Barbie and her friends spent some time with traditional baby dolls, they pretended to be adults when they played with paper dolls, dressing and undressing the cardboard figures for hours on end, creating a make-believe world of dates, proms, weddings, and outings. But when Handler broached the idea of creating an adult plastic doll, complete with different outfits, the men at Mattel brushed her off, claiming that the doll would require an Asian manufacturer to keep costs down. "That was the *official* reason," she later wrote. "But I really think that the squeamishness of those designers—every last one of them male—stemmed mostly from the fact that the doll would have *breasts* . . . . Elliott claimed that 'no mother will ever buy her daughter a doll with a chest.'" Handler eventually prevailed and proved them wrong. Mattel began manufacturing Barbie, and by 1993 company sales exceeded $1 billion.

But success mattered little in June 1970. "Losing a breast," she wrote twenty years later, "made me feel dewomanized. I'd been proud of the way I looked. I was well built and my designer clothes showed off my body. Now I felt the surgeon had taken the part of me that made me feminine and attractive . . . . I'd like to chop off parts of that doctor."

Handler's breast was gone, but not her entrepreneurial spirit; soon she detected a business opportunity. Several weeks after the mastectomy, she went to a Beverly Hills lingerie shop in search of a breast prosthesis. Clerks handled her request with hushed whispers, as if they were negotiating an illegitimate deal, shunted her over to a shrouded dressing area, and furtively handed over a pocketed, surgical brassiere and an egg-shaped, liquid-filled glob. "After struggling to get the prosthesis into the bra," she recalled, "I put my clothes on and studied my reflection in the mirror. The prosthesis looked awful. It was no match for the real thing on the right." Early prostheses were sized independently, not in conjunction with bra sizes, and they were interchangeable. "Every woman knows that her two breasts are as different as her two feet," Handler complained. "We wouldn't think of putting the same shoe on both the right and left foot, would we? It was obviously designed by a man who didn't have to wear it."

After five years of searching in vain for the right prosthesis, she approached Peyton Massey, a talented prosthetist, who did a plaster cast of her chest and designed a special silicone prosthesis to fit. Still, the design had problems, not the least of which was a temperature inversion. "It had been cold in his laboratory on the day he had made my plaster cast," Handler said, "and the artificial breasts he made for me had firm nipples while the nipple on my remaining breast was usually soft and flat! Once again,

I found myself wearing layers of clothes to hide my differences." The second prototype looked better, and Handler decided, "Wow, I should be making these for other women." With more than 100,000 women undergoing mastectomies each year, a market existed. "Peyton," she announced to Massey, "I'm going into the breast business."

She founded Nearly Me, Inc., a company committed to breast prostheses that weighed the same as the absent breast, were available in standard bra sizes, fit conveniently into regular brassieres, came in left and right versions, and could be purchased over-the-counter at less than $100 each. During the next sixteen years, Nearly Me mushroomed into the major supplier of breast prostheses. "Nearly Me . . . restored my *own* shattered sense of self . . . dealing all day long with women who had also undergone mastectomies helped me come to terms with the loss of my own breast, helped me change my opinion that I'd been 'dewomanized.' Women taught me that breasts do not make the woman."

Handler's positive self-image developed just in time. In 1989, nearly nineteen years after her first mastectomy, she lost her other breast. Although reconstruction surgery was available, she crusaded as an inveterate opponent of the procedure. Critics accused her of condemning breast reconstruction out of self-interest. Surgical implants would eliminate Nearly Me's market. But Handler's objections were sincere. After spending ten years fitting women with prostheses, she had seen tens of thousands of reconstructed breasts. "I can't tell you how many times . . . that a woman with an implant would come into the fitting room with a 'mess' on her chest and a plea for help." The breasts were often mismatched and, all too often, the silicone implant had shifted out of place, "usually climbing up high on the chest wall." Other women developed thick fibrous tissue around the implants, making the breast hard to the touch. A number of clients complained that the implants were leaking. "I also knew women who had gotten terrible infections from all those surgeries." Handler thought something was terribly wrong. "It's hard for me to believe that if I saw all these awful things, the medical community and the silicone manufacturers were not seeing them too."[18]

Millions of implant recipients shared her worries. Over time, the implants often leaked into the bloodstream, allegedly triggering immune-related disorders. Women with high silicone levels in their blood complained of fatigue, headaches, arthritis, rashes, and other ailments. Some worried that silicone was a carcinogen. Breast implant manufacturers and the surgeons who had installed them faced economic disaster. They had operated on more than two million women to augment breast size or to repair mastectomies, and in the 1990s they confronted a litigious nightmare. More than 400,000 former patients complained about crippling side effects of the surgery and demanded compensation for pain and suffering. Had she undergone breast reconstruction, Ruth Handler might have been one of them. Manufacturers like Dow Corning, Bristol Myers Squibb, Surgitek, and Replicon denied any connection between the implants and the illnesses, and they buttressed their contention with a number of scientific studies.

But in 1992 the Food and Drug Administration noted a connection compelling enough to ban silicone implants for cosmetic reasons, though not for breast reconstruction. Manufacturers halted production after a Houston jury ordered Dow Corning to pay $4.25 billion in damages to more than 400,000 women. Physicians could still use saline implants, but saline-based products usually lasted for only five years, requiring repeat operations. Instead, surgeons turned increasingly to a patient's own tissue from the abdomen or back to use in the reconstruction of a breast, rather than relying on silicone or saline.[19]

The controversy erupted again in the summer of 1995 when a Harvard University study found no correlation between silicone implants and connective tissue diseases. Between 1976 and 1990, Harvard tracked 87,501 nurses who had completed detailed health questionnaires and participated in follow-up interviews. In the group, 516 suffered from connective tissue diseases, and 1,183 had received silicone implants. Of the 516 women with connective tissue problems, only three had silicone implants, supporting the claim that the risk was no greater for implant recipients than for the population at large. Nor was there any increased susceptibility to cancer. Reactions were predictable. Mark Schusterman, chair of the plastic surgery department at M. D. Anderson Cancer Center in Houston, said that the report "is just one more good scientific study to refute the claims of non-scientific studies on the subject. It has been shown that they are safe when properly used." Shaun Ruddy, a rheumatologist at the Medical College of Virginia, added, "I would think that if there had not been the endless litigation that it is unlikely that anyone would choose to study this issue further." Dow Corning's attorney testified that "maybe you can argue about one or two, but now there are seven or eight respected studies. When are we going to finally say the curtain has fallen on this, that they are safe?" But 400,000 victims and their highly-paid class-action attorneys were not about to back down. Too much was at stake, and too many genuinely believed that the implants had permanently damaged their health. Richard Laminack, a Houston attorney representing implant clients, blasted the study as hopelessly biased and poorly designed. The manufacturers, he claimed, had financed the research and prejudiced the findings. *Nobody*, in fact, was about to back down.[20]

While many people blamed chemical companies and industrial pollution for the breast cancer epidemic, others looked to chromosomes. By the early 1990s, most oncologists had concluded that the secrets to understanding cancer would be found at the molecular level, lined up on an obscure chromosome deep inside the nucleus of human cells. Inherited susceptibility probably explained a small percentage of all breast cancers. What causes the rest? In 1996 Gabriel Hortobagyi, chairman of medical breast oncology at M. D. Anderson Cancer Center, said, "Most of us believe that every breast cancer is the result of some genetic injury." But there will probably never be, at least in the foreseeable future, a telltale "smoking gun," the discovery of a single explanation for the rising incidence of the disease. Prevention, which breast cancer advocates have set as their ultimate objective, will be a daunting task. Breast cancer's etiology is rooted in a host of genetic, social, and environmental variables.[21]

Genes confront millions of variables in the environment. Lurking in human cells are bits of aberrant DNA, mutated over millennia and programmed some day to explode into tumors. Susceptibility, however, does not necessarily dictate outcome. Genetic predispositions may have once been just that—inclinations never fulfilled, passed from one generation to the next over the ages while remaining safely dormant except for the unfortunate few. But after the Industrial Revolution, dormant impulses may have become transfigured into deadly imperatives, awakened by modern chemistry and rapid social change. Ecogenetics—the idea of genetic possibilities becoming probabilities in a carcinogenically-charged environment—is emerging as a new paradigm in breast cancer etiology.

In modern society, women function in a chemically synthetic world, submerged in an ocean of industrial and pharmaceutical products. A few synthetic chemicals are known carcinogens. Ever since 1775, when Percival Pott identified coal dust as the source of scrotal cancer in chimney sweeps, scientists have recognized the carcinogenic potential of some industrial products. Since then, other cancer-causing agents have been identified, including tobacco, asbestos, nickel ores, analine dyes, paraffin, uranium, radium dial paint, and betanaphthylamine. Women are exposed to tens of thousands of other synthetic chemicals, of which only a few have been positively identified as carcinogens. Pharmaceutical companies have created a chemical blizzard of their own, releasing thousands of medicines into a drug-dependent society anxious to feel good, physically and emotionally. The Food and Drug Administration requires elaborate, long-term testing to determine product safety, but occasionally carcinogenic inventions—like saccharine and diethylstilbesterol—slip through.

In their emphasis on preventing breast cancer, advocates have focused on the synthetic chemical environment as the most likely cause of the disease. To be sure, scientists have discovered several carcinogens out there, only a few of which, such as estrogen and DDT, can even be weakly linked to breast cancer. Activists take little comfort in the lack of suspects, however, and wonder about the carcinogenic potential of long-term, multiple-chemical exposures. Even if no individual product explains the rising incidence, some combination of two or three or fifty synthetic chemicals might be responsible. Discovering such a carcinogenic concoction will be a monumental task, since the number of permutations based on various combinations of exposure is infinite.

Though ecogenetics drives the debate over the origins of the disease, breast cancer is not just a matter of ecology and chromosomes. Ecogenetics must be placed in a larger social and cultural context. Breast cancer is as much a disease of modern society as of mutated DNA and chemical carcinogens. Recent social changes may have upset nature's evolutionary balances, destabilizing a biochemical machine millions of years in the making. Other factors are at work, many of which will be difficult to control, since they revolve around inextricable connections between biology, evolution, and destiny. Through the ages, since the emergence of humans as a species, evolution crafted an intricate biochemical system. It took millions of years for the female body to achieve its hormonal symmetry. Alterations in long established biological processes are fraught with danger; nature can respond capriciously to sudden changes in its systems. In the past two centuries, cultural and economic changes have confronted evolution's momentum. Walking today in an unfamiliar biochemical wilderness, women's bodies are reacting unpredictably. Breast cancer may very well be one of those reactions.

Until only recently in the history of the species, women married young and bore children early in their reproductive cycle. Evolution designed their hormonal systems for early reproduction and frequent pregnancies, an experience most women had before the advent of artificial birth control. But in the last century, especially in the developed world and particularly among the middle and upper classes, women have married later, postponed childbirth, and borne fewer children. In 1970, 9 percent of thirty-five-year-old women in the United States had not borne children. By 1990 the number had increased to 20 percent. Anne of Austria knew that nuns often fell victim to breast cancer; the modern equivalent of nuns may very well be women who decide not to have children or who postpone childbirth until late in the reproductive cycle.[22]

Evolution also designed the breast to nurse newborns. For millions of years, women nursed babies. During the reproductive cycle, a typical premodern woman might have given birth six or seven times and nursed each baby, spending ten to fifteen years with an infant at her breast. Nursing babies interrupted estrogen production, saving the breast from the monthly tissue changes undergone during menstruation. Such was the biological pattern encoded into a woman's hormonal system. But in the twentieth century, many women abandoned breast-feeding. Some did so for cosmetic reasons, fearing that the sucking child would distort the shape of breasts and render them less sexually appealing. Other women, enslaved by a Victorian squeamishness, gave up breast-feeding because it seemed socially inappropriate. Many feminists associated breast-feeding with social and economic impotence, since it bound women to the home instead of the workplace. Rejecting breast-feeding seemed an act of liberation. Actually, the reasons mattered little; the consequences did. Breasts without function can be dangerous. Women who do not breast-feed may well be more at risk of falling victim to premenopausal cancer.

Throughout human history, women lived marginal lives economically. For millions of years they foraged for food, surviving on a minimal number of calories and barely keeping ahead of starvation. Their food tended to be low in fat, since they had access to relatively little animal fat. Even the wild game they managed to kill was grass-fed and very lean. Obesity was unknown. But in the last two hundred years, calorie consumption has increased enormously, as have average body weights. Breast cancer is more common in obese women than in slender women, perhaps because fatty tissues stimulate estrogen production and alter breast tissue development.

Improved nutrition has also changed biorhythms. Adolescent young women today undergo menarche—their first period—at a much younger age than they did in the past. Three centuries ago in New England, most young women did not have their first period until their later teens. Today, the average age is around twelve and dropping steadily. Epidemiologists know that women who begin ovulating early in their lives have a higher incidence of breast cancer, perhaps because of the extra time their tissues are exposed to estrogen. Hormone replacement therapy also extends that period of exposure, providing more opportunities for cells to begin dividing uncontrollably.

Finally, women live longer. Over the millennia, women rarely outlived men because of the dangers of childbirth. Until late in the nineteenth century, most women did not live to see their forty-fifth birthday. They never experienced menopause, dying before their ovaries shut down estrogen production. But the medical triumph over infectious diseases and technological improvements in prenatal care gave women longer lives. As women age, their chances of getting sick with breast cancer escalate, most likely because they are exposed to more carcinogens over a longer period of time and because of the body's own programmed system for self-destruction. For those women who live longer, postpone childbirth, decline to nurse babies, and put on extra pounds, the risks of developing breast cancer will continue to grow, regardless of scientific progress. Breast tissues experience dramatic change with each menstrual cycle, and modern women may have hundreds more monthly periods than their ancestors did, increasing the odds for genetic damage to breast cells. Add to that biochemical mix the availability of birth control pills, fertility drugs, and estrogen replacement therapy, all of which might feed malignant tissues. Society may have become biology and biology destiny.[23]

At least according to the cancer establishment. Late in 1995 the National Cancer Institute published the latest of its inquiries into the etiology of breast cancer. The women most at risk carried a genetic predisposition, but the next most vulnerable group consisted of women whose personal biology and lifestyle choices had merged in a conjunction of dis-

uge of interview requests. Pleas from desperate terminally ill patients inundated such major cancer centers. Alternative therapists—herbalists, naturopaths, nutritionists, and homeopaths—began touting Folkman's ideas, claiming they could achieve the same results with natural therapies. A meticulous scientist given to understatement, Folkman was embarrassed by all the attention. He knew all too well the dangers of hyperbole, raising patients' expectations to impossible heights, guaranteeing disappointment, and generating acrimony in the academic community. Watson wrote Folkman an apologetic letter denying he had ever made such an outlandish statement, but the *New York Times* stood by the story, and Folkman had to endure the spotlight.

He stood up pretty well. Early in his career, Folkman had focused on angiogenesis—how rapidly growing tumors hungry for oxygen and nutrients draw into them, like a magnet attracting iron flakes, new blood vessels. When growing tumors begin gasping for oxygen, they secrete special molecules that inspire nearby endothelial cells to divide more rapidly and migrate toward the tumor, where they metamorphose—in a process known as angiogenesis—into new blood vessels, sating the voracious malignancy. Folkman searched for drugs that could inhibit angiogenesis, and by the 1980s and 1990s a series of pharmaceutical and genetic engineering companies joined the hunt. Such a drug, by blocking the generation of new capillaries, could starve a tumor or at least prevent it from growing. "If we could slow tumor growth and prolong life with a drug that had little toxicity," said Lee Ellis of M. D. Anderson Cancer Center, "we'd be doing far better than we are today." But like so much of the hype in the history of cancer, Watson's predictions proved cruelly premature. Other researchers had difficulty replicating Folkman's results, creating even more controversy, and even though anti-angiogenesis did show definite promise, it would be of little use to advanced cancer patients praying for a scientific miracle. The amount of time between a scientific breakthrough and clinical treatment could be years.[1]

In the meantime, women would continue to die. Breast cancer, as Anne of Austria would have certainly testified, is no respecter of persons and strikes the rich and famous with as much ferocity as it hits the poor and obscure. Actresses Bette Davis and Ingrid Bergman succumbed to breast cancer, as did romance novelist Jacqueline Susann and mob moll and JFK mistress Judith Exner. Virginia Clinton, the president's mother, also joined the list. When celebrities fall victim to the disease, society does take notice.

Jill Ireland's breast cancer garnered extraordinary attention. A successful English actress married to Charles Bronson, she was known to millions of moviegoers for her blonde hair, sensual smile, and lithesome athleticism. One morning in May 1984, she discovered a lump near her right armpit. Ray Weston, her gynecologist, referred Ireland to Mitchell Karlan, a Beverly Hills surgeon who performed a biopsy. The lump was malignant, and Ireland underwent a modified radical mastectomy. Karlan showed up the next day to discuss another hurdle—a lymph node report. Good news, he told Charlie and Jill, would be no sign of cancer—solid evidence that the cancer exited her body in the amputated breast. "If we find cancer in less than five nodes," he went on, "we think it's not too bad a prognosis. But if five or more have been affected, then it's bad. The statistics are not good." Jill felt "scared but optimistic" during the next four days. But the news was not good—eight positive nodes.

The choice narrowed to death or chemotherapy. In June 1984, three weeks after the mastectomy, oncologist Michael Van Scoy Mosher administered state-of-the-art therapy: consecutive injections of fluorouracil, Adriamycin, and Cytoxan. Jill experienced mild nausea and swelling in the mouth and throat, but by the next day felt fine. Two weeks later, while shampooing in the shower, her hair came out in clumps. The treatments continued every three weeks for six months. The second dose resulted in severe burning sensations. The third left large sores in her mouth and severe nausea. Two days after the fourth chemotherapy session, Jill noticed a burning sensation in her left breast and found another lump. Karlan aspirated it, drawing clear liquid from a benign cyst. "God loves you," he sighed. "It's just a cyst." The remaining treatments caused flu-like aches and pains. She finished the last treatment on December 13, 1984. By Christmas, Jill was in excellent spirits.

She adjusted well to surgery and chemotherapy. She mourned the loss of her breast but did not consider it an emotional catastrophe. Karlan changed the dressing two days after the operation, giving Ireland her first look at the wound. She expected something ugly, but all she saw was nothing—a flat chest, smooth, beautiful skin, and a horizontal scar, nothing dramatic or even ugly. "I don't consider myself ugly," she later wrote. "I don't consider the scar unsightly either." Two weeks after the surgery,

Bronson and Ireland made love. "I realize," she later wrote, "how lucky I was that Charlie and I could pick up and resume a normal, healthy sex life. That was not to be one of my problems."

Friends suggested that Ireland also pursue alternative medicine. Finding practitioners was easy. Beverly Hills was the New Age capital of the world, the city where leisure, money, and hopes for immortality met in a great narcissistic conjunction, producing tens of thousands of wealthy people obsessed with postponing old age and death. Jill visited O. Carl Simonton, the psychotherapeutic author of *Getting Well Again,* who told her that she was "living a very unhealthy lifestyle. If you don't change it and start honoring yourself and taking care of your needs, you will die." She believed, and he prescribed daily sessions of meditation in which she symbolically imagined her immunological system destroying the cancer cells.

Jill spoke with a "holistic counselor" almost daily. Susan Colin, who proudly displayed a master's degree diploma on the wall of her office and advertised as a "meditation therapist," had trained under Simonton. She coached Jill's meditation techniques, asking her again and again, "Are you ready to give up your cancer by changing your lifestyle?" Colin also convinced Ireland of the "healing power of quartz crystals." She would "hold a crystal in her hand, drawing the healing energy into her." Jill wore crystal pendants and pins, placed crystals in her pockets and purses, fondled crystals while watching television or driving in the car, and tucked crystals under her pillow at night, hoping against hope that crystals killed cancer.

She spent several hours a week with Bernard Dowson, an "electromagnetic therapist" who promised a cure if she would drink, eight times a day, his "electromagnetically-charged" water and rest on his special vibrating table, which shot charged "waves" into her body to "rebalance" cells. Dowson performed acupuncture on her right ear and collected weekly samples of hair, saliva, and fingernail clippings to assess her "vitality and energy potential." Every week, as Jill wrote out a check, Dowson assured her that she was getting better and better all the time.

Ireland also had regular $100-per-hour sessions with Chakrapani, "one of India's best astrologists." He read her astrological charts, convinced Jill of her strength and energy, warned her to take care of herself, and promised that she would live to be an old woman. During their first reading, she asked Chakrapani if she would be debilitated in old age. He prophesied, "You will never live as a helpless woman." "Never?" Jill replied.

"Never," he intoned. He was worth every penny. "I'd just bought myself a long, healthy life, cheap at any price," Jill later wrote.

I Ching also gave her a sense of power. A book of oracles going back three thousand years in China, *I Ching* enjoyed a small cult following in California. Each morning, followers took three coins, threw them into the air, and studied the pattern they formed on the floor. After repeating the procedure six times, sketching the complete pattern, and analyzing the final shape, the faithful looked up the shape in the *I Ching* book, which told them about the day and their future. For Jill Ireland, it all made sense.

She changed her diet. Since some experts believed that cancer is more likely to afflict obese people, Jill cut back on fatty foods, avoiding red meat and rich sauces. Some dietitians also saw processed foods as carcinogens, so Jill filled her diet with whole grains and fresh vegetables. Others preached the evils of sugar; she cut back on sweets. She added bulk to her diet to prevent colon cancer. To avoid dangers of chemical fertilizers and insecticides, Jill switched to organically grown foods and a macrobiotic diet. In a matter of months, she was an expert on the literature of nutritional cures. She felt confident and empowered.

Jill's health held for two years. She had the usual minor aches and pains of a fifty-year-old woman, but in cancer patients, morbid possibilities accentuate every discomfort. Back strain, chemotherapy-induced ringing in the ears, and swelling under her right arm from poor postmastectomy drainage frustrated Ireland, but her physicians patiently reassured her. She had a scare in September 1985 when she noticed a new lump in her left breast, not far from the earlier cyst. The growth proved benign, leaving her with a one-inch scar and a profound sense of relief. She had parts in two films—*Assassination* (1986) and *Caught* (1987)—co-produced *Murphy's Law* (1987), and made a number of personal appearances. Her 1987 autobiography, *Life Wish*, became a best-seller, prompting a tour of the United States and Great Britain, where she promoted early detection. Jill volunteered in Reach to Recovery, a breast cancer support group, served as National Crusade Chairman for the American Cancer Society, and received the Medal of Courage Award from President Ronald Reagan.

But in April 1988, an ache in her right shoulder punctured Jill's tranquility. Oncologist Mosher took blood tests in search of cancer enzymes, but the results were negative. So were x-rays. But the pain sharpened—keeping her awake at night in spite of sleeping pills. Three months later a cherry-sized lump popped up under Jill's right collarbone. It was malignant. The cancer had escaped Karlan's knife and Mosher's poisons. Subsequent bone and liver scans proved negative. Perhaps the cancer was confined to the lymph nodes. Mosher ruled out chemotherapy, opting instead for radiation. A Beverly Hills radiotherapist outlined the "radiation field" with a purple magic marker. The field included the right side of Jill's neck, right collarbone, right shoulder and underarm, and upper right chest. The treatments she had over the next seven weeks were not painful, but during the course of the therapy her chest, underarm, and neck reddened into a first-degree burn. The soft tissues swelled, and a troublesome case of phlebitis afflicted her. She was frustrated, "constantly being on the edge of feeling never terribly ill but never terribly well . . . . I can't help wondering if this is the way it is going to be for me."

It was. When the radiation treatments ended, relief never came. Jill tried to push nagging doubts out of her mind but later recalled, "I was never without a small, evil companion who had to accompany me on the happiest occasions . . . . I found it hard to believe that, as my surgeon assured me, radiation could cause such devastations, but it was preferable to the alternative." By February 1989, even after a relaxing week at a Palm Springs spa, she felt sick, frightened now about a deep, hacking cough. Early in March, Ray Weston ordered x-rays and blood tests. Two days later, he called Ireland at home and told her, "They've found a tumor in your lung." Jill went into a rage, cursing hysterically and sobbing uncontrollably. Taken aback, Weston asked her to "calm down. They're only small tumors." Incredulous, she sarcastically replied, "No tumors are small tumors. It's like being a little bit pregnant. You know that." The breast cancer had metastasized to her sternum, liver, pelvis, thyroid, lymph nodes, shoulders, and lungs.

Ireland scrapped the alternative therapies. She had neither the time nor the energy for homeopaths, wave therapists, macrobiotic dietitians, or palm readers. In an interview with *Good Housekeeping*, she remembered, "When I first learned I had cancer, I hit the disease running. My emotional powers were galvanized into making myself a stronger, healthier me. I was sure I could do it. I meditated and dieted. I researched every book on the subject . . . . Never was I more aware of my own life force . . . . But now I don't have the same enthusiasm for the cures and endless searching. I fought my big war and it seems I can't go back and use those same weapons again. I'm aware that I must handle cancer differently this time.

Ireland entered the murky world of experimental oncology. Mosher had given her two years, give or take some months; the only chance for more time lay in extreme measures. He recommended Adriamycin, which she had received back in 1984, and vincristine, a derivative of the periwinkle plant. Because the previous chemo had collapsed her veins, she had a catheter implanted in her chest so Mosher could pump the chemicals directly into her heart. At the Arlington Cancer Center, Ireland submitted to more radiotherapy and hyperthermia treatments. The radiotherapy was "palliative"—designed to relieve pain and buy time by spot-treating bone, lung, and thyroid metastases. Purple lines from the multiple radiation fields crisscrossed her body, and she went through the buzzing treatments under the gigantic machine several times a day. The radiotherapy was not really painful. Hyperthermia was. It raised Jill's body temperature to near lethal levels, just short of destroying her brain and kidneys, and dramatically elevated the temperature of her chest cavity, all in a desperate quest to kill the lung tumors. The doctors tunneled four long metal rods under the skin of her torso and heated them to 160 degrees. The only way she could tolerate the three-hour treatments was in a morphine stupor.

The treatments fell short. New tumors sprouted all over, in spite of a modified radical mastectomy, fluorouracil, Adriamycin, Cytoxan, vincristine, hyperthermia, radiation, O. Carl Simonton, *I Ching,* quartz crystals, and Chakrapani. Fluids collected in her lungs, making breathing difficult, and she lost even more weight. With the cures worse than the disease, Jill went home to die. Bronson, the tough-guy vigilante of *Death Wish,* nursed her tenderly to the end. "I never saw a couple who loved each other more," said a family friend. Jill spent her final days writing and visiting with friends and family. On May 5, 1990, she made her last public appearance, attending her son's wedding. Twelve days later, lulled into peace by a morphine drip, she died, one of 45,000 women who did not survive breast cancer that year.[2]

Other women in the 1990s, however, had more reason for hope than ever before. New developments had emerged in breast cancer incidence, treatment, and survival. In the 1980s and early 1990s, steadily increasing rates of breast cancer had convinced many women's health advocates that an epidemic was in the making, caused perhaps by an environmental wilderness of toxic wastes and synthetic chemicals. After all, the number of new cases of invasive breast carcinoma had leaped from 105,000 in 1980 to 138,000 in 1990 to more than 180,000 in 1994. Most biostatisticians attributed the rising incidence rate to an aging population and to earlier diagnoses because of more frequent breast self-examinations and the increasingly widespread use of mammograms. But suddenly—and *suddenly* has never been a common word in the lexicon of breast cancer science or technology—the epidemic appeared to be contained. In 1995, the incidence of breast cancer peaked and plateaued, and by the end of the 1990s, hints of a modest, but very real, decline appeared. In 1999, the American Cancer Society estimated there were 179,000 new cases. Since no dramatic environmental initiatives or changes could explain the decline, the statisticians claimed victory. Earlier diagnosis and an aging population, more than anything else, had explained the epidemic of the 1970s and 1980s.[3]

Equally comforting, a consensus had emerged about treatment. Ever since the 1950s, when surgeons abandoned the superradical mastectomy, the logic of maintaining survival rates for breast cancer patients gained momentum. In April 1995, the *New England Journal of Medicine* proclaimed that an intellectual revolution had forever altered breast cancer treatment. "It has been almost exactly 100 years," the editor noted, "since William Stewart Halsted published his seminal report on the use of radical mastectomy . . . . [His] ideas and his operation dominated our thinking about the treatment of breast cancer until approximately twenty-five years ago, when a major paradigmatic shift began." Back in 1979, the National Cancer Institute had taken on Halsted once and for all, conducting a randomized study comparing lumpectomy combined with axillary dissection and radiotherapy with modified radical mastectomies in 247 women. Ten-year survival rates confirmed the growing consensus that less radical procedures were sufficient in early stage disease. More than 77 percent of the women receiving lumpectomy plus radiation were still alive after ten years, compared to 75 percent of the mastectomy group. More aggressive forms of local control could not improve survival rates because breast cancer was not a local disease. The paradigm shift was complete. William Stewart Halsted moved from surgical texts to history books.[4]

Surgery and radiotherapy remained standard options, but both had also reached their intellectual limits. After a century of increasingly aggressive surgical protocols, the scientific tide turned. Damage control and quality of life, not long-term cures, now dominated surgery and radiotherapy. Instead of removing and radiating more tissue in order to pro-long life, surgeons and radiotherapists collaborated to remove less—to do less damage—while maintaining existing long-term survival rates. The future of breast cancer was not in local control but in systemic treatments for systemic disease. Molecular biology was the key. Electron microscopes and pharmaceutical laboratories, not scalpels and linear accelerators, filled the research horizon.[5]

The long-term benefits of chemotherapy had become abundantly clear. Preliminary studies in the 1970s and 1980s had clearly shown that various chemotherapy regimens could postpone recurrences for many women, but a few critics argued that disease-free survival and long-term survival were not at all the same. In the 1990s, however, convincing proof emerged that chemotherapy extended life. And, because of growing convictions that the disease was systemic from the very beginning, the practice of confining chemotherapy only to women with advanced, metastatic tumors gave way to treating women with early stage breast cancer as well. After a hundred years of surgery and radiotherapy, the quest for a cure was back in the apothecary. The drugs were no less exotic than centuries before, but their effects were predictable, if not for individuals then certainly for statistical aggregates.

Women undergoing chemotherapy after surgery improved their odds. Oncologists around the world reported consistently similar results. In the same issue where it underscored the merits of lumpectomies and radiation, the *New England Journal of Medicine* described Gianni Bonadonna's extended clinical trial at the National Tumor Institute in Milan. The Italian experiment divided 386 women into two groups. All the women had positive lymph nodes and had undergone radical mastectomies, but half also received follow-up treatments of combined Cytoxan, methotrexate, and fluorouracil. Twenty years later, 34 percent of the chemotherapy patients were still alive, compared with only 25 percent of the others. Chemotherapy worked.[6]

The adoption of lumpectomies and radiotherapy where appropriate was certainly the most important manifestation of the "do less harm" notion, but other technologies in the 1990s reinforced it. Ever since Halsted pioneered the radical mastectomy, which removed axillary lymph nodes in the armpit as well as the diseased breast, cancer survivors spent the rest of their lives battling lymphedema, a painful and uncomfortable condition in which lymphatic fluids collect in the upper arm because they have nowhere else to go. But in the 1990s, the "sentinel node biopsy" reduced that problem. Surgeons and radiologists injected a radioactive tracer and then massaged and compressed the breast to push the tracer out into the lymphatic system. X-rays could then determine into which lymph nodes the tracer had drained, most likely the same track any spreading cancer cells had taken. Instead of pursuing a "slash and burn" policy of gouging out all of the nodes, surgeons could remove only the "sentinel" node and prevent lymphedema. Dr. Patrick Borden of Memorial Sloan-Kettering Cancer Center in New York City, without exaggeration, said of sentinel node biopsy, "Aside from the lumpectomy, this is the century's most important development in breast surgery."

New surgical twists on the old mastectomy in the 1990s left patients with much better cosmetic results. At the University of Texas M. D. Anderson Cancer Center in Houston, surgeon Eva Singletary helped pioneer the "skin-sparing mastectomy." Singletary cut out the nipple and areolae and then scooped out breast tissue while leaving behind all of the skin that had covered the breast. She filled the empty pouch of breast skin with fatty tissues from the patient's abdomen and then, with tattooed abdominal skin, fashioned a new nipple and areolae. The result was the removal of dangerous breast tissues without changing the breast texture or appearance.

Some of the problems inherent in mammograms were also solved in the 1990s. Because standard mammograms miss approximately 10 percent of malignant lesions, they are hardly foolproof. Also, because 75 percent of the tumors mammograms identify are benign, a host of unnecessary biopsies are performed. But new high-resolution ultrasound scanners are now capable of picking up tumors as small as two millimeters and distinguishing between potentially dangerous solid mass tumors and harmless cysts, greatly reducing the number of women who have to undergo surgical biopsies.

Surgical biopsies have also changed. Until the mid-1990s, women with suspicious lumps had to endure a "needle localization" procedure in which surgeons, using x-rays of the breast as a map, implanted a strip of wire near the tumor. But it was hit or miss, especially when the tumors were embedded deep in the breast or near the chest wall. Pinpointing tumors with any precision often required a grueling period of jabbing and probing. Then, in a second procedure under a general anesthetic, the surgeon removed a sample of the tumor for pathological examination. But the advent of the MIBB—the minimally invasive breast biopsy—changed all that. After administering a local anesthetic, a surgeon wielding a digital x-ray camera that also houses a biopsy needle, locates the tumor, lines up the needle, and pushes a button that plunges the needle through the breast and straight into the mass. Patients walk away from the thirty-minute procedure wide-awake with no surgical scar and only a minor bruise that heals quickly.[7]

Scientists also uncovered some of breast cancer's furtive biochemical secrets. At the National Institute of Medical Research in Strasbourg, France, Pierre Chambon learned that breast tumor cells release a growth protein into surrounding, healthy connective tissues. For unknown reasons, those connective cells begin producing the enzyme metalloproteinase that degrades the protein matrix holding the tumor cells in place. Metalloproteinase then chews holes in blood and lymph vessels, allowing tumor cells to escape local confinement and travel to distant sites. Chambon speculated that if metalloproteinase could be suppressed chemotherapeutically, metastasis could be prevented.

On the other side of the Atlantic, at Children's Hospital in Boston, Michael O'Reilly isolated a tumor growth–inhibiting factor in breast cancer patients. Angiostatin, a naturally growing hormone, is produced by the primary breast tumor. It moves freely throughout the circulatory system, suppressing the growth of microscopic metastases. Ironically, once the primary tumor is surgically removed, drying up the source of angiostatin, the tiny, invisible tumors go into high-gear, uncontrolled growth spurts, eventually overwhelming the patient. Thirty years before, George Crile thought he had seen a link between removal of a primary tumor and growth in micrometastases. Now there was a biochemical explanation for his anecdotal musings. Isaiah Fidler, a metastasis expert at M. D. Anderson Hospital, said that O'Reilly's discovery was "of immense importance . . . . It has far-reaching implications for the therapy of cancer metastases because it is based on profound understanding of the biology of the process. Now the challenge is to translate it into a clinical reality. This is just the beginning." If angiostatin could be artificially produced and introduced to breast cancer patients after surgery, perhaps metastases could be prevented or at least postponed.[8]

Epilogue: The New Millennium

A few of breast cancer's genetic secrets were also being exposed. That breast cancer ran in families had been common knowledge for centuries, and differences in the tumors of white and black women also hinted at genetic etiologies. Although white women are more likely to get breast cancer, black women are much more likely to die from it. Epidemiologists long believed that social and economic factors explained the discrepancy, since black women have less access to health care than white women or wait too long to see a doctor. But in the mid-1990s, pathologists determined that the tumors of black women were faster growing, more aggressive, and less likely to possess hormone receptors than tumors in white women. Brenda Edwards, an epidemiologist at the National Cancer Institute, acknowledged the racial differential. "There's a difference and I don't think we can ignore it."[9]

The search for the elusive breast cancer gene was the late-twentieth-century equivalent of the nineteenth century's scramble to discover the headwaters of the Nile River. When she announced her discovery in October 1990, Mary-Claire King became an instant celebrity in the small world of molecular biologists. Along the e-mail grapevine of the great genetics laboratories—where scientists, computers, and electron microscopes map human genes—the news was electrifying. She had achieved the impossible. She had isolated a gene causing breast cancer and located it somewhere on chromosome 17.

The quest for the genetic holy grail consumed the first twenty years of Mary-Claire King's career. A native of Evanston, Illinois, King was forty-four years old when she told the world about chromosome 17. A mathematician turned geneticist, she graduated from Carleton College in 1966 and then earned a Ph.D. at the University of California at Berkeley in 1973. Recognizing her potential, Berkeley's geneticists offered her a position on the faculty, and during the next seventeen years, she wrote eighty scientific articles, earning tenure, a full professorship, and a national reputation.

The inherited susceptibility for breast cancer became the fulcrum of King's career. Beginning in the 1970s, she collected tissue samples from more than four hundred women in twenty-three breast cancer–ridden families. No fewer than 146 of the women had been diagnosed with the disease. She started tracking protein markers common to breast cancer DNA and, after the development of polymerase chain reaction (PCR) analysis in the mid-1980s, worked her way down to fifty million base pairs on chromosome 17. At the October 1990 meetings of the American Society of Human Genetics, she announced the discovery and fired the starting gun in a race to find the gene. Identifying the gene would be a public relations windfall for the lucky laboratory that achieved it. By 1993, after eliminating tens of millions of possibilities, the search had narrowed to a region of only 300,000 base pairs. The race quickened. King's Berkeley team went into high gear, working around the clock in top secrecy. So did everybody else. But in September 1994, Mark Skolnick at the University of Utah convened a press conference and explained how they had cloned and sequenced "BRCA1," a mutated gene responsible for six thousand cases of breast cancer each year in the United States. One in every two hundred women carries the gene, and 80 to 90 percent of them will get breast cancer. Mary-Claire King took the news in stride. "I keep asking myself, am I suddenly going to feel terrible about this?" she told a reporter from *Science*. "But I don't. I think it's great."

The Utah geneticists also noted a curious wrinkle to the discovery. For centuries, male physicians had speculated about biological, and even emotional, connections between breasts, ovaries, and the uterus. Skolnick's team had finally identified a connection, although he could not explain the reason for it: between 40 and 50 percent of women carrying the breast cancer gene will someday be diagnosed with ovarian cancer.[10]

A consortium at the Institute of Cancer Research in Surrey, England, closed in on another culprit. Carefully analyzing tissue samples from fifteen families with long histories of breast cancer, Michael Stratton and Douglas Easton focused on chromosome 13, where they found BRCA2 in September 1994. One in every two hundred women carries the gene, and more than 85 percent of them will develop breast cancer. Unlike carriers of BRCA1, however, they do not possess an elevated risk for ovarian cancer.[11]

Several months later, a global team led by Yosef Shiloh of Tel Aviv University isolated another breast cancer gene. After an eighteen-year search, they located what became known as the ATM gene. When inherited from both parents, the gene causes ataxia telangiectasia, a debilitating and ultimately fatal disease affecting one in every forty thousand people. Epidemiologists early in the 1970s had noticed a higher incidence of cancer among relatives of ataxia victims, and the search for the genetic connection began. Individuals inheriting just one ATM gene have high rates of cancer, especially certain lymphomas, leukemias, and breast cancer. A woman carrying the ATM gene has a 400 to 500 percent increased risk for breast cancer. Shiloh speculated that the ATM is the source of perhaps 8,000 new cases of breast cancer each year in the United States.[12]

A year after Skolnick's lab located BRCA1, the molehill of genetic evidence began growing into what would become a mountain. A team of Israeli and American scientists, after testing 858 Ashkenazi Jewish women (Jews of central and eastern European descent), reported that one in every one hundred possessed the gene, an incidence rate twice as high as that of the general population. In the October 1995 issue of *Nature Genetics,* they provided an explanation for why Jewish women, on Long Island and elsewhere, had unusually high rates of breast cancer. The implications were enormous. Perhaps the high incidence of breast cancer on Long Island had more to do with the percentage of Jewish women living there than with pollution. Also, it had become possible to screen a high-risk group for breast cancer, but since no cure exists for the disease, and there is no way to prevent it, what are BRCA1 carriers to do? Would insurance companies cancel the health policies of carriers? Might companies fire employees with the gene in order to keep health insurance costs down? Francis S. Collins, head of the National Center for Human Genome Research, worried about women with the gene. "You're not entitled to select your genes. They shouldn't be used against you."[13]

Discovery of breast cancer genes also forced genetic carriers to consider prophylactic mastectomies. *New York Times* writer Jane Brody in 1993 described a forty-three-year-old publishing executive's decision to undergo bilateral mastectomies after a mammography revealed a precancerous lesion in one breast. Her physician recommended no treatment, just careful monitoring. "After a few months," the woman recalled, "this watch-and-wait technique was making me increasingly nervous. I felt like I was sitting on a powder keg and I just couldn't live with that." She opted for bilateral mastectomies and breast reconstruction. Gina Kolata, another *New York Times* journalist, argued that some women "are irrationally afraid of keeping their breasts." Juliet Whitman, whose *Breast Cancer Journal: A Century of Petals* recounted her own struggle with the disease, knew the feeling. "My breasts were dangerous. They could harbor my death. At times I wished I'd had the courage to have them cut off."[14]

Some women did. Because of a history of breast lumps or because

Bathsheba's Breast

they carried the BRCA1 gene, they took the extraordinary step of under-going bilateral prophylactic mastectomies—having both breasts removed before any tumors had appeared. Physicians had warned that such a rad-ical step would provide no guarantees, that breast cancer could germinate in the breast tissues that escaped the scalpel. But in 1999 and in 2001, so-phisticated studies revealed that prophylactic mastectomy worked, that women undergoing the surgery stood a 90 percent chance of avoiding breast cancer. It was a high price to pay for prevention.[15]

At the turn of the millennium, hopes of curing all cancers had all but faded from the medical scene. The disease was so complex, so diverse, and so intricately and subtly connected to genetic and environmental variables that finding a cure, even after an investment of hundreds of billions of dol-lars, still seemed remote. But hope of controlling the disease, of turning it from an acute killer to a chronic malaise, had never been higher. In 1999 Stephen Baylin, associate director for research of the Johns Hopkins On-cology Center in Baltimore, remarked, "One aims for the cure, certainly, but we would do well to simply delay the progression of cancer. You could live with cancer, as long as you knew it wouldn't spread. I think that offers the greatest hope in the near future, to slow the progress of cancer."[16]

Breast cancer appeared to be a good example. In 1990, approximately 26 per 100,000 women in the United States died of breast cancer, a mor-tality rate only marginally better than it had been in the 1930s. But then, in the United States and Great Britain, the tide seemed to turn. In 1991, mortality rates for breast cancer peaked and then began a slow, annual de-cline of 2 percent per year until 1995, when the death rate fell at an even faster clip. By the end of the 1990s, 14,000 fewer women were dying an-nually of breast cancer in the United States and Great Britain than had died in 1989. Richard Peto, an epidemiologist at Oxford University, re-marked, "This is the first time that improvements in the treatment of any type of cancer have ever produced such a rapid fall in national death rates. They really are remarkable trends." Between 1989 and 1996, the breast can-cer death rate for U.S. women between the ages of twenty-nine and sixty dropped from approximately 40 in every 100,000 to less than 34, a decline of historic proportions. It was hardly a cure. In 2000, 85 percent of all American women diagnosed with breast cancer would be alive five years later. But only 71 percent would be alive in ten years, and only 57 percent in fifteen years. After an interval of twenty years, the survival rate was only

declining AIDS death rates, breast cancer had climbed to the top of the public health ladder. Every October, during Breast Cancer Awareness Month, millions of women wear pink ribbons to raise awareness of the disease, and tens of thousands run in Race for the Cure events to raise money. In less than a generation, advocacy groups and survivors have given breast cancer a much higher profile, forcing politicians to invest hundreds of millions of dollars in the crusade. Hardly a day passes without announcements of new discoveries, new ironies, new obituaries. Millions of women have become preoccupied with their own odds of contracting the disease. Those with a family history of breast cancer worry about whether or not they possess a genetic predisposition to the disease and how they should approach the problem. Articles about how to prevent breast cancer have proliferated in women's magazines. A host of advocates and promoters, cherry-picking data from scientific journals, tout the merits of regular exercise, low-fat diets, organically-grown foods, daily doses of aspirin, stress management, and multivitamin regimens, and in doing so manage to titillate the media and sell copy.

Breast cancer in the 1990s had lost much of its stigma and had even muscled its way into popular culture. In June 1996 novelist Danielle Steele's nineteenth book climbed up the fiction best-seller lists on a ladder provided by Doubleday, *Today, CBS This Morning, Good Morning America, Regis and Kathy Lee,* and dozens of local market talk shows. *Lightning* was romance fiction at its glitziest. The heroine, Alexandra Parker, is a successful career woman in her early forties. Endowed with genius, beauty, and wit, she is a brilliant litigator at New York's most prestigious law firm. She and her husband Sam are breathlessly in love after seventeen years of marriage, still anxious to hop between their silky Pratesi sheets at every opportunity. He jets from New York to London to Paris to Tokyo, negotiating tricky real estate deals, bond schemes, and futures trades, raising venture capital and matching investors with opportunities. The envy of New York's social register, Sam and Alexandra enjoy a seven-figure income, a beautiful daughter Annabelle, a Park Avenue penthouse, a summer home in the Hamptons, and a marriage made in heaven. "We're both so powerful in our own ways," Alex assures Sam. "We're strong people, with good jobs, we move a lot of people around, make a lot of decisions that affect money and people and corporations." They are, indeed, beautiful people in complete control of their destiny.

Until a routine mammogram reveals a tumor in Alex's left breast. She endures a mastectomy, divorce, reconstruction surgery, and eventual reconciliation, not the usual formula for romance novels but close enough. How times have changed. A mass market romance novel about breast cancer. For eons mastectomy had been synonymous with castration and death, a mutilating horror robbing victims of gender and life. Women with the disease treated it as a scandalous secret and revealed it grudgingly. Healthy women talked about it surreptitiously, in hushed tones, as if mentioning breast cancer might be carcinogenic. But in 1996, supermarket book racks, convenience store carousels, Wal-Mart and Kmart best-seller sections, and Bookstop, Barnes & Noble, Borders, Crown, Walden, and B. Dalton shelves featured a glamorous, sexy, one-breasted heroine.[22]

In 1997 CBS included breast cancer in the scripts of *Murphy Brown*, its hippest, top-rated situation comedy. Candice Bergen played Murphy Brown, the outspoken, wisecracking producer for a local television news station. Always trendy, *Murphy Brown* in 1991 had elicited attacks from Vice-President Dan Quayle when the unmarried heroine became pregnant and then a single mother. Quayle used the program to bemoan the decline of the American family, sparking a vigorous national debate and sending *Murphy Brown*'s Nielsen ratings into the stratosphere. Early in the 1997 prime-time season, Murphy Brown noticed a lump in her breast and underwent a mastectomy, and the show's writers then exploited the disease for months of comic relief, poignant introspection, and public health crusading. How times had changed—breast cancer as the focus of a situation comedy.[23]

Perhaps the glossy, color covers of *People Weekly* on October 26, 1998, and *Parade* on January 31, 1999, heralded the new era in the public perception of breast cancer. The women beam happily out on America, as if each had just won the lotto or Publishers Clearinghouse sweepstakes. Among them are actresses Ann Jillian, Marcia Wallace, Diahann Carroll, Jill Eikenberry, Kate Jackson, and Shirley Temple Black; journalists Linda Ellerbee and Betty Rollin; singers Carly Simon and Olivia Newton-John; Supreme Court Justice Sandra Day O'Connor; first ladies Nancy Reagan and Betty Ford; cuisine guru Julia Child; Olympic gold medalist Peggy Fleming; and feminist leader Gloria Steinem. As breast cancer survivors, they all share a unique sisterhood that transcends money, fame, time, and space.[24]

Epilogue: The New Millennium

Notes

Prologue: Across Time

1. Aeschylus, "The Persians," in Robert Potter, trans. and ed., *The Plays of Aeschylus* (London, 1895), 1.

2. Bill Hewitt, "Prisoner at Earth's End," *People Weekly,* November 1, 1999, 133–34.

3. Jerri Nielsen, *Ice Bound: A Doctor's Incredible Battle for Survival at the South Pole* (New York, 2001), 144.

4. Richard Crawley, trans. and ed., *The History of Herodotus* (New York, 1952), 118.

5. Nielsen, *Ice Bound,* 144, 207–8.

6. *New York Times,* July 13, 1999.

7. *Mail on Sunday* [London], August 15, 1999; Hewitt, "Prisoner," 135.

8. Nielsen, *Ice Bound,* 273.

9. Hewitt, "Prisoner," 130; *New York Times,* October 16, 1999; "I'd Like to Learn My Fate," *Newsweek,* October 25, 1999, 40; *New York Times,* October 20, 1999.

10. Nielsen, *Ice Bound,* 358.

11. Jeff Giles, "Lady McCartney," *Newsweek,* May 4, 1998, 64–67.

Chapter One: Dark Ages

1. Peter Allen Braithwaite and Dace Shugg, "Rembrandt's Bathsheba: The Dark Shadow of the Left Breast," *Annals of the Royal College of Surgeons of England,* 65 (1983): 337–38; T. C. Greco, "Rembrandt e il cancro della mammella," *Ospital Italien Chirurgía* 22 (February 1970): 141–44. Stoffels actually died during a bubonic plague epidemic, but friends had noticed a long, general decline

in her health, with severe weight loss and listlessness—certainly a "long illness." See Charles Fowkes, *The Life of Rembrandt* (London, 1978), 128–33; and Simon Schama, *Rembrandt's Eyes* (New York, 1999), 551–52.

2. James V. Ricci, *Aetios of Amida* (Philadelphia, 1950); Francis Adams, ed., *The Seven Books of Paulus Aegineta* (London, 1844–1847), Book 6, Section 45; Betty B. Gallucci, "Selected Concepts of Cancer as a Disease: From the Greeks to 1900," *Oncology Nursing Forum* 12 (July-August 1985): 67–68; Joseph H. Farrow, "Antiquity of Breast Cancer," *Cancer* 28 (December 1971): 1369–71; Harold Lamb, *Theodora and the Emperor* (New York, 1963), 1–46; Averil Cameron, ed., *Procopius* (New York, 1967), 319–21.

3. George Miller, "'Airs, Waters and Places' in History," *Journal of the History of Medicine* 17 (January 1962): 129–40; F. B. Lund, "The Life and Writings of Hippocrates," *Boston Medicine and Surgical Journal* 191 (1924): 1009–14. For a recent look at Hippocrates, see Owsei Temkin, *Hippocrates in a World of Pagans and Christians* (Baltimore, 1991).

4. Thomas Gaille, *The Institucion of Chyrurgerie* (London, 1567), 367.

5. Francis Adams, ed., *The Seven Books of Paulus Aegineta* (London, 1844), Book 6, Section 45.

6. D. G. Lytton and L. M. Resuhr, "Galen on Abnormal Swellings," *Journal of the History of Medicine and the Allied Sciences* 33 (October 1978): 531–49.

7. R. E. Siegal, *Galen's System of Physiology and Medicine* (Basel, 1968) and C. R. Singer, *Greek Biology and Medicine* (Oxford, 1922).

8. See F. G. Brunner, *Pathologie und Therapie der Geschwulste in der Antiken Medizin bei Celsus und Galen* (Zurich, 1977). For a biography of Galen, see G. S. Sarton, *Galen of Pergamon* (Lawrence, Kans., 1954).

9. See Owsei Temkin, *Galenism: Rise and Fall of a Medical Philosophy* (New York, 1973).

10. An excellent biography is Ruth Kleinman, *Anne of Austria. Queen of France* (Columbus, Ohio, 1985).

11. W. H. Lewis, *The Splendid Century: Life in the France of Louis XIV* (New York, 1953), 118–23.

12. On the death of Louis XIII, see Elizabeth Wirth Marvick, "The Character of Louis XIII: The Role of His Physician," *Journal of Interdisciplinary History* 4 (Winter 1974): 347–74.

13. For a description of the court of Louis XIV, see Robert K. Massie, *Peter the Great: His Life and World* (New York, 1980), 157–62. Also see Richard Bonney, *Political Change in France under Richelieu and Mazarin, 1624–1661* (Oxford, 1978) and John B. Wolf, *Louis XIV* (New York, 1968).

14. The descriptions of Anne's disease and her reactions to it are available

because of the remarkable notes and memoirs of François Bertaut de Motteville, who spent a quarter of a century at the side of Anne of Austria. The quotations are taken from Ruth Kleinman, "Facing Cancer in the Seventeenth Century: The Last Illness of Anne of Austria, 1664–1666," *Advances in Thanatology* 4 (1977): 37–55, and from Kleinman, *Anne of Austria*. Also see P. F. Lefevre, "Comment Anne d'Autriche devint femme (25 janvier 1619), d'après le Journal d'Héroard et les relations des Ambassadeurs," *Histoire des Sciences Medicales* 25 (1991): 185–90.

15. Quoted in Sherwin B. Nuland, *Doctors* (New York, 1988), 98–99. Also see W. B. Hamby, *Ambroise Paré, Surgeon of the Renaissance* (St. Louis, 1967).

16. Wallace B. Hanks, *The Case Reports and Autopsy Records of Ambroise Paré* (Springfield, Ill., 1960), 15–16.

17. Lewis, *The Splendid Century,* 177–78.

18. Ibid., 180–81.

19. For discussions of *artes moriendi,* see Philippe Aries, *Western Attitudes toward Death from the Middle Ages to the Present* (New York, 1974). J. A. Sharpe's "'Last Dying Speeches': Religion, Ideology and Public Execution in Seventeenth Century England," *Past and Present* 107 (February 1985): 144–67, provides an English perspective. For an eighteenth-century French point of view, see John McManners, *Death and the Enlightenment: Changing Attitudes to Death among Christians and Unbelievers in Eighteenth-Century France* (New York, 1981).

20. Wilmer Cave Wright, ed., *De Morbis Artificum by Bernardino Ramazzini: The Latin Text of 1713* (London, 1940), 191. Also see P. T. Mustacchi, "Ramazzini and Rigoni-Stern on Parity and Breast Cancer," *Archives of Internal Medicine* 108 (October 1961): 639–42.

21. Nicholas L. Petrakis, "Historic Milestones in Cancer Epidemiology," *Seminars in Oncology* 6 (December 1979): 433–44.

22. Robert Jackson, "St. Peregrine, O.S.M.—Patron Saint of Cancer Patients," *Canadian Medical Association Journal* 111 (October 19, 1971): 824, 827.

23. H. Pomeroy Brewster, *Saints and Festivals of the Christian Church* (New York, 1926), 94–96.

24. Josephine A. Dolan, *History of Nursing* (Philadelphia, 1963), 69–127; Vern L. Bullough and Bonnie Bullough, *The Care of the Sick* (New York, 1978), 26–48.

25. David Hugh Farmer, *The Oxford Dictionary of Saints* (New York, 1982), 4–5; Edward F. Lewison, "Saint Agatha: The Patron Saint of the Breast in Legend and Art," *Bulletin of the History of Medicine* 24 (September-October 1950): 411; *The New Catholic Encyclopedia* (New York, 1967), 1: 196–97, 8: 1062.

26. Camille Piton, *Le Costume civil en France du XIIIe au XIXe siecle* (Paris, n.d.), 216–48.

1. Quoted in Douglas Southall Freeman, *George Washington: A Biography* (New York, 1954), 6: 228–29.

2. Frederick Benays, "Washington and his Mother," *American History Illustrated* 26 (July-August 1991): 44–47.

3. Benjamin Rush, *Letters,* ed. L. H. Butterfield (Princeton, 1951) 1: 518. For the life of Benjamin Rush, see Carl Singer, *Revolutionary Doctor: Benjamin Rush, 1746–1813* (New York, 1966).

4. Quoted in Sherwin B. Nuland, *Doctors: The Biography of Medicine* (New York, 1986), 175–76; Ann Dally, *Women under the Knife: A History of Surgery* (New York, 1991), 1, 11, 35–42.

5. See C. D. O'Malley, *Vesalius of Brussels* (Berkeley, Calif., 1964), and Jerome J. Bylebyl, *William Harvey and His Age: The Professional and Social Context of the Discovery of Circulation* (Baltimore, 1979).

6. S. R. Gloyne, *John Hunter* (London, 1950); W. I. B. Onuigbo, "False Firsts in Cancer Literature," *Oncology* 25 (1971): 165.

7. Michael Potter, "Percivall Pott's Contribution to Cancer Research," *National Cancer Institute Monograph,* No. 10 (1963): 1–13; M. D. Kipling and H. A. Waldron, "Percivall Pott and Cancer Scroti," *British Journal of Indian Medicine* 32 (August 1975): 244–50.

8. Nuland, *Doctors,* 145–70.

9. Giovanni Battista Morgagni, *The Seats and Causes of Diseases Investigated by Anatomy,* trans. by Benjamin Alexander (New York, 1960), Letter L, Article 41.

10. Daniel De Moulin, "Historical Notes on Breast Cancer, with Emphasis on The Netherlands. I. Pathological and Therapeutic Concepts in the Seventeenth Century," *The Netherlands Journal of Surgery* 32 (March 1980): 129–34.

11. Jacob Wolff, *Die Lehre von der Krebskrankheit* (Jena, 1907), 1: 63–64.

12. Quoted in Daniel De Moulin, "Historical Notes on Breast Cancer, with Emphasis on The Netherlands. II. Pathophysiological Concepts, Diagnosis and Therapy in the Eighteenth Century," *The Netherlands Journal of Surgery* 33 (June 1981): 207; Wilmer Cave Wright, ed., *De Morbis Artificum by Bernardino Ramazzini: The Latin Text of 1713* (New York, 1940), 191.

13. W. A. Cooper, "The History of the Radical Mastectomy," *Annals of Medical History* 3 (1941): 36–42.

14. Henri F. le Dran, "Mémoire avec un précis de plusieurs observations sur le cancer," *Memoires de Academie Royale Chirgicales* 3 (1757): 1–54; Bernard Fisher

and Mark C. Gebhardt, "The Evolution of Breast Cancer Surgery: Past, Present, and Future," *Seminars in Oncology* 5 (December 1978): 385–94.

15. Alan D. Steinfeld, "A Historical Report of a Mastectomy for Carcinoma of the Breast," *Surgery, Gynecology & Obstetrics* 141 (October 1975): 616–17.

16. American Philosophical Society, *Transactions* 2 (1784): 216.

17. James Nooth, *Observations on the Treatment of Scirrhous Tumors of the Breast* (London, 1806), 13.

18. M. B. Shimkin, "An Historical Note on Tumor Transplantation in Man," *Cancer* 35 (February 1975): 540–41; W. H. Woglom, *The Study of Experimental Cancer: A Review* (New York, 1913), 43.

19. Rush, *Letters,* 1: 251.

20. Ibid., 1: 518; Benjamin Rush, "An Account of the Late Dr. Hugh Martin's Cancer Powder, with Brief Observations on Cancers," American Philosophical Society, *Transactions* 11 (1786): 212–17.

21. Lynne Withey, *Dearest Friend: A Life of Abigail Adams* (New York, 1981).

22. Linda Mayo, "Miss Adams in Love," *American Heritage* 16 (February 1965): 36–49.

23. The discussion and the quotations on Nabby's illness, unless other noted, are taken from Phyllis Lee Levin, *Abigail Adams: A Biography* (New York, 1987), 448–50, 458–60, and David McCullough, *John Adams* (New York, 2001), 601–2, 613, 628. The reader should also note that for narrative purposes, in describing the operation, I have generalized beyond the source itself, adding details about early-nineteenth-century mastectomies that were common to most surgeries but *not* necessarily to Nabby's.

24. Rush, *Letters,* 2: 1104.

25. Ibid., 1106.

Chapter Three: William Stewart Halsted and the Radical Mastectomy

1. Harold Ellis, "The Treatment of Breast Cancer: A Study in Evolution," *Annals of the Royal College of Surgeons of England* 69 (September 1987): 212–13.

2. Paul Huard, "Velpeau, cancérologue," *Congrès National des Societies Savantes* 2 (1968): 159–62; Charles H. Moore, "On the Influence of Inadequate Operations on the Theory of Cancer," *Med.-Chir. Transactions* 59 (1867): 245–80; A. P. M. Forrest, "Breast Cancer: 121 Years On," *Journal of the Royal College of Surgeons, Edinburgh* 34 (October 1989): 239.

3. John H. Talbott, *A Biographical History of Medicine* (New York, 1970), 556–57; Charles Underwood, "John Brown Talks of Breast Cancer," *Journal of the Medical Association of Georgia* 76 (May 1987): 308–9.

4. Bradford Smith, *Yankees in Paradise: The New England Impact on Hawaii* (Philadelphia, 1956), 244–46.

5. K. C. Carter, ed., *Ignac Semmelweis: The Etiology, Concept, and Prophylaxis of Childbed Fever* (Madison, 1983); Sherwin B. Nuland, "The Enigma of Semmelweis: An Interpretation," *Journal of the History of Medicine and Allied Sciences* 34 (July 1979): 255–72; W. W. L. Glenn, "Some Evidence of the Influence of the Development of Aseptic Techniques on Surgical Practice," *Surgery* 43 (1958): 688–98.

6. R. B. Fisher, *Joseph Lister* (New York, 1977); Lester S. King, "Germ Theory and Its Influence," *Journal of the American Medical Association* 249 (February 11, 1983): 794–98; Rhoda Truax, *The Doctors Warren of Boston: First Family of Surgery* (Boston, 1968), 266–67.

7. John C. Warren, *Surgical Observations on Tumours with Cases and Operations* (London, 1839), 259–61.

8. Lorenz Heister, "Van de kanker der boorsten," in H. T. Ulhoorn, ed., *Heelkindige onderwijzingen* (Amsterdam, 1718), 2: 845–56; Kenneth K. Meyer and William C. Beck, "Mastectomy Performed by Lawrence Heister in the Eighteenth Century," *Surgery, Gynecology & Obstetrics* 159 (October 1984): 391–94; C. M. Verkoorst, "De levensbeschrijving van de Zeeuwse arts Paulus de Wind (1714–1771) doorzijn zoon Samuels," *Archief Meded Kon Zeeuwsch Genootsch Wetensch* 11 (1974): 21–31; W. Brockband and F. Kenworthy, eds., *Diary of Richard Kay, 1716–51* (Manchester, 1968), 142–43.

9. Daniel De Moulin, "Historical Notes on Breast Cancer, with Emphasis on The Netherlands. II. Pathophysiological Concepts, Diagnosis and Therapy in the Eighteenth Century," *The Netherlands Journal of Surgery* 33 (October 1981): 215.

10. Julia Epstein, "Writing the Unspeakable," *Representations* 16 (Fall 1986): 131–65; Kay Torrey, "Fanny Burney's Mastectomy," *Border Crossing, Meridian* 10 (1991): 79–85; Robert G. Richardson, *Larrey, Surgeon to Napoleon's Imperial Guard* (London, 1974), 23; Ann Dally, *Women under the Knife: A History of Surgery* (New York, 1991), 104–9.

11. Quoted in Sherwin B. Nuland, *Doctors: The Biography of Medicine* (New York, 1988), 289–90; H. J. Bigelow, "Insensibility during Surgical Operations Produced by Inhalation," *Boston Medical and Surgery Journal* 35 (1846): 309–17.

12. Martin S. Pernick, *A Calculus of Suffering: Pain, Professionalism, and Anesthesia in Nineteenth-Century America* (New York, 1985), 47–48, 151–57; Daniel De Moulin, "A Historical-Phenomenological Study of Bodily Pain in Western Man," *Bulletin of the History of Medicine* 48 (Winter 1974): 549–70.

13. Susan M. Love, *Dr. Susan Love's Breast Book* (Reading, Mass., 1991),

97–120; V. T. DeVita, Jr., S. R. Helman, and S. A. Rosenberg, eds., *Cancer: Principles and Practice of Oncology* (Philadelphia, 1989), 1: 1204–6; Warren, *Surgical Observations*, 204.

14. Elizabeth Silverthorne, *Ashbel Smith of Texas: Pioneer, Patriot, Statesman, 1805–1886* (College Station, Tex., 1982), 111; Madge Thornall Roberts, *Star of Destiny: The Private Life of Sam and Margaret Houston* (Denton, Tex., 1993), 141–52; William Seale, *Sam Houston's Wife: A Biography of Margaret Lea Houston* (Norman, Okla., 1970), 120–27.

15. Brian Bracegirdle, "J. J. Lister and the Establishment of Histology," *Medical History* 21 (1977): 187–91.

16. Hans G. Schlumberger, "Origins of the Cell Concept in Pathology," *Archives of Pathology* 37 (May 1944): 396–407; Arsen Fiks, "Cytosarcoma Phylloides of the Mammary Gland—Muller's Tumor," *Virchows Archiv: A Pathological Anatomy and Histology* 392 (1981): 1–6; "Sero-Cystic Diseases of the Breast—Brodie's Tumor," *Cancer Bulletin* 11 (May-June 1961): 58–59.

17. E. H. Ackerknecht, *Rudolf Virchow—Doctor, Statesman, Anthropologist* (Madison, 1953); J. Walter Wilson, "Virchow's Contribution to the Cell Theory," *Journal of the History of Medicine* 2 (Spring 1947): 163–78.

18. S. J. Crowe, *Halsted of Johns Hopkins* (New York, 1957); W. G. MacCallum, *William Stewart Halsted, Surgeon* (Baltimore, 1930).

19. Edward F. Lewison, "Breast Cancer Surgery from Halsted to 1972," *Proceedings of the National Cancer Conference* 6 (1972): 276.

20. W. S. Halsted, "The Treatment of Wounds with Especial Reference to the Value of the Blood Clot in the Management of the Dead Space," *Johns Hopkins Hospital Reports* 2 (1890): 225–28; William Meyer, "An Improved Method of the Radical Operation for Carcinoma of the Breast," *Medical Record* 46 (1894): 746–50.

21. W. S. Halsted, "The Results of Operations for the Cure of Cancer of the Breast Performed at the Johns Hopkins Hospital from June, 1889, to January, 1894," *Johns Hopkins Hospital Reports* 4 (1894–95): 1–60.

22. Quoted in Nuland, *Doctors*, 409.

23. Ibid., 410.

24. W. S. Halsted, "The Results of Radical Operations for the Cure of Carcinoma of the Breast," *Annals of Surgery* 46 (1901): 1–7.

25. Ibid.

26. Paul Starr, *The Social Transformation of American Medicine* (New York, 1982), 32, 49–51; Dally, *Women under the Knife*, 42–44, 60–62.

1. See Jean Strouse, *Alice James: A Biography* (Boston, 1980), 300–315.

2. E. S. Judd, "Tumors of the Breast, with Special Reference to Obtaining Better Results in Malignant Cases," in *Collected Papers by the Staff of St. Mary's Hospital and Mayo Clinic, 1905–1909* (Rochester, Minn., 1910), 368.

3. Quoted in James Patterson, *The Dread Disease: Cancer and Modern American Culture* (Cambridge, Mass., 1987), 74.

4. Samuel Hopkins Adams, "What Can We Do About Cancer?: The Most Vital and Insistent Question in the Medical World," *Ladies Home Journal*, May 1913, 21; Patterson, *The Dread Disease*, 67.

5. Harry C. Saltzein, "The Average Treatment for Cancer," *Journal of the American Medical Association* 91 (August 18, 1928): 465–68; James Wright, "The Development of the Frozen Section Technique, the Evolution of Surgical Biopsy, and the Origins of Surgical Pathology," *Bulletin of the History of Medicine* 59 (Fall 1985): 285–326.

6. Bernard Fisher and Mark C. Gebhardt, "The Evolution of Breast Cancer Surgery: Past, Present, and Future," *Seminars in Oncology* 5 (December 1978): 386–89.

7. Wilson I. B. Onuigbo, "The Paradox of Virchow's Views on Cancer Metastasis," *Bulletin of the History of Medicine* 36 (September-October 1962): 444–49; Wilson I. B. Onuigbo, "Joseph Coats of Glasgow and the Theory of Cancer Metastasis," *Scottish Medical Journal* 15 (August 1970): 281–84; E. E. Grundmann, "Die Vorstellungen von Julius Cohnheim zur Geschwulstentstehung und Metastasierung im Blickwinkel Neuer Forschungsergebnisse," *Zentralblatt für Allgemeine Pathologie und Pathologische Anatomie* 130 (1985): 323–31.

8. William Sampson Handley, *Cancer of the Breast and Its Operative Treatment* (London, 1906).

9. W. S. Halsted, "The Results of Radical Operations for the Cure of Carcinoma of the Breast," *Annals of Surgery* 46 (1907): 1.

10. Quoted in Fisher and Gebhardt, "Evolution of Breast Cancer Surgery," 385.

11. W. S. Halsted, "The Treatment of Wounds with Especial Reference to the Value of the Blood Clot in the Management of Dead Spaces," *Johns Hopkins Hospital Reports* 2 (1890–1891): 255; C. W. G. Westerman, "Thoraxexcisie bij recidief can carcinoma mammae," *Ned Tijdschr Geneeskd* 54 (1910): 1686.

12. N. S. R. Maluf, "The History of Blood Transfusion," *Journal of the History of Medicine and Allied Sciences* 9 (January 1954), 59–107.

13. Helmuth M. Bottcher, *Wonder Drugs: A History of Antibiotics* (New York, 1964).

14. E. Harris Pierce and John W. Kirklin, "The Operability Rate of Carcinoma of the Breast," *Annals of Surgery* 145 (February 1957): 207–9.

15. C. E. Gardner, G. H. McSwain, and J. D. Moody, "Removal of Internal Mammary Lymphatics in Carcinoma of the Breast," *Surgery* 30 (1951): 271; George T. Pack and Irving M. Ariel, "A Half Century of Effort to Control Cancer," *International Abstracts of Surgery* (May 1955): 425–28.

16. R. S. Handley and A. C. Thackery, "The Internal Mammary Lymph Chain in Carcinoma of the Breast: A Study of 50 Cases," *Lancet* 2 (1949): 276–78; Jerome Urban, "Radical Mastectomy in Continuity with En Bloc Resection of the Internal Mammary Lymph-Node Chain," *Cancer* 5 (September 1952): 992–1008.

17. Urban, "Radical Mastectomy," 992–1008.

18. Quoted in Ann Dally, *Women under the Knife: A History of Surgery* (New York, 1991), 84.

19. A. S. Schinzinger, "Ueber Carcinoma mammae," Verhandlungen der Deutschen Gesellschaft für Chirurgie, 18 Kongress, Berlin, 24–27 April 1889, 29.

20. G. T. Beatson, "On the Treatment of Inoperable Cases of Carcinoma of the Mamma: Suggestion for a New Method of Treatment, with Illustrative Cases," *Lancet* 2 (1896): 165.

21. Stanley Boyd, "On Oophorectomy in Cancer of the Breast, *British Medical Journal* 2 (1900): 1161; N. C. Lake, "The East Operating Theatre," *Charing Cross Gazette* 58 (1960): 27; "Inoperable Breast Cancer and Oophorectomy," *British Medical Journal* 1 (1989): 1222.

22. See the proceedings of the meeting of the Royal Medical and Surgical Society of January 1905, reported in *Lancet* 1 (1905): 228; H. H. Simmer, "Oophorectomy for Breast Cancer Patients: Its Proposal, First Performance, and First Explanation as an Endocrine Ablation," *Clio Medica* 4 (December 1969): 227–49.

23. Henry Morris, "A Discussion in the Treatment of Inoperable Cancer," *British Medical Journal* 2 (1902): 1293.

24. Ira S. Goldenberg, "Hormones and Breast Cancer: Historical Perspectives," *Surgery* 53 (1963): 285–88.

25. J. M. Grodin, P. K. Siiteri, and P. C. MacDonald, "Source of Estrogen Production in Postmenopausal Women," *Journal of Clinical Endocrinology and Metabolism* 36 (February 1973): 207–14.

26. "Charles Brenton Huggins," *CA—A Cancer Journal for Clinicians* 22

(July-August 1972): 230–31; "Some Aspects of Hormonal Therapy," *Cancer Bulletin* 18 (July-August 1966): 70–72.

27. C. B. Huggins and W. W. Scott, "Bilateral Adrenalectomy in Prostatic Cancer," *Annals of Surgery* 122 (December 1945): 1031; C. B. Huggins and D. M. Bergenstal, "Inhibition of Human Mammary and Prostatic Cancers by Adrenalectomy," *Cancer Research* 12 (February 1952): 134.

28. Rolf Luft and Herbert Olivecrona, "Experiences with Hypophysectomy in Man," *Journal of Neurosurgery* 10 (May 1953): 301–16; Charles E. MacMahon and John L. Cahill, "The Evolution of the Concept of the Use of Surgical Castration in the Palliation of Breast Cancer in Pre-Menopausal Females," *Annals of Surgery* 184 (December 1976): 713–16.

29. Patterson, *The Dread Disease,* 51.

30. For a brilliant discussion of the rise to power of the medical establishment, see Paul Starr, *The Social Transformation of American Medicine* (New York, 1982): 79–144.

31. Morris Manges, "The General Practitioner's Response in the Early Diagnosis of Cancer," *American Journal of Surgery* 29 (1915): 377–79.

Chapter Five: New Beginnings: Assault on the Radical Mastectomy

1. *U.S. News and World Report,* April 2, 1950, 13; *Life,* May 5, 1958, 102–12; James T. Patterson, *The Dread Disease: Cancer and Modern American Culture* (Cambridge, Mass., 1987), 145–48.

2. "Wilhelm Konrad Röntgen (1845–1923)," *CA—A Cancer Journal for Clinicians* 22 (May-June 1972): 151–52.

3. Paul C. Hodges, *The Life and Times of Emil H. Grubbe* (Chicago, 1964): 3–30; "Roentgen, Forssell, and Madame Curie," *Cancer Bulletin* 14 (May-June 1962): 47–48; Jerome M. Vaeth, "Historical Aspects of Tylectomy and Radiation Therapy in the Treatment of Cancer of the Breast," *Frontiers of Radiation Therapy and Oncology* 17 (1983): 1–10.

4. Françoise Giroud, *Marie Curie: A Life* (New York, 1986).

5. Manuel Lederman, "The Early History of Radiotherapy: 1895–1939," *International Journal of Radiation Oncology, Biology, and Physics* 7 (1981): 639–48.

6. Geoffrey Keynes, *The Gates of Memory* (London, 1981); Reginald Murley, "Breast Cancer: Keynes and Conservatism," *Transactions of the Medical Society of London* 99 (1982): 1–13; Harold Ellis, "The Treatment of Breast Cancer: A Study in Evolution," *Annals of the Royal College of Surgeons of England* 69 (September 1987): 212–15; L. J. Berglung, "Sir Geoffrey Keynes—den brosrtbevarande kirurgins foregangsman," *Lakartidningen* 88 (May 8, 1991): 1805–6.

7. Dale E. Trout, "The History of High Energy Radiation Sources for Cancer Therapy," *Cancer Bulletin* 8 (January-February 1956): 8–12.

8. Maurice Lenz, "The Early Workers in Clinical Radiotherapy of Cancer at the Radium Institute of the Curie Foundation, Paris, France," *Cancer* 32 (September 1973): 519–23.

9. Robert McWhirter, "The Treatment of Cancer of the Breast," *Proceedings of the Royal Society of Medicine* 41 (1948): 118–32.

10. D. H. Patey and W. H. Dyson, "The Prognosis of Carcinoma of the Breast in Relation to the Type of Operation Performed," *British Journal of Cancer* 2 (1948): 7–10.

11. Ibid.

12. Quoted in W. S. Brainbridge, *The Cancer Problem* (New York, 1914): 2.

13. Eduard Bloch, "My Patient, Hitler," *Collier's,* March 15, 1941, 4, 35–38; March 22, 1941, 72–75.

14. John Toland, *Adolf Hitler* (New York, 1976) 1: 75–79.

15. Jerzy Einhorn, "Nitrogen Mustard: The Origin of Chemotherapy for Cancer," *International Journal of Radiation Oncology, Biology, and Physics* 11 (July 1985): 1375–78.

16. Saul A. Schepartz, "History of the National Cancer Institute and the Plant Screening Program," *Cancer Treatment Reports* 60 (August 1976): 975–78; Carl G. Kardinal, "Cancer Chemotherapy in Historical Perspective," *Journal of the Louisiana State Medical Society* 145 (April 1993): 175–77.

17. Paul DeKruif, "Fifty Thousand Could Live," *Reader's Digest,* November 1944, 89–93; Harry Schacht, "Cancer and the Atom," *Harper's,* August 1949, 83–87.

18. *New York Times,* October 3, 1953.

19. Carl G. Kardinal, "Cancer Chemotherapy: Historical Aspects and Future Considerations," *Postgraduate Medicine* 77 (May 1, 1985): 165–74.

20. "Breaking the News," *Time,* July 17, 1950, 45; *Los Angeles Times,* July 10, 1950.

Chapter Six: Beauty and the Breast: The Great American Obsession

1. Carol Felsenthal, *Alice Roosevelt Longworth* (New York, 1988): 234, 249.

2. Max Cutler, "Conservative Radical Mastectomy," *Journal of the International College of Surgeons* 44 (December 1965): 697–98.

3. Jerome A. Urban, "Extended Radical Mastectomy for Breast Cancer," *American Journal of Surgery* 106 (September 1963): 399–404; Jerome A. Urban, "Clinical Experience and Excision of the Internal Mammary Lymph Node

29. D. H. Patey and W. H. Dyson, "The Prognosis of Carcinoma of the Breast in Relation to the Type of Operation Performed," *British Journal of Cancer* 2 (1948): 10; Urban, "Extended Radical Mastectomy," 399–404.

30. Felsenthal, *Alice Roosevelt Longworth*, 250.

Chapter Seven: Out of the Closet: Breast Cancer in the 1970s

1. James Patterson, *The Dread Disease: Cancer and Modern American Culture* (Cambridge, Mass., 1987), 248–49; Richard A. Rettig, *Cancer Crusade: The Story of the National Cancer Act of 1971* (Princeton, 1977).

2. *New York Times*, October 2, 1971; Lester David, "A Brave Family Faces Up to Breast Cancer," *Today's Health*, June 1972, 16–21, 71.

3. Shirley Temple Black, *Child Star: An Autobiography* (New York, 1988).

4. Shirley Temple, "Don't Sit Home and Be Afraid," *McCall's*, February 1973, 82, 112–14.

5. "Verleihunh des 7. Dr.-Josef-Steiner Krebsforschungspreises 1992 an Prof. Dr. Bernard Fisher und an Prof. Dr. Gianni Bonadonna," *Schweiz. med. Wschr.* 122 (1992): 1814–15.

6. *New York Times*, April 4, 1994.

7. Bernard Fisher and Edwin R. Fisher, "Transmigration of Lymph Nodes by Tumor Cells," *Science* 152 (June 3, 1966): 1397–98; Bernard Fisher and E. R. Fisher, "The Interrelationship of Hematogenous and Lymphatic Tumor Cell Dissemination," *Surgery, Gynecology, & Obstetrics* 122 (April 1966): 791–98.

8. "The Breast Cancer Debate," *Newsweek*, November 16, 1970, 121; Albert Maisel, "Controversy over Breast Cancer," *Reader's Digest*, December 1971, 151–55.

9. Temple, "Don't Sit Home and Be Afraid," 112–14.

10. Gerald Caplan, "An Outpouring of Love for Shirley Temple," *McCall's*, March 1973, 48–53.

11. Lawrence W. Bassett and Richard H. Gold, "The Evolution of Mammography," *American Journal of Radiology* 150 (March 1988): 493–98; Paul Peter Rosen, "Specimen Radiography and the Diagnosis of Clinically Occult Mammary Carcinoma: A Brief Historical Review," *Pathology Annual* 15 (1980): 225–37.

12. Betty Ford, "I Feel Like I've Been Reborn," *McCall's*, February 1975, 98–99, 142–43.

13. "Happy's Brush with Cancer," *Newsweek*, October 28, 1974, 26–29; *New York Times*, October 18–20, 1974.

14. "Happy's Brush with Cancer," 28–29.

15. *New York Times*, November 25, 1974.

16. Ibid., November 27, 1974.

17. Ibid., November 25, 1974; Margaretta Rockefeller and Eleanor Harris, "If It Should Happen to You," *Reader's Digest,* May 1976, 131–34.

18. Betty Rollin, *At First You Cry* (Philadelphia, 1976).

19. Bernard Fisher and Mark C. Gebhardt, "The Evolution of Breast Cancer Surgery: Past, Present, and Future," *Seminars in Oncology* 5 (December 1978): 385–94.

20. Roberta Altman and Michael J. Sarg, *The Cancer Dictionary* (New York, 1992).

21. Malin Dollinger, Ernest H. Rosenbaum, and Greg Cable, *Everyone's Guide to Cancer Therapy* (New York, 1991), 52–54.

22. J. M. Bull, D. C. Tormey, S. H. Li et al., "A Randomized Comparative Trial of Adriamycin versus Methotrexate in Combination Drug Therapy," *Cancer* 41 (May 1978): 1649–57; Carl G. Kardinal, "Cancer Chemotherapy: Historical Aspects and Future Considerations," *Postgraduate Medicine* 77 (May 1, 1985): 165–74; Lerner, *Breast Cancer Wars,* 136–37, 251–55.

23. "Easing Out Radical Mastectomies," *Science News* 115 (June 16, 1979): 389.

24. "Minnie Riperton," *Ebony,* December 1976, 33–42; "She Never Sang the Blues," *Ebony,* August 1979, 95–100; J. W. Eley, H. A. Hill, V. W. Chen et al., "Racial Differences in Survival from Breast Cancer: Results of the National Cancer Institute Black/White Cancer Survival Study," *Journal of the American Medical Association* 272 (September 28, 1994): 947–54.

Chapter Eight: Patient Heal Thyself: Quacks and Cures in the Age of Narcissism

1. Stephen Barrett and William T. Jarvis, *The Health Robbers: A Close Look at Quackery in America* (New York, 1993), 97.

2. Morris Fishbein, "History of Cancer Quackery," *Perspectives in Biology and Medicine* 8 (Winter 1965): 139–66.

3. James Harvey Young, *The Medical Messiahs: A Social History of Health Quackery in Twentieth-Century America* (Princeton, 1967), 360–90.

4. Patricia Spain Ward, "Who Will Bell the Cat? Andrew C. Ivy and Krebiozen," *Bulletin of the History of Medicine* 58 (Spring 1984): 28–52.

5. Michael B. Shimkin, "End Results in Cancer of the Breast," *Cancer* 20 (1967): 1039–43; John S. Stehlin, Richard A. Evans, Augusto E. Gutierrez et al., "Treatment of Carcinoma of the Breast," *Surgery, Gynecology, & Obstetrics* 149 (December 1979): 911–22; "Treatment of Early Carcinoma of the Breast," *British Medical Journal* 2 (May 20, 1972): 417–18.

6. J. L. Hayward, "The Guy's Trial of Treatments of Early Breast Cancer," *World Journal of Surgery* 1 (May 1977): 314–16; Umberto Veronesi, "Conserva-

tive Treatment of Breast Cancer: A Trial in Progress at the Cancer Institute of Milan," *World Journal of Surgery* 1 (May 1977): 324–26.

7. Albert Maisel, "Controversy over Breast Cancer," *Reader's Digest,* December 1971, 153.

8. Jan Stjerneswärd, "Decreased Survival Related to Irradiation Postoperatively in Early Operable Breast Cancer," *Lancet* (November 30, 1974): 1285–86; Thomas L. Dao and John Kovaric, "Incidence of Pulmonary and Skin Metastases in Women with Breast Cancer Who Received Postoperative Irradiation," *Surgery* 52 (July 1962): 203–12.

9. Susan Nessim and Judith Ellis, *Cancervive: The Challenge of Life After Cancer* (Boston, 1991), 203; Smita Bhatia, Leslie L. Robison, Odile Oberlin et al., "Breast Cancer and Other Second Neoplasms after Childhood Hodgkin's Disease," *New England Journal of Medicine* 334 (March 21, 1996): 745–51.

10. Los Angeles *Herald-Examiner,* November 3, 1980.

11. I. Thomas and P. Newman, "Flinty Grandmother Battles for the Victims of Utah's Nuclear Tragedy," *People Weekly,* October 1, 1979, 26–29; K. G. Jackovich and M. Sennet, "Children of John Wayne, Susan Hayward and Dick Powell Fear That Fallout Killed Their Parents," *People Weekly,* November 10, 1980, 42–47; *Variety,* April 21, 1980, 33.

12. Roberta Altman and Michael J. Sarg, *The Cancer Dictionary* (New York, 1992), 53–55.

13. Barrett and Jarvis, *The Health Robbers,* 92–94.

14. Gerald E. Markle and James C. Peterson, *Politics, Science, and Cancer: The Laetrile Phenomenon* (New York, 1980), 11–60.

15. Barrett and Jarvis, *The Health Robbers,* 97.

16. Ibid., 92–94.

17. Daniel Yergin, "Supernutritionist," *The New York Times Magazine,* May 20, 1973, 32–33, 58–64, 71; Frederick Hoffman, *Cancer and Diet* (New York, 1937): 167–68, 652–62.

18. William J. Broad, "Pop Nutrition Books Face Legal Hurdles," *Science* 205 (September 14, 1979): 1113.

19. Adelle Davis, *Let's Get Well* (New York, 1965), 298–306.

20. *New York Times,* June 1, 1974.

21. William Parker, *Cancer: A Study of 397 Cases of the Human Breast* (New York, 1885), 34–35.

22. Daniel De Moulin, "Historical Notes on Breast Cancer, with Emphasis on The Netherlands. I. Pathological and Therapeutic Concepts in the Seventeenth Century," *The Netherlands Journal of Surgery* 32 (March 1980): 130–31; James Paget, *Surgical Pathology* (London, 1870), 122; Wilhelm Reich, *Cancer*

Biopathy (New York, 1938); Myron Sharif, *Fury on Earth: A Biography of Wilhelm Reich* (New York, 1983), 298–303; Samuel J. Kowal, "Emotions as a Cause of Cancer: 18th and 19th Century Contributions," *Psychoanalytic Review* 42 (1955): 217–27.

23. *New York Times,* November 3, 1957.

24. Christopher Lasch, *The Culture of Narcissism: American Life in an Age of Diminishing Expectations* (New York, 1978), 7–12.

25. Quoted in ibid., 14.

26. Susan Sontag, *Illness as Metaphor* (New York, 1978), 51. Also see Lawrence LeShan, *Cancer as a Turning Point* (New York, 1989).

27. Gina Kolata, "Texas Counselors Use Psychology in Cancer Therapy," *Smithsonian,* August 1980, 49–57.

28. O. Carl Simonton and Stephanie Matthews-Simonton, *Getting Well Again* (New York, 1980), 230–31.

29. Norman Cousins, *Anatomy of an Illness* (New York, 1979), 27–48.

30. Bernie S. Siegel, *Love, Medicine & Miracles* (New York, 1986), 171.

31. Quoted in Barrett and Jarvis, *The Health Robbers,* 96.

32. R. B. Shekelle, W. J. Raynor, A. M. Ostfeld et al., "Psychological Depression and 17-Year Risk of Death from Cancer," *Psychosomatic Medicine* 43 (April 1981): 117–25; Marcia Angell, "Disease as a Reflection of the Psyche," *New England Journal of Medicine* 312 (June 13, 1985): 1570–72; V. W. Persky, J. Kempthorne-Rawson, and R. B. Shekelle, "Personality and Risk of Cancer: 20-Year Follow-Up of the Western Electric Study," *Psychosomatic Medicine* 49 (September-October 1987): 435–49; G. A. Kaplan and P. Reynolds, "Depression and Cancer Mortality and Morbidity: Prospective Evidence from the Alameda County Study," *Journal of Behavioral Medicine* 11 (February 1988): 1–13; R. C. Hahn and D. B. Petitti, "Minnesota Multiphasic Personality Inventory–Rated Depression and the Incidence of Breast Cancer," *Cancer* 61 (February 15, 1988): 845–48; A. B. Zonderman, P. T. Costa, and R. R. McRae, "Depression as a Risk for Cancer Morbidity and Mortality in a Nationally Representative Sample," *Journal of the American Medical Association* 262 (September 1, 1989): 1191–95; Bernard H. Fox, "Depressive Symptoms and Risk of Cancer," *Journal of the American Medical Association* 262 (September 1, 1989): 1231; J. Kaprio, M. Koskenvuo, and H. Rita, "Mortality after Bereavement: A Prospective Study of 95,647 Widowed Persons," *American Journal of Public Health* 77 (March 1987): 283–87; K. J. Helsing, G. W. Comstock, and M. Szklo, "Causes of Death in a Widowed Population," *American Journal of Epidemiology* 116 (September 1982): 524–32; Dana H. Bovbjerg, "Psychoneuroimmunotherapy: Implications for Oncology?" *Cancer* 67 (February 1 Supplement 1991): 828–32; Barron H. Lerner, "Can Stress

Cause Disease? Revisiting the Tuberculosis Research of Thomas Holmes, 1949–1961," *Annals of Internal Medicine* 124 (April 1, 1996): 674–80.

33. B. H. Fox, "Premorbid Psychological Factors as Related to Cancer Incidence," *Behavioral Medicine* 1 (March 1978): 133; David K. Wellisch and Joel Yager, "Is There a Cancer-Prone Personality," *CA—A Journal for Clinicians* 33 (May/June 1983): 145–53.

34. Kolata, "Texas Counselors Use Psychology in Cancer Therapy," 56; Karen Ritchie, "Guilt and the Cancer Patient," *Cancer Bulletin* 43 (September-October 1991): 430.

35. American Cancer Society, "Unproven Methods of Cancer Management: O. Carl Simonton, M.D.," *CA—A Cancer Journal for Clinicians* 32 (January-February 1982): 58–61; American Medical Association, *Reader's Guide to Unproven Health Methods* (New York, 1993), 142–43.

36. Louis D. Rubin, Jr., "Susan Sontag and the D Camp Followers," *Sewanee Review* 82 (Summer 1974): 503–10.

37. Ellen Willis, "The Cancer Ward," *Rolling Stone*, January 26, 1978, 27.

38. Carol Kahn, "Alone against Illness," *Family Health*, November 1978, 50–53. Sontag, *Illness as Metaphor*, 57–69.

39. Sontag, *Illness as Metaphor*.

40. Kahn, "Alone against Illness," 53.

Chapter Nine: Choices: Medical Treatment in the Age of Liberation

1. The material in this chapter on Rose Kushner's life is taken from her book *Breast Cancer: A Personal History and Investigative Report* (New York, 1975).

2. Ibid., 30.

3. Arthur L. Herbst, Howard Ulfelder, and David C. Poskanzer, "Adenocarcinoma of the Vagina: Association of Maternal Stilbesterol Therapy with Tumor Appearance in Young Women," *New England Journal of Medicine* 284 (April 22, 1971): 878–81.

4. Paul Kuehn, *Breast Cancer Care Options for the 1990s* (South Windsor, Conn., 1991), 62.

5. Carol Ann Rinzler, *Estrogen and Breast Cancer* (New York, 1993), 80–82.

6. Elfriede Fasal and Ralph S. Paffenbarger, "OC as Related to Cancer and Benign Lesions of the Breast," *Journal of the National Cancer Institute* 55 (October 1975): 767–73.

7. Ralph S. Paffenbarger, Jr., Elfriede Fasal, Martha E. Simmons, and James Kampert, "Cancer Risk as Related to Use of Oral Contraceptives during Fertile Years," *Cancer* 39 (April Supplement, 1977): 1887–91; M. C. Pike, B. E. Hen-

derson, J. T. Casagrande et al., "Oral Contraceptive Use and Early Abortion as Risk Factors for Breast Cancer in Young Women," *British Journal of Cancer* 43 (1981): 72–76; M. C. Pike, B. E. Henderson, M. D. Krailo et al., "Breast Cancer in Young Women and Use of Oral Contraceptives: Possible Modifying Effect of Formulation and Age at Use," *Lancet* (October 22, 1983): 926–29.

8. B. V. Stadel and J. J. Schlesselman, "Oral Contraceptive Use and the Risk of Breast Cancer in Women with a 'Prior' History of Benign Breast Disease," *American Journal of Epidemiology* 123 (March 1986): 373–82.

9. Clair Chilvers, K. McPherson, J. Peto et al., "Oral Contraceptives and Breast Cancer Risk in Young Women," *Lancet* (May 6, 1989): 973–82; Hakan Olsson, Torgil R. Moller, and Jonas Ranstam, "Early Oral Contraceptive Use and Breast Cancer among Premenopausal Women: Final Report from a Study in Southern Sweden," *Journal of the National Cancer Institute* 81 (July 5, 1989): 1000–1004; C. T. Paul, D. C. G. Skegg, G. F. S. Spears et al., "Oral Contraceptives and Breast Cancer: A National Study," *British Medical Journal* 293 (September 20, 1986): 723–26; Isabelle Romieu, Walter C. Willett, Graham A. Colditz et al., "Prospective Study of Oral Contraceptive Use and Risk of Breast Cancer in Women," *Journal of the National Cancer Institute* 81 (September 6, 1989): 1313–21; Richard W. Sattin, George L. Rubin, Phyllis A. Wingo et al., "Oral-Contraceptive Use and the Risk of Breast Cancer," *New England Journal of Medicine* 315 (August 14, 1986): 405–11.

10. Rinzler, *Estrogen and Breast Cancer,* 92–93.

11. Karen Steinberg, Stephen B. Thaker, S. Jay Smith et al., "A Meta-Analysis of the Effect of Estrogen Replacement Therapy on the Risk of Breast Cancer," *Journal of the American Medical Association* 265 (April 17, 1991): 1985–90.

12. Rose Kushner, "My Side," *Working Woman,* May 1983, 160–61.

13. Elwood V. Jensen, "Historical Perspective: Hormone Dependency of Human Breast Cancers," *Cancer* 46 (Supplement, December 15, 1980): 2759–61.

14. V. Craig Jordan, "The Development of Tamoxifen for Breast Cancer Therapy: A Tribute to the Late Arthur L. Walpole," *Breast Cancer Research and Treatment* 11 (1988): 197–209.

15. George P. Rosemond, Willis P. Maier, and Thomas J. Brobyn, "Needle Aspiration of Breast Cysts," *CA—A Journal for Clinicians* 23 (January–February 1973): 33–46; Gordon F. Schwartz, "A Plea for Sensible Breast Biopsy," *Medical Opinion* (March 1975): 1–4.

16. Shirley Temple, "Don't Sit Home and Be Afraid," *McCall's,* February 1973, 82, 112–14; Kushner, "My Side," 160–61.

17. Bernard Fisher, M. Bauer, R. Margolese et al., "Five-Year Results of a Randomized Clinical Trial Comparing Total Mastectomy and Segmental Mas-

tectomy with or without Radiation in the Treatment of Breast Cancer," *New England Journal of Medicine* 312 (March 14, 1985): 665–73; Bernard Fisher, Carol Redmond, and Roger Poisson, "Eight-Year Results of a Randomized Clinical Trial Comparing Total Mastectomy and Lumpectomy with or without Irradiation in the Treatment of Breast Cancer," *New England Journal of Medicine* 320 (March 30, 1989): 822–28; Bernard Fisher, Carol Redmond, N. V. Dimotrov et al., "A Randomized Clinical Trial Evaluating Sequential Methotrexate and Flourouracil in the Treatment of Patients with Node-Negative Breast Cancer Who Have Estrogen-Receptor-Negative Tumors," *New England Journal of Medicine* 320 (February 23, 1989): 473–78; Bernard Fisher, J. Costantino, Carol Redmond et al., "A Randomized Clinical Trial Evaluating Tamoxifen in the Treatment of Patients with Node-Negative Breast Cancer Who Have Estrogen-Receptor-Positive Tumors," *New England Journal of Medicine* 320 (February 23, 1989): 479–84; *New York Times,* April 25–26, 1979; Bernard Fisher, "Breast-Cancer Management: Alternatives to Radical Mastectomy," *New England Journal of Medicine* 301 (August 9, 1979): 326–28; Lerner, *Breast Cancer Wars,* 227.

18. Ronald Reagan, *An American Life* (New York, 1990), 693–95; *New York Times,* October 18, 1987; Nancy Reagan, *My Turn: The Memoirs of Nancy Reagan* (New York, 1989), 297–98; Ann Butler Nattinger, Raymond G. Hoffmann, Alicia Howell-Petz et al., "Effect of Nancy Reagan's Mastectomy on Choice of Surgery for Breast Cancer by US Women," *Journal of the American Medical Association* 279 (March 11, 1998): 762–66.

19. Nattinger, Hoffmann, Howell-Petz et al., "Effect of Nancy Reagan's Mastectomy," 726–66; D. S. Lane, A. P. Polednak, and M. A. Burg, "The Impact of Media Coverage of Nancy Reagan's Experience on Breast Cancer Screening," *American Journal of Public Health* 79 (November 1989): 1551–52.

20. *New York Times,* January 10, 1990.

Chapter Ten: The Breast Cancer Wars

1. Christine Gorman, "Do Abortions Raise the Risk of Breast Cancer?" *Time,* November 7, 1994, 61; Rita Rubin, "Linking Abortion and Breast Cancer," *U.S. News and World Report,* November 7, 1994, 70; "Do Abortions Heighten Breast Cancer Risk?" *Science News* 146 (November 5, 1994): 294; J. R. Daling, K. E. Malone, L. F. Voight et al., "Risk of Breast Cancer among Young Women: Relationship to Induced Abortion," *Journal of the National Cancer Institute* 86 (November 2, 1994): 1584–93; Lynn Rosenberg, "Induced Abortion and Breast Cancer: More Scientific Data Are Needed," *Journal of the National Cancer Institute* 86 (November 2, 1994): 1569–70; M. C. Pike, B. E. Henderson, J. T. Casagrande et al., "Oral Contraceptive Use and Early Abortion as Risk Factors

for Breast Cancer in Young Women," *British Journal of Cancer* 43 (1981): 72–76; L. I. Remennick, "Induced Abortion as Cancer Risk Factor: A Review of Epidemiological Evidence," *Journal of Epidemiology and Community Health* 44 (December 1990): 259–64; Bill Turque, "Aborted Revolution?" *Newsweek,* December 12, 1994, 40; Abortion Industry Monitor, *Before You Choose: The Link between Abortion & Breast Cancer* (1995).

2. *New York Times,* January 13 and September 21, 1994.

3. *New York Times,* February 9, 1992; Eileen Mechas and Denise Foley, *Unequal Treatment* (New York, 1994), 79–80. For a look at how women's health has tended to be ignored by academic medicine, see Sue V. Rosser, *Women's Health: Missing from U.S. Medicine* (New York, 1994).

4. Susan Ferraro, "The Anguished Politics of Breast Cancer," *The New York Times Magazine,* August 15, 1993, 58–62.

5. Ibid.; "Confronting Breast Cancer: An Interview with Susan Love," *Technology Review* 96 (May/June 1993): 45–53.

6. Carol Ann Rinzler, *Estrogen and Breast Cancer* (New York, 1993), 114; E. J. Freuer, L.-M. Wun, C. C. Boring et al., "The Lifetime Risk of Developing Breast Cancer," *Journal of the National Cancer Institute* 85 (June 2, 1993): 892–97.

7. Quoted in Robert N. Proctor, *Cancer Wars: How Politics Shapes What We Know and Don't Know About Cancer* (New York, 1995), 250–51.

8. John C. Bailar III, "Re-Thinking the War on Cancer," *Issues in Science and Technology* (Fall 1987): 16–21; John C. Bailar III and Elaine M. Smith, "Progress against Cancer?" *New England Journal of Medicine* 314 (May 8, 1986): 1226–32.

9. David Spiegel, J. R. Bloom, H. C. Kraemer et al., "Effect of Psychosocial Treatment on Survival of Patients with Metastatic Breast Cancer," *Lancet* 2 (October 14, 1989): 881–91. For a survey of breast cancer politics, see Maureen Hogan Casamayou, *The Politics of Breast Cancer* (Washington, D.C., 2001).

10. Ferraro, "The Anguished Politics of Breast Cancer," 25–26, 58–62.

11. Ibid.; *New York Times,* February 9, 1992, and December 12, 1995; Eliot Marshall, "The Politics of Breast Cancer," *Science* 259 (29 January 1993): 616–17; Maureen Henderson, "Current Approaches to Breast Cancer Prevention," *Science* 259 (29 January 1993): 630–32; Jan Blustein, "Medicare Coverage, Supplemental Insurance, and the Use of Mammography by Older Women," *New England Journal of Medicine* 332 (April 27, 1995): 1138–43; Alisa Solomon, "The Politics of Breast Cancer," *The Village Voice,* May 14, 1991, 22–27; Jane Erikson, "Breast Cancer Activists Seek Voice in Research Decisions," *Science* 269 (September 15, 1995): 1508–9.

12. *New York Times,* October 26–27, 2000.

13. Ibid., December 29, 1994; *Houston Chronicle,* July 5, 1995.

14. *New York Times,* March 24 and April 16, 1999.

15. Ann Butler Nattinger, Mark S. Gottlieb, Judith Veum et al., "Geographic Variation in the Use of Breast-Conserving Treatment for Breast Cancer," *New England Journal of Medicine* 326 (April 23, 1992): 1102–7; D. A. August, T. R. Rea, and V. K. Sondak, "Age Related Differences in Breast Cancer Treatment," *Annals of Surgical Oncology* 1 (January 1994): 45–52; Virginia L. Ernster, John Barclay, Karla Kerlikowske et al., "Incidence of and Treatment for Ductal Carcinoma In Situ of the Breast," *Journal of the American Medical Association* 275 (March 27, 1996): 913–18.

16. *Chicago Tribune,* August 18–19, 1993.

17. DeAnn Lazovich, Emily White, David B. Thomas et al., "Underutilization of Breast-Conserving Surgery and Radiation Therapy among Women with Stage I or II Breast Cancer," *Journal of the American Medical Association* 266 (December 25, 1991): 3433–38.

18. "Confronting Breast Cancer: An Interview with Susan Love," 45–53; *New York Times,* May 5, 1993.

19. Proctor, *Cancer Wars,* 261, 265; John C. Bailar III, "Mammography: A Contrary View," *Annals of Internal Medicine* 84 (January 1976): 77–84.

20. Barbara J. Culliton, "Breast Cancer: Second Thoughts about Routine Mammography," *Science* 193 (August 13, 1976): 555–58; G. J. Subak-Sharpe, "Is Mammography Safe? Yes, No, and Maybe," *New York Times Magazine,* October 24, 1976, 42–44; Walter Ross, *Crusade: The Official History of the American Cancer Society* (New York, 1986), 102–11, 227; Proctor, *Cancer Wars,* 261–66; Leslie Laurence and Beth Weinhouse, *Outrageous Practices: The Alarming Truth about How Medicine Mistreats Women* (New York, 1994), 114; *New York Times,* December 5, 14, 27, 30, 1993; Barron H. Lerner, *The Breast Cancer Wars: Hope, Fear, and the Pursuit of a Cure in Twentieth-Century America* (New York, 2001), 246–48.

21. *New York Times,* January 1, April 7, and April 30, 1992, and June 29, 1994; Michael De Gregorio and Valerie J. Wiebe, *Tamoxifen & Breast Cancer* (New Haven, 1993), 72–83; Laurence and Weinhouse, *Outrageous Practices,* 120–25.

22. Peter B. Chowka, "The National Cancer Institute and the Fifty-Year Cover-Up," *East West,* January 1978, 22–27; Bailar and Smith, "Progress against Cancer?" 1226–32; Proctor, *Cancer Wars,* 4–6; Tim Beardsley, "A War Not Won," *Scientific American* 270 (January 1994): 130–38.

23. David Plotkin, "Good News and Bad News about Breast Cancer," *The Atlantic Monthly,* June 1996, 55–56.

24. *New York Times,* September 30, 1994; L. M. Wun and E. J. Feuer, "Are Increases in Mammographic Screening Still a Valid Explanation for Trends in

Breast Cancer Incidence in the United States?" *Cancer: Causes & Control* 6 (March 1995): 135–44.

25. *New York Times*, August 15–16, 1993; *Houston Chronicle*, January 13, 1995.

26. Laurence and Weinhouse, *Outrageous Practices*, 136–37; Erikson, "Breast Cancer Activists Seek Voice in Research Decisions," 388–92; Lerner, *Breast Cancer Wars*, 232–33.

27. Marcia Angell and Jerome P. Kassirer, "Setting the Record Straight in the Breast-Cancer Trials," *New England Journal of Medicine* 330 (May 19, 1994): 1448–50.

28. *New York Times*, January 3, 1992.

29. *Baltimore Sun*, March 13, 1994; *New York Times*, April 4 and June 14, 1994; *Houston Chronicle*, May 1, 1994.

30. *New York Times*, April 29, 1996.

31. Ferraro, "The Anguished Politics of Breast Cancer," 58–62; *Houston Chronicle*, August 17, 1993; Matuschka, "A Vessel of Great Nourishment," *American Journal of Nursing* 94 (May 1994): 29.

Chapter Eleven: Biology, Society, and Destiny

1. J. W. Berg and R. V. P. Hutter, "Breast Cancer," *Cancer* 75 (January 1, 1995, 1 Suppl.): 257–69.

2. H. K. Sonoo and J. S. Kurebayashi, "Recent Development of Endocrine Treatment for Breast Cancer," *Japanese Journal of Cancer & Chemotherapy* 20 (December 1993): 2289–99; H. B. Muss, "Endocrine Therapy for Advanced Breast Cancer: A Review," *Breast Cancer Research & Treatment* 21 (1992): 15–26; *Houston Chronicle*, April 30, 1996; Linda S. Cook, Noel S. Weiss, Stephen M. Schwartz et al., "Population-Based Study of Tamoxifen Therapy and Subsequent Ovarian, Endometrial, and Breast Cancers," *Journal of the National Cancer Institute* 87 (September 20, 1995): 1359–64.

3. Virginia L. Ernster, John Barclay, Karla Kerlikowske et al., "Incidence of and Treatment for Ductal Carcinoma In Situ of the Breast," *Journal of the American Medical Association* 275 (March 27, 1996): 913–18.

4. A. P. Forrest and F. E. Alexander, "A Question That Will Not Go Away: At What Age Should Mammographic Screening Begin?" *Journal of the National Cancer Institute* 87 (August 16, 1995): 1195–97; *Houston Chronicle*, January 25, 2002.

5. David Plotkin, "Good News and Bad News about Breast Cancer," *Atlantic Monthly*, June 1996, 72.

6. E. J. Barrett-Connor and N. J. Friedlander, "Dietary Fat, Calories, and the Risk of Breast Cancer in Postmenopausal Women: A Prospective Population-Based Study," *Journal of the American College of Nutrition* 12 (August 1993):

390–99; T. R. Byers, "Nutritional Risk Factors for Breast Cancer," *Cancer* 74 (1 Suppl., July 1, 1994): 288–95; G. R. Howe, "Dietary Fat and Breast Cancer Risks: An Epidemiologic Perspective," *Cancer* 74 (3 Suppl., August 1, 1994): 1078–84; "Dietary Fat, Breast Cancer Link Is Challenged," *Harvard Health Letter* (May 1999): 8.

7. *New York Times,* February 5, 1992; *Houston Chronicle,* September 2, 1995.

8. "A Real Midlife Crisis," *Newsweek,* June 26, 1995, 62–63; Graham A. Colditz, Susan E. Hankinson, David J. Hunter et al., "The Use of Estrogens and Progestins and the Risk of Breast Cancer in Postmenopausal Women," *New England Journal of Medicine* 332 (June 15, 1995): 1589–93.

9. Janet L. Stanford, Noel S. Weiss, Lynda F. Voigt et al., "Combined Estrogen and Progestin Hormone Replacement Therapy in Relation to Risk of Breast Cancer in Middle-Aged Women," *Journal of the American Medical Association* 274 (July 12, 1995): 137–42. In 2002, however, *JAMA* insisted that there was a link between estrogen replacement therapy and breast cancer. See Chi-Ling Chen, Noel S. Weiss, Polly Newcomb et al., "Hormone Replacement Therapy in Relation to Breast Cancer," *The Journal of the American Medical Association* 287 (February 13, 2002): 734–41.

10. M. V. Dhodapkar, J. N. Ingle, and D. L. Ahmann, "Estrogen Replacement Therapy Withdrawal and Regression of Metastatic Breast Cancer," *Cancer* 75 (January 1, 1995): 43–46; R. L. Theriault and R. V. Sellin, "A Clinical Dilemma: Estrogen Replacement Therapy in Postmenopausal Women with a Background of Primary Breast Cancer," *Annals of Oncology* 2 (November-December 1991): 709–17.

11. *New York Times,* April 15, 1964; H. Patricia Hynes, *The Recurring Silent Spring* (New York, 1989), 2–4, 16–20, 30–34; Mary A. McCay, *Rachel Carson* (New York, 1993), 2–5, 40–44; Rachel Carson, *Silent Spring* (New York, 1962), 219–43; Martha Freeman, ed., *Always, Rachel: The Letters of Rachel Carson and Dorothy Freeman, 1952–1964* (Boston, 1995).

12. Samuel Epstein, *Politics of Cancer* (New York, 1978); Robert N. Proctor, *Cancer Wars: How Politics Shapes What We Know and Don't Know About Cancer* (New York, 1995), 57–64.

13. Bruce Ames, "Mother Nature Is Meaner Than You Think," *Science* 84 (July-August 1984): 98; Elizabeth Whelan, *Toxic Terror* (Ottawa, Ill., 1985); Edith Efron, *The Apocalyptics: Cancer and the Big Lie* (New York, 1984), 83.

14. Liane Clorfene-Casten, "The Environmental Link to Breast Cancer," *Ms.,* May/June 1993, 52–54; Susan Rennie, "Breast Cancer Prevention: Diet vs. Drugs," *Ms.,* May/June 1993, 38–51; Monte Paulsen, "The Cancer Business," *Mother Jones,* June 1994, 41; "Breast Cancer, Inc.," *Houston Press,* August 12–18,

1993, 19–27; Amanda Spake, "Is the Modern World Giving Us Cancer?" *Health,* October 1995, 52–56.

15. *New York Times,* January 8, 1992, and August 15, 1993.

16. Ibid., April 13 and 18, 1994; *Houston Chronicle,* October 29, 1995.

17. *New York Times,* April 22, 1993, and April 20, 1994.

18. Ruth Handler, *Dream Doll: The Ruth Handler Story* (Stamford, Conn., 1994).

19. Meryl Gordon, "Going for the Perfect Breast," *Elle,* September 1993, 366.

20. *Houston Chronicle,* June 22, 1995; Jorge Sánchez-Guerrero, Graham A. Colditz, Elizabeth W. Karlson et al., "Silicone Breast Implants and the Risk of Connective-Tissue Disease and Symptoms," *New England Journal of Medicine* 332 (June 22, 1995): 1666–70.

21. "Confronting Breast Cancer: An Interview With Susan Love," 45–53; *Houston Chronicle,* April 29, 1996.

22. F. G. Cunningham and K. J. Levano, "Childbearing Among Older Women—The Message Is Cautiously Optimistic," *New England Journal of Medicine* 333 (October 12, 1995): 1002–3.

23. David Plotkin, "Good News and Bad News About Breast Cancer," 53–82.

24. Ibid.; M. P. Madigan, R. G. Zeigler, J. Benichou et al., "Proportion of Breast Cancer Cases in the United States Explained by Well-Established Risk Factors," *Journal of the National Cancer Institute* 87 (November 15, 1995): 1681–85.

25. *NBC Nightly News,* January 4, 1996; author interview with Sheila O'Day.

Epilogue: The New Millennium

1. *New York Times,* May 3–7, 1998; *Washington Times,* July 12, 1999; Robert Cooke, *Dr. Folkman's War: Angiogenisis and the Struggle to Defeat Cancer* (New York, 2001).

2. For Jill Ireland's battle with cancer, see "Facing Breast Cancer with Courage," *Harper's Bazaar,* August 1985, 196–98; Jill Ireland, *Life Wish* (New York, 1987); Jill Ireland, "A Battle with Breast Cancer Puts a Star's Life into Focus," *People Weekly,* March 16, 1987, 57–58; Vernon Scott, "I Will Live," *Good Housekeeping,* May 1989, 183, 238, 240–41; Holly Miller, "Battling the Beast Within," *Saturday Evening Post,* July-August 1989, 44–45, 104; "Jill Ireland," *Hollywood Reporter,* May 19, 1990; Susan Schindehette, "Jill Ireland Loses a Battle with Cancer, but Leaves an Inspiring Legacy of Love and Courage," *People Weekly,* June 4, 1990, 121–24; Jill Ireland, "Why Me," *Life,* June 1989, 108–9; Barbara Kantrowitz, "Shattered for the Second Time," *Newsweek,* May 8, 1989, 66; *The Times* [London], May 19, 1990.

3. *The Kansas City Star,* May 16, 2000; *Houston Chronicle,* March 13, 1998.

4. I. Craig Henderson, "Paradigmatic Shifts in the Management of Breast Cancer," *New England Journal of Medicine* 332 (April 6, 1995): 951–52; Aron Goldhirsch, William C. Wood, Hans-Jorg Senn et al., "Meeting Highlights: International Consensus Panel on the Treatment of Primary Breast Cancer," *Journal of the National Cancer Institute* 87 (October 4, 1995): 1441–45.

5. J. A. Jacobsen, D. N. Danforth, and K. H. Cowan, "Ten Year Results of a Comparison of Conservation with Mastectomy in the Treatment of Stage I and II Breast Cancer," *New England Journal of Medicine* 332 (April 1995): 907–11.

6. Gianni Bonadonna, Pinuccia Valagussa, Angela Moliterni et al., "Adjuvant Cyclophosphamide, Methotrexate, and Flourouracil in Node-Positive Breast Cancer," *New England Journal of Medicine* 332 (April 1995): 901–6.

7. Geoffrey Cowley and Anne Underwood, "Defeating Breast Cancer," *Newsweek Special Issue,* Spring/Summer 1999, 40–44.

8. *Houston Chronicle,* October 21, 1994.

9. *New York Times,* August 3, 1994; G. M. Swanson, N. E. Ragheb, C. S. Lin et al., "Breast Cancer among Black and White Women in the 1980s: Changing Patterns in the United States by Race, Age, and Extent of Disease," *Cancer* 72 (August 1, 1993): 788–98; R. M. Elledge, G. M. Clark, G. C. Chamness et al., "Tumor Biologic Factors and Breast Cancer Prognosis among White, Hispanic, and Black Women in the United States," *Journal of the National Cancer Institute* 86 (May 4, 1994): 705–12; Edwin T. Johnson, *Breast Cancer, Black Woman* (New York, 1993); Sylvia Dunnavant, *Celebrating Life: African-American Women Speak Out About Breast Cancer* (New York, 1995); Jill Moormeier, "Breast Cancer in Black Women," *Annals of Internal Medicine* 124 (May 15, 1996): 897–905.

10. *Houston Chronicle,* September 24, 1994; *New York Times,* May 5, 1993.

11. Yoshio Miki, Jeff Swenson, Donna Shattuck-Eidens et al., "A Strong Candidate for the Breast and Ovarian Cancer Susceptibility Gene BRCA1," *Science* 266 (October 7, 1994): 66–71; "Breast Cancer Gene Offers Surprises," *Science* 265 (September 23, 1994): 1796–99.

12. Richard Wooster, Susan L. Neuhausen, Jonathan Mangion et al., "Localization of a Breast Cancer Susceptibility Gene, BRCA2, to Chromosome 13q12–13," *Science* 265 (September 30, 1994): 2088–90.

13. *Houston Chronicle,* June 23, 1995; Sigrid Sjogren, Mats Inganas, Torbjorn Norberg et al., "The p53 Gene in Breast Cancer: Prognostic Value of Complementary DNA Sequencing versus Immunohistochemistry," *Journal of the National Cancer Institute* 88 (February 21, 1996): 173–82; B. Kuska, "BRCA1 Alteration Found in Eastern European Jews," *Journal of the National Cancer Institute* 87 (October 18, 1995): 1505.

14. Brody quoted in Robert N. Proctor, *Cancer Wars: How Politics Shapes*

What We Know and Don't Know about Cancer (New York, 1995), 242; Juliet Whitman, *Breast Cancer Journal: Century of Petals* (Golden, Colo., 1993), 103; *Houston Chronicle,* September 29, 1995; David E. Goldgar and Philip R. Reilly, "A Common BRCA1 Mutation in the Ashkenazim," *Nature Genetics* 11 (October 1995): 113–14; Lynn C. Hartmann, Daniel J. Schaid, John E. Woods et al., "Efficacy of Bilateral Prophylactic Mastectomy in Women with a Family History of Breast Cancer," *New England Journal of Medicine* 340 (January 14, 1999): 77–84.

15. Hartmann, Schaid, Woods et al., "Efficacy of Bilateral Prophylactic Mastectomy," 77–84; Hanne Meijers-Heijboer, Bert Van Geel, Wim L. J. van Putten et al., Breast Cancer after Prophylactic Bilateral Mastectomy in Women with a BRCA1 or BRCA2 Mutation," *New England Journal of Medicine* 345 (July 19, 2001): 159–64.

16. *Washington Times,* July 12, 1999.

17. *Medical Industry Today,* May 16, 2000, 1–3; *Atlanta Constitution,* May 19, 2000; *Electronic Telegraph,* Issue 1820 (May 19, 2000); *Washington Times,* July 12, 1999.

18. Christopher I. Li, Kathleen E. Malone, Noel S. Weiss et al., "Tamoxifen Therapy for Primary Breast Cancer and Risk of Contralateral Breast Cancer," *Journal of the National Cancer Institute* 93 (July 4, 2001): 1008–13.

19. *London Telegraph,* May 21, 2000; Richard Peto, Jillian Boreham, Mike Clarke et al., "UK and USA Breast Cancer Deaths Down 25% in Year 2000 at Ages 20–69 Years," *Lancet* 355 (May 20, 2000): 1822; Phyllis McIntosh, "The New Weapons against Breast Cancer," *Remedy* 6 (January/February 1999): 20–26.

20. Robert Bazell, *Her-2: The Making of Herceptin, a Revolutionary Treatment for Breast Cancer* (New York, 1998); McIntosh, "New Weapons," 23.

21. *London Telegraph,* June 24, 1999.

22. Danielle Steele, *Lightning* (New York, 1995).

23. B. Brophey, "Murphy & Me," *TV Guide,* September 27, 1997, 24–27.

24. *People Weekly,* October 26, 1998; *Parade,* January 31, 1999.

Index

About the Author

James S. Olson is Distinguished Professor and Chair in the Department of History at Sam Houston State University, Huntsville, Texas. He is the author of *Honest Graft: The World of George Washington Plunkitt; The Cuban-Americans; Saving Capitalism: The Reconstruction Finance Corporation and the New Deal, 1933–1940; Catholic Immigrants in America;* and *The Ethnic Dimension in American History.* He is the coauthor, with Randy Roberts, of *Winning is the Only Thing: Sports in America Since 1945; Where the Domino Fell: America and Vietnam, 1945–1990; John Wayne: American* (which won the National Book Award of the Popular Culture Association); and *A Line in the Sand: The Alamo in Blood and Memory,* winner of the Outstanding Achievement in Historical Research Award from the Texas Historical Foundation.